ALLERGIES AND INFECTIOUS DISEASES

SALMONELLA

CLASSIFICATION, GENETICS AND DISEASE OUTBREAKS

Allergies and Infectious Diseases

Additional books in this series can be found on Nova's website
under the Series tab.

Additional E-books in this series can be found on Nova's website
under the E-book tab.

Public Health in the 21st Century

Additional books in this series can be found on Nova's website
under the Series tab.

Additional E-books in this series can be found on Nova's website
under the E-book tab.

ALLERGIES AND INFECTIOUS DISEASES

SALMONELLA

CLASSIFICATION, GENETICS AND DISEASE OUTBREAKS

ADELAIDE S. MONTE
AND
PAULO EDUARDO DE SANTOS
EDITORS

Nova Science Publishers, Inc.
New York

LIBRARY OF CONGRESS CATALOGING-IN-PUBLICATION DATA

Library of Congress Control Number: 2012930423

ISBN: 978-1-61942-928-4

Published by Nova Science Publishers, Inc. † New York

CONTENTS

PREFACE

Salmonella are ubiquitous enteric bacteria, responsible for thousands of deaths worldwide. In this book, the authors present current research in the study of the classification, genetics and disease outbreak cases relating to salmonella. Topics include the pre- and post-harvest intervention strategies for controlling salmonella contamination in broiler production; *Salmonella enterica* survival to biocides and antibiotics; salmonella newport contamination in produce; genome comparisons of salmonella; salmonella in sub-Antarctica and Antarctica; and hazard of salmonella in the intact shell egg.

Chapter 1 - Contamination of poultry with *Salmonella* occurs prior to entry into the processing facility and by cross-contamination in the processing plant. Breeder flocks, hatcheries, contaminated feed and water, and environmental sources/vectors such as litter, humans, and insects are potential pre-harvest sources of *Salmonella* contamination in poultry. Knowledge of key pre-harvest factors responsible for *Salmonella* colonization would help integrators and poultry producers in defining critical, pre-harvest control points on the farm. Intervention at these points could reduce or eliminate horizontal transmission and *Salmonella* positive birds arriving at the processing plants. It is difficult to improve the microbiological quality of chickens once they have reached the processing plant. Several physical and chemical decontamination procedures have been applied to poultry carcasses and have been useful in reducing the level and frequency of *Salmonella* on poultry carcasses at the processing plants. A combination of pre- and post-harvest intervention strategies can reduce or eliminate *Salmonella* on fresh poultry delivered to consumers, thereby significantly reducing the medical and productivity costs associated with salmonellosis.

Chapter 2 - Many strains of *Salmonella enterica* represent zoonotic pathogens which are capable of causing disease in humans. One major source of food poisoning is *Salmonella enterica* serovar Enteritidis which is often found associated with chicken meat, meat products and eggs. A number of virulence factors enable this bacterium to colonize and systemically infect poultry. In this review the authors will concentrate on the *S.* Enteritidis Type III Secretion System (T3SS) located on *Salmonella* Pathogenicity Island-1 and highlight its role in invasion of chickens. The structural components of the complex secretion apparatus and the secreted effector proteins will be introduced. Aspects of T3SS assembly, its expression regulation under different conditions as well as its involvement in colonization and invasion of poultry will be discussed in the context of the recent findings.

Chapter 3 - It is well known that the main microbiological hazard derived from egg consumption is the presence of *Salmonellae*, being the serovars *S.* Enteritidis and *S.*

Typhimurium the most frequently implicated in the outbreaks. Although bacteria can reach the inside of the eggs by transovarian or through the shell pores, the main way of contamination probably occurs from organisms located in the shell, which can attain the inner part of the egg when it is broken for cooking other foods, e.g. custard, salads, desserts. In developed countries, the outbreaks of salmonellosis increased until 2004, observing a clear decline afterward, which is attributed to the success of implementing programs to control *Salmonella* in poultry populations. In spite of this, salmonellosis is still the main cause of foodborne illness. Therefore, the decontamination of shell eggs remains of public health concern yet. Many chemical (e.g. washing, hydrogen peroxide, ozone and electrolyzed water) and physical (e.g. water boiling, pasteurization, ionizing and ultraviolet radiation, pulsed light, high pressure,) methods for shell eggs sanitation have been envisaged, being the pasteurization that of the most concern. Many heat treatment conditions have been proposed to remove *Salmonellae* from eggshells, but none have been completely satisfactory due to the adverse effects of the heat on the functional properties of the white and yolk. An attempt to develop a procedure to reach this goal has been recently performed by the authors' group. The ability of thermoultrasonication (ultrasounds and heat simultaneously applied) to eliminate *Salmonella* from eggshell was studied, using *S.* Enteritidis and *S.* Senftenberg as models. The thermoultrasonication dramatically reduced the heat resistant of *Salmonella*. E.g., the D-value of *S.* Enteritidis at 55 °C (2.89 minutes for the heat treatment alone) was reduced a 77.16 %, i.e. it passed to 0.66 minutes when the thermoultrasonication was applied. In the case of *S.* Senftenberg the reduction was lower. The same figures at 57 °C were 10.54 and 3.92 minutes, respectively. No effects of the thermoultrasonication on several attributes (shelf-life, loss of freshness, eggshell breaking strength, emulsifying and foaming abilities, etc.) were observed. The fundamentals of the new process for shell egg sanitation have been established at a laboratory scale. As an ultrasonic treatment added to an existing heat process would increase its bactericidal efficiency, the process might have important practical implications for the egg industry. It is now necessary to validate the process at a higher scale to confirm the results.

Chapter 4 - Nowadays, *Salmonella* spp. is still considered one of the major foodborne pathogens, being responsible for thousands of deaths worldwide and widespread economic losses every year. *Salmonella enterica* strains have proven to be highly adaptable and able to survive in the external environment, and their ability to respond effectively to environmental changes is important in their survival in the food chain. Moreover, like many other microorganisms, *S. enterica* is able to adhere and form biofilms on several different surfaces, which increases its inherent resistance and, thus, significantly affects plant sanitation and product safety. Bacterial resistance to antimicrobial agents in general, as well as the underlying mechanisms, have been widely studied by several authors. Additionally, a number of scientists have recently expressed concern that the common and indiscriminate use of biocides may be a contributing factor to the development and selection of antibiotic-resistant strains, giving rise to a phenomenon known as "cross-resistance". In this context, the present chapter intends to review the scientific results concerning the mechanisms by which *S. enterica* planktonic and biofilm cells may become resistant to biocides action, as well as the relation between biocide and antibiotic resistance by this foodborne pathogen. Moreover, genomic aspects involved in such adaptive and resistant behaviours will also be considered.

Chapter 5 - Culture-based methods for detection of *Salmonella* spp. in food demand the performance of several steps in stages (preenrichment, enrichment, selective plating, identification, and confirmation). This results in significant time-to-detection, media and reagents and labor needed. As a consequence of the need for rapid and specific detection techniques, molecular-based rapid detection methods such as real time polymerase chain reaction (RT-PCR), nucleic acid sequence based amplification (NASBA) or immunoassays have been developed. These methods, however, may still be negatively affected by interference from inhibitors, may be qualitative in nature or require extraction of target molecules (DNA, rRNA, mRNA) prior to analysis allowing for possible contamination or amplification of target sequences from non-viable cells. Alternative rapid detection techniques for *Salmonella* spp. in food have been developed which accomplish identification and enumeration of whole-cell targets. Fluorescence *in situ* hybridization (FISH) employs sequence-specific rRNA-targeted fluorescently-labeled oligonucleotide probes to specifically hybridize whole permeabilized bacterial cells. FISH can be coupled with fluorescence microscopy, flow cytometry or capillary electrophoresis to achieve detection and enumeration. Bacteriophage-based detection techniques for *Salmonella* spp. which make use of the inherent specificity of phages for their target bacterial host have also been described. In addition, biosensor-based detection may offer simplicity and high throughput capability for whole-cell detection of *Salmonella* spp. in food. These alternative methods for whole-cell detection of *Salmonella* spp. have shown potential as sensitive, specific, and quantitative methods for detection and identification of this pathogen in foods. The advantages and disadvantages of these methods as well as the current status of development and future directions are discussed here.

Chapter 6 - *Salmonella enterica* is the most frequent source of bacterial foodborne illness in the U.S., causing an estimated 1.4 million cases of salmonellosis annually. Historically, infection by *Salmonella* occurs after eating undercooked meats, poultry and eggs. However, over the past decade, the consumption of raw ready-to-eat produce has been implicated in several severe and widespread outbreaks within the U. S. Most notably, an *S. enterica* Saintpaul outbreak associated with jalapeño and Serrano peppers sickened over 1400 individuals during the summer of 2008. One *Salmonella* serovar in particular, *Salmonella enterica* Newport, has been associated perennially with contamination events involving fresh tomatoes and prepared fresh foods containing tomatoes. *S.* Newport is a non-typhoidal salmonellae classified taxonomically as subspecies (i.e. “group”) I *Salmonella enterica enterica*. Prior to its emergence in produce and in produce growing environments, *S.* Newport was found predominantly in swine, cattle and other livestock commodities. *S.* Newport association with tomatoes retains a geographically skewed distribution. Metagenomic analyses of tomato phyllopsheres, based on 16S rDNA sequences and deep genome sequencing of tomato microbial communities, point to resident colonization on tomatoes from the Mid-Atlantic growing regions but not other predominant fresh tomato growing regions such as Florida or California, signaling niche adaptation of *S.* Newport in some growing environments but not others. Genetic analysis of *S.* Newport has revealed specific differences among strains from disparate locales. Pulsed-field gel electrophoresis, for example, has yielded several pulsotypes of environmental *S.* Newport primarily associated with the Virginia eastern shore, a prominent fresh tomato production region of the county. Whole-genome sequencing affirmed these phylo-geographic differences within the serovar. Surprisingly, certain genotypes of *S.* Newport have been isolated from this region that genetically match previous outbreaks where tomatoes were a suspected vehicle. *S.* Newport can be readily detected in the environment of the Virginian eastern shore growing region using both molecular (i.e. PCR) and microbiological (i.e. FDA-BAM) screening methods.

Taken together, these issues highlight the important intersection of microbiological, genetic, and ecological investigation for fully understanding the complex life cycle of this dangerous foodborne pathogen.

Chapter 7 - *Salmonella* was identified as the first cause of food-borne diseases in the last decade in Brazil. Currently, Brazil is an important producer of pork and is the major poultry and beef exporter in the world. Brazilian animal products have been recognized worldwide, and to attend international standards the Brazilian food industries have been putting considerable effort in order to prevent food contamination, especially by *Salmonella*. A representative part of the Brazilian eggs, beef, poultry, and pork meats is produced in the State of Rio Grande do Sul (RS), in southern Brazil, where *Salmonella* was pointed out as the first cause of food-borne diseases for almost two decades. In this region, homemade mayonnaise was identified as the food preparation mostly involved with salmonellosis, and both meat and meat products were also identified as frequent vehicles for salmonellosis. A specific strain of *Salmonella* Enteritidis (named SE86) was identified as the responsible agent in more than 95 % of investigated food-borne diseases throughout the last decade. SE86 strains isolated from several outbreaks demonstrated the same DNA banding patterns when typed by PCR-methods and PFGE, suggesting that it is spread out through RS. SE86 demonstrated high percentages of sensitivity to many antibiotics; however, an increasing resistance to nalidixic acid and ampicillin has been identified. After exposure to sub-letal pHs, SE86 demonstrated a greater acid adaptation and also to be more acid-and-thermal-resistant than *S.* Typhimurium and *S.* Bredeney also isolated in RS State. Acid-adapted SE86 presents higher virulence than non-acid-adapted SE86 and acid-adapted *S.* Typhimurium in germ-free mice. This strain has shown to be able to form biofilms on stainless steel and polypropylene, and was more resistant to 200 and 400 ppm sodium hypochlorite than others *Salmonella* serovars, but was not more resistant than other *S.* Enteritidis isolated in countries such as Albania, Morocco, Pakistan and Zimbabwe. SE86 mutants (*dps, rpoS*) were constructed in order to investigate the involvement of these genes with oxidative stress caused by sodium hypochlorite exposure. The results demonstrated that both genes are expressed during such exposure; however, *dps* was expressed in much higher amounts, increasing survival rates of SE86. Poultry meat produced in RS State demonstrated *Salmonella* prevalence of 4.4 % to 15 %, whilst expressively higher percentages of *Salmonella* were found in pork meat samples. Strains isolated from poultry and pork belonged to diverse serovars and, in general, demonstrated different patterns and higher antimicrobial resistance than SE86 isolated from salmonellosis.

Chapter 8 - *Salmonella spp.* are ubiquitous enteric bacteria. These gram-negative rods are the etiologic agents of food-borne salmonellosis and other food borne diseases **(1, 2)**. It is also the agents that cause typhoid and paratyphoid fevers. An estimated 2 to 4 million cases of salmonellosis occur annually in the United States **(3).** In Tunisia, bacteriological results showed that the rate of *salmonella* contamination remains quite high. In fact, the infection progresses, mostly under sporadic and rarely in an epidemic mode. *Salmonella spp.* can survive for long periods in natural waters, and the persistence of specific and epidemic strains is of great concern in public health. However, information on the diversity and occurrence of *Salmonella* strains is very scarce (4, 5), and as a consequence, the ecology of these species remains unknown. *Salmonella* bacteria cause, also, much of the food poisoning in the world, including an estimated 1,400,000 cases of salmonellosis in the United States each year. Although foods of animal origin (eggs, poultry, beef, dairy products…) are the vehicles of transmission in most *Salmonella* outbreaks, contaminated fresh fruits and vegetables are now recognized as the main cause of salmonellosis (1, 2). The purpose of the present review was to provide information on the diversity of *Salmonella* strains isolated from environmental, animal, food and human samples which allows to follow trends in *Salmonella enterica* seotypes that provide information about source of infection and the efficacy of prevention and control measures. *Salmonella* is an important source of food-borne disease in humans throughout the world. An important change in the epidemiology of *Salmonella* occurred since the mid 1980s, when *Salmonella Enteritidis* (*S. Enteritidis*) became a major contaminant of eggs and egg products, hereby causing a worldwide pandemic. In France, salmonellosis is also the largest documented cause of foodborne infections (6). A total of 21 *S. Muenster* isolates had been received by the the French Food Safety Agency (Afssa) between January 2006 and February 2008. Among them, four were food isolates (poultry); the other 17 strains were from different origins (meat and bone meal, environmental isolates). In Canada, in 1982, a documented food poisoning outbreak caused by *S. Muenster* occurred and implicated cheddar cheese made from unpasteurised milk as the source of infection (7). On March 2008, the National Reference Centre (NRC) for *Salmonella* reported three laboratory-confirmed cases of *S. Muenster* to the (Institut de veille sanitaire, InVS). In Tunisia, during the study period (1994-2004), Nazek and coll showed that the top three *Salmonella* serotypes frequentely isolated with interchangeable ranking were: *Anatum, Enteritidis* and *Corvallis* (8). Aknown food origine was reported for all *Salmonella* isolates: red meat for *S.enterica* and *S.Anatum*. Whereas, *S.Enteritidis*, *Corvallis* and *Anatum* were most commonly isolated from poultry. The highest serotype commonly isolated from vegetables and fruits were *S.enterica* serotypes: *Anatum, Enteritidis* and *Corvallis*. Serotypes most frequentely isolated from milk and dairy products was *S.enterica* serotype *Anatum*. Finally, on November 2007, the Singapore Ministry of Health was notified of an outbreak of food poisoning. This outbreak was the largest common source outbreak of gastroenteritis caused by *Salmonella enterica* subspecies *enterica* serotype *Enteritidis* in Singapore. The epidemiological evidence implicates cream cake as the vehicle of transmission (9). In addition to food contamination, *Salmonella* species are pathogenic bacteria often detected in wastewater, freshwater, marine coastal water, and groundwater. Municipal sewage and storm water runoff become the conduits for the passage of pathogens into surface waters (10, 11). Serotype *Typhimurium* was dominant in all river samples and in marine and freshwater sediments. A high occurrence of this serotype has already been reported for polluted freshwaters (12, 13). In contrast, serotype *Newport* was the dominant serotype in wastewater, and consequently, it was also found in river samples. In Tunisia, Nazek and coll. reported that *S.enterica* serotype *Corvallis* was the most frequentely reported *Salmonella* serotype, accounting for 17.3% of all environmental isolates. Whereas, *S.enterica* serotype *Enteritidis* and *S.enterica* serotype *Anatum* came in second and third position, respectively, with non consistent trends during the study period (8). The most frequent source of isolation was tap water samples (8). Another study analyzing 60 wastewater samples showed that in entrance point 66.6% of samples were contaminated with *Salmonella* whereas, in exit points, a percentage of 20% were found. In entrance points, three serotypes of *Salmonella spp*. were detected: *Typhimurium*, *Enteritidis* and *Montevideo*; however, in exit points only the *Typhimurim* serotype was isolated (14). In 1999 and 2000, in Spain, the most frequent serotypes isolated from wastewater were *S. Enteritidis* and *S. Anatum* (15). Regarding *Salmonella* strains isolated from animal, the most frequently isolated *Salmonella* serotype during the study period was *S.enterica* serotype

Enteritidis followed by *S.enterica* serotype *Corvallis*. For *Enteritidis* serotypes, the source of isolation was poultry (70%), cattle (69%) and fish and shellfish (22%). While, *S.enterica* serotype *Amesterdam* and *S. enterica* serotype *Corvallis* were in a lead for cattles (8). *Salmonella* strains present a great impact on human health. In Tunisia, during 11 year surveillance periode (1994-2004), the top three reported *Salmonella* serotypes (*Enteritidis, Corvallis and Linvingstone*) accounted for 48.4% of all human isolates (8). *S.enterica* serotype *Enteritidis* came in first position during the study period, except for the years 2001, 2002, and 2003 where it came in the second position, prececed by *S.enterica* serotype *Livingstone* (8). The next not frequently reported serotype was *Corvallis*. Data from 2000 to 2004 suggest that *Salmonella Corvallis* infections are decreasing. *S. enterica* serotype *Linvingstone* was the third most common serotype (8). The most frequent source of isolation was stool samples (95% of *Salmonella* serotypes that were most commonly isolated) (8).Human infection due to *Salmonella enterica* serovar *Senftenberg* is infrequent in the United States. This bacterium colonizes the gastrointestinal tract of birds and mammals, and has been isolated from sewage systems, poultry processing plants, and different animal feeds (16, 17). *S. Senftenberg* infections in humans have been documented, mainly in Africa (18, 19) and India (20, 21), as well as in 1 US outbreak of gastroenteritis (22). Nonintestinal infectious syndromes due to *S. Senftenberg* were also reported in the Indian study (23, 24). At the end of February 2005, the National Institute for Health Surveillance was informed by the National Reference Centre for *Salmonella* of an increase of *Salmonella enterica* serotype *Agona* isolated in infants in January-February 2005. This is the first documented outbreak of *Salmonella Agona* in France. This investigation shows that regular microbiological examinations of formula were insufficient to detect low-grade or inhomogeneous contamination (http://www.invs.sante.fr). The authors' study highlighted the role of *Salmonella* as a pathogen widely dispersed in nature. These organisms can cause disease states that range from self-limited diarrhea to bacteremia considered as a public health problem. Thus, routine controls of all food, animal and human samples must be done in order to prevent community wide outbreaks of *salmonellosis*. The availability of routine molecular typing techniques in outbreak settings would facilitate tracing the source of infection and confirming epidemiological linkages of the *Salmonella* strains isolated from humans, food, animals and the environment.

Chapter 9 - Salmonellosis is of public health concern, accounting for about a quarter of all bacterial foodborne infections. According to the CDC, Salmonella enterica serovar Typhimurium is the most common Salmonella serotype reported. Of great concern is the possession and dissemination of antimicrobial resistance among Salmonella strains. Many antimicrobial resistance genes associated with Salmonella are found on conjugative plasmids. The misuse of antimicrobials in medical and animal-production settings may provide selective pressures that contribute to the proliferation of antimicrobial resistance, primarily by plasmid transfer. This study aims to present a selective pressure (i.e., varying antibiotic concentrations of four antibiotics) on the plasmid transfer rates of Salmonella via conjugation in-vitro. The four antimicrobials were selected for their plasmid-encoded resistance genes, activity against gram negative bacteria, and FDA approval for use in animal production. Successful conjugation pairs of S. Typhimurium isolates were mated under varying pressure conditions, plated on double antibiotic plates to select for transconjugants, and then conjugation rates were calculated. Preliminary results indicate a difference in conjugation rates across the four antimicrobials and within antimicrobials of varying concentration. Final results of the study may be useful in identifying antibiotics that may be more or less likely to initiate plasmid transfer between S. Typhimurium isolates in-vitro.

Chapter 10 - Human salmonellosis infections are usually acquired via the food chain as a result of the ability of *Salmonella* serovars to colonize and persist within the gastrointestinal tract of food-producing animals and the avian reproductive tract, being able to contaminate, survive and grow inside eggs. This review gives an overview of the cellular and molecular processes involved in the colonization of hen's eggs and in *Salmonella* persistence in the harsh conditions of the egg albumen with special focus on serovar Enteritidis, which shows a particular tropism and ability to persist in chicken oviducts and ovaries and to contaminate, survive and grow inside eggs. The trans-ovarian (also referred to as vertical transmission) and the trans-shell (referred to as horizontal transmission) routes of colonization of the egg are briefly described. In addition, several gene candidates involved in bacterial survival in the egg albumen are identified as potential biomarkers, appropriate for the design of ambitious strategies for the prevention of salmonellosis.

Chapter 11 - Members of *Salmonella* are able to infect a wide range of hosts with some subspecies and serovars being host-specific while others are wide host range organisms. Salmonella is most commonly associated with humans, food animals (bovine, swine and poultry) and reptiles such as turtles, lizards, and iguanas. The exact nature of this diversity towards host susceptibility is still unclear. In the present study, whole genomes and subsequent protein homologues from Salmonella Pathogenicity Islands 1 and 2 of several *Salmonella* serovars were analyzed for their structure-function constraints to identify evolutionary pressures. Whole genome alignment showed no explicit pattern of rearrangement, phylogenetic trees of pathogenicity islands genes revealed that the branch lengths were very small, and functional constraint analysis revealed that most of these genes were operating under negative selection. The results indicate that genes of Salmonella Pathogenicity Island 1 and 2 are functionally conserved across serovars, regardless of host range. Thus, the present result suggests that genes located in the pathogenic islands may not be sufficient solely for host specificity and pathogenesis, and other accessory proteins from different strains as well as host factors may play an important role in influencing the severity of the outcome of the diseases.

Chapter 12 - The *Salmonella*/microsome assay is a technique for detection of mutagens based on the principle that mutagens can cause the the reversion of genetic engineered mutations that suppress biosynthesis of histidine in strains of *Salmonella typhimurium*. It started and has been employed since the beggining of the 70's to investigate chemical and biological samples (urine, feces and plasma) and is currently the most used to evaluate the presence of mutagenic compounds in environmental samples (soil, water, atmospheric material and sediment). Due to its importance, it is nowadays included in environmental legislation in several countries. Several improvements were introduced to enhance the sensibility of the test and broaden its applicability and reliability. Even about to complete its forty-year birthday, the assay keeps receiving improvements, including the development of new sensitive strains for detection of groups of compounds and new ways of evaluation and interpretation of the results. This chapter brings a brief review covering the forty years of the *Salmonella*/microsome assay studies and future perspectives and trends of this important mutagenicity assay.

Chapter 13 - *Salmonella enterica* subspecies *enterica* has been isolated from every region around the world and is considered as a potential pathogen for many animal species. The epidemiology, reservoirs and transmission of *Salmonella* is very complex owing to humans, animals and environment are involved. The purpose of this work was to review the current knowledge of *Salmonella* in the wildlife of sub-Antarctic and Antarctic region. For a long time Antarctic was a region that remained isolated from human contact, but in recent years the human presence has notably increased and as consequence, the danger of introduction of microorganisms to the Antarctic fauna. One of the most extensively studied bacterial species in the region is *Salmonella*, because of its characteristics mentioned above. *Salmonella* infections in Antarctic wildlife were first reported in 1970. Since then, several studies have been conducted, which showed that *Salmonella enterica* subspecies *enterica* isolated from sub-Antarctic and Antarctic fauna belonged to the most prevalent serovars in humans and domesticated animals, with the exception of few rare or exotic serovars. Some of *Salmonella* serovars found in Antarctic wildlife were: Enteritidis, Typhimurium, Newport, Infantis which are among the main serovars isolated from salmonellosis cases in humans and animals in the world. *Salmonella* infections in sub-Antarctic and Antarctic wildlife were reported in the following animals: *Adelie* penguins (*Pygoscelis adelie*), south polar skuas (*Catharacta maccormicki*), gentoo penguins (*Pygoscelis papua*), fur seal (*Arctocephalus gazelle*), black-browed albatross (*Diomedea melanophrys*), sea lions (*Phocarctos hookeri*), southern petrels (*Macronectes giganteus*), kelp gulls (*Larus dominicanus*), Weddell seals (*Leptonychotes weddelli*), emperor penguin (*Aptenodytes forsteri*). All of these animal species were *Salmonella* carriers and none of them had clinical signs of salmonellosis. Different routes of introduction of *Salmonella* to Antarctic region have been proposed: by human carriers, by contaminated foods, by infected birds, sewage from some land-based operations or from discharge of this material from ships sailing in waters of the region. One of the most possible routes of introduction is by birds, because many Antarctic birds have long routes of migration. Studies on *Salmonella* carried out in Antarctic region allow the scientific community to know the sanitary status of Antarctic fauna and also, they can be used as an indicator to know the local ecosystem status. Up to now, in spite of the different studies that have been performed in sub-Antarctic and Antarctic, it was impossible to determine if *Salmonella* was introduced or was and indigenous bacterium in the Antarctic ecosystem.

In: Salmonella: Classification, Genetics and Disease Outbreaks ISBN: 978-1-61942-928-4
Editors: Adelaide S. Monte, Paulo Eduardo De Santos

Chapter 1

PRE-AND POST-HARVEST INTERVENTION STRATEGIES FOR CONTROLLING SALMONELLA CONTAMINATION IN BROILER PRODUCTION

Rajesh Nayak[1], Corliss A. O'Bryan[2], P. Brett Kenney[3], Philip G. Crandall[2] and Steven C. Ricke[2,*]

[1]U.S. Food and Drug Administration, National Center for Toxicological Research, Division of Microbiology (HFT-250), Jefferson, AR, US
[2]Center for Food Safety, University of Arkansas, Fayetteville, AR, US
[3]Division of Animal and Nutritional Sciences, West Virginia University, Morgantown, WV, US

ABSTRACT

Contamination of poultry with *Salmonella* occurs prior to entry into the processing facility and by cross-contamination in the processing plant. Breeder flocks, hatcheries, contaminated feed and water, and environmental sources/vectors such as litter, humans, and insects are potential pre-harvest sources of *Salmonella* contamination in poultry. Knowledge of key pre-harvest factors responsible for *Salmonella* colonization would help integrators and poultry producers in defining critical, pre-harvest control points on the farm. Intervention at these points could reduce or eliminate horizontal transmission and *Salmonella* positive birds arriving at the processing plants. It is difficult to improve the microbiological quality of chickens once they have reached the processing plant. Several physical and chemical decontamination procedures have been applied to poultry carcasses and have been useful in reducing the level and frequency of *Salmonella* on poultry carcasses at the processing plants. A combination of pre- and post-harvest intervention strategies can reduce or eliminate *Salmonella* on fresh poultry delivered to consumers, thereby significantly reducing the medical and productivity costs associated with salmonellosis.

---

* Corresponding author: Department of Food Science, University of Arkansas, 2650 N Young Ave. Fayetteville, AR 72704-5690; E-mail: sricke@uark.edu.

The views presented in this Chapter do not necessarily reflect those of the U.S. Food and Drug Administration.

INTRODUCTION

The Centers for Disease Control and Prevention (CDC) estimates that 31 major pathogens cause 9.4 million episodes of foodborne illness each year, leading to almost 56,000 hospitalizations and 1,351 deaths (Scallan et al., 2011). Non-typhoidal *Salmonella* are the second leading cause of these illnesses, after noroviruses, and the cause of most (35%) hospitalizations (Scallan et al., 2011). Scharff (2010) estimated the health care burden of all foodborne illnesses for the U.S. economy to be $152 billion just for the costs of the acute illnesses and a few of the long-term health-related costs. Of those costs, nontyphoidal *Salmonella* spp. account for almost $15 billion (Scharff, 2010).

Foodborne *Salmonella* outbreaks have been associated with a variety of food items, including meat, poultry, eggs, fruits, and vegetables (CDC 2007, 2009a, 2009b). Chicken, shell eggs and foods containing these items are commonly identified as vehicles in outbreaks of *Salmonella* infections (Chittik et al., 2006). Chickens can be contaminated with *Salmonella* because *Salmonella* is able to colonize the bird intestinal tract and thus enter the human food chain through carcass contamination or by systemic infection and ensuing shell egg contamination (Dunkley et al., 2009; Foley et al., 2011; Harvey et al., 2011; Howard et al., 2011; Ricke 2003). Colonized chickens can spread *Salmonella* to clean birds, or chickens may acquire *Salmonella* from feed or rodents (Cox et al., 2000; White et al., 1997). Other sources of pre-harvest contamination include breeder flocks, hatcheries, contaminated water, and environmental sources/vectors such as litter, humans, and insects (Jones et al., 1991; Bailey, 1993; Hoover et al., 1997; Nayak et al., 2003; Park et al., 2008).

Birds may be contaminated with *Salmonella* prior to entry into the processing facility; therefore a possibility exists for cross-contamination to *Salmonella*-free birds in the processing plants. It is difficult to improve the microbiological quality of chickens in the processing plant, but several physical and chemical decontamination procedures have been applied to poultry carcasses in an attempt to reduce and/or eliminate *Salmonella* contamination (Berrang et al., 2011). None of these treatments have been completely successful in eliminating *Salmonella;* hence, it is necessary to develop new methods to eliminate the pathogen from poultry carcasses. To achieve this objective, a clearer understanding of the mechanism of *Salmonella* attachment to poultry skin/tissue is necessary.

To achieve a significant reduction in the level of *Salmonella* contamination among broiler carcasses, only *Salmonella*-free chickens must be delivered to the processing plants. A reduction of *Salmonella* on poultry carcasses necessitates comprehensive control at the farm where birds are brooded and raised before shipment to processing plants. Knowledge of key pre-harvest factors influencing *Salmonella* colonization would assist integrators and poultry producers in defining pre-harvest critical control points on the farm. Intervention at these points could reduce or eliminate horizontal transmission and reduce the number of *Salmonella* positive birds arriving at processing plants. Treatment of carcasses with novel chemicals such as trisodium phosphate (Vareltzis et al., 1997; Xiong et al., 1998), cetylpyridinium chloride (Xiong et al., 1998), hydrogen peroxide (Lillard and Thomson, 1983) or electrolyzed water (Park et al., 2002), could be useful in reducing the level and frequency of *Salmonella* on poultry carcasses at the processing plants. A combination of pre- and post-harvest intervention strategies can ultimately deliver *Salmonella* free, fresh poultry to consumers, thereby significantly reducing the medical and productivity costs associated with salmonellosis.

SALMONELLA PROFILE

Characteristics

Salmonella spp. are members of the family *Enterobacteriaceae,* and are facultatively anaerobic, gram-negative rods (D'Aoust and Maurer, 2007). Most salmonellae are motile by means of peritrichous flagella, with the exception of serovars Pullorum and Gallinarum, which are non-motile; in addition, non-motile strains can develop due to dysfunctional flagellae (D'Aoust and Maurer, 2007). The members of the genus have been thought to share many characteristics that form the basis for biochemical identification of *Salmonella.* It is traditionally believed that a typical *Salmonella* isolate produces acid and gas from glucose in triple sugar iron (TSI) agar medium, does not utilize lactose or sucrose in TSI or in differential plating media such as brilliant green, xylose lysine desoxycholate, or Hektoen enteric agars, produces an alkaline reaction from decarboxylation of lysine to cadaverine in lysine iron agar (LIA) and generates hydrogen sulfide gas in TSI and LIA media (Andrews and Hammack 2011; D'Aoust and Purvis 1998). However, it has become apparent within the last few years that there is much more biochemical diversity in the genus (D'Aoust and Maurer, 2007). Biotypes that are lactose and or sucrose positive, that cannot decarboxylate lysine, that possess urease activity, that produce indole, or that readily grow in the presence of KCN have all been identified (D'Aoust and Maurer, 2007). The diagnostic value of biochemical tests has been questioned (Hoofrar et al., 1999), and these tests will most likely be replaced with molecular methods that target stable genetic loci that are unique to the genus (Hoofrar et al., 2000).

Molecular Characterization

Biochemical identification of *Salmonella* has traditionally been confirmed by serotyping involving agglutination of bacterial surface antigens with *Salmonella*-specific antibodies. Over 2,000 serotypes of *Salmonella* have been identified (D'Aoust and Maurer, 2007). Serotyping of *Salmonella* involves the agglutination of surface antigens with *Salmonella*-specific antibodies (Tankouo-Sandjong et al., 2007). The process is complex, labor intensive and time consuming. Surface antigens targeted include O lipopolysaccharides (LPS) on the external surface of the bacterial outer membrane, H antigens associated with the peritrichous flagella, and the capsular (Vi) antigens found only in *S.* Typhi, *S.* Paratyphi C, and *S.* Dublin (Chart et al., 2007).

Besides being time consuming, serotyping cannot reflect molecular characterization at the nucleic acid level. Therefore, various genotyping methods have been developed to characterize the molecular epidemiology of *Salmonella*, and to delineate their sources and transmission pathways, and identify reservoirs of contamination (Kaldhone et al., 2008; Nayak et al., 2004; Nayak and Stewart-King, 2008). One of these methods is pulsed-field gel electrophoresis (PFGE) (Schwartz and Cantor, 1984; Smith and Cantor, 1987; Smith et al., 1988) which provides a method of molecular fingerprinting useful for epidemiological studies (Maslow et al., 1993). PFGE works by cutting bacterial DNA into small pieces and then subjecting these pieces to gel electrophoresis. The DNA pieces are separated according to size, with smaller pieces of DNA migrating farther down the gel than bigger pieces, creating a pattern of bands sometimes referred to as a "fingerprint". The DNA restriction patterns generated by PFGE are stable and reproducible both within and between laboratories (Ribot et al., 2006). However, limitations exist including being time consuming and requiring a high-level of skill. Additionally, some *Salmonella* serotypes, such as Enteritidis, are highly clonal and have a limited number of PFGE patterns so that it is difficult to discriminate between isolates to detect clusters and outbreaks (Olsen et al., 1994).

Another molecular method is restriction fragment length polymorphism (RFLP; Matsui et al., 2001). The basic technique involves fragmenting a sample of DNA using a restriction enzyme, which can recognize and cut DNA wherever a specific short sequence occurs, in a process known as a restriction digest. The resulting DNA fragments are then separated by length using gel electrophoresis, and transferred to a membrane using a Southern blot procedure. Hybridization of the membrane to a labeled DNA probe then determines the lengths of the fragments which are complementary to the probe (Geilhausen et al., 1990). Analysis by RFLP is also slow and labor intensive, requiring a large amount of sample DNA. The combined process of probe labeling, DNA fragmentation, electrophoresis, blotting, hybridization, washing, and autoradiography can take up to a month (Genge, 2002). In addition, Tompkins et al. (1986) reported that many *Salmonella* strains have identical restriction endonuclease digestion patterns and are difficult to differentiate by simple restriction analysis.

Ribotyping involves the fingerprinting of genomic DNA restriction fragments that contain all or part of the genes coding for the 16S and 23S rRNA. DNA is extracted from a colony of bacteria fragmented as is done for RFLP. The DNA is subsequently transferred to a membrane and probed with a region of the rRNA operon to reveal the pattern of rRNA genes (Grimont and Grimont, 1986). Variations among bacteria in both the position and intensity of rRNA bands can be used for their classification and identification. Ribotyping has been automated by the development of machinery to perform the entire procedure automatically, data is stored electronically and the banding pattern from a particular organism can be compared to the entire databank stored in the computer (Olive and Bean, 1999). In contrast to PFGE, the time required to perform automated ribotyping is minimal, and results can be obtained in as little as 4 hours. Ribotype analysis is capable of subtyping some of the isolates that fall within some common serotypes and phage types (Landeras et al., 1996; Thong et al., 1995). However, other researchers have identified isolates that belong to different phage types yet demonstrate identical ribotypes (Mendoza and Landeras, 1999; Liebisch and Schwarz, 1996; Fontana et al., 2002).

Multilocus sequence typing (MLST), developed as an alternative method to analyze bacterial population structure and discrimination among strains (Harbottle et al., 2006; Maiden et al., 1998), is increasingly being used as an evolutionary and epidemiological tool for a number of bacterial pathogens (Sukhnanand et al., 2005; Torpdahl et al., 2005; Urwin and Maiden, 2003). MLST compares DNA sequences from portions of housekeeping or virulence genes and/or rRNA sequences (Maiden et al., 1998). Kotetishvili et al. (2002) characterized more than 230 *Salmonella* isolates by MLST based on sequences from the 16S

RNA, *pduF*, *glnA* and *manB* genes. The MLST results were compared to PFGE and serotype analysis, and MLST could differentiate strains better than PFGE, though not all genes performed equally. Only *manB* demonstrated clusters among the clinical and environmental strains. The 16S rRNA locus showed significant homogeneity among the isolates and grouped most isolates together. MLST develops accurate strain discrimination and data is accurate between laboratories, but there is a need for development of affordable automated sequence machinery and laboratory technicians will need to become familiar with DNA sequence analysis and statistical software (Winokur, 2003).

COLONIZATION OF *SALMONELLA* IN BROILERS

Sources and Transmission

The primary sites of *Salmonella* colonization in broilers are the ceca, large intestine, and crop (Bryan and Doyle, 1995; Corrier et al., 1991; Fanelli et al., 1971; Hargis et al., 1995; McMeekin et al., 1984; Snoeyenbos et al., 1982; Nayak et al., 2003; Nayak and Stewart-King, 2008). Several factors affect the susceptibility of poultry to *Salmonella* colonization, including (1) age of birds; (2) *Salmonella* serotype and initial challenge dose level; (3) stress from environment, transport, and overt or subclinical disease; (4) feed additives such as antimicrobials and anticoccidials; (5) survival of *Salmonella* through the gastric barrier; (6) competition with gut microflora; (7) location of a hospitable colonization site; and (8) host genetic background (Bailey, 1987; Ricke, 2003). There are also several potential sources of *Salmonella* contamination in an integrated poultry operation (Holder, 1998; Hoover et al., 1997; Nayak and Stewart-King, 2008). *Salmonella* can be disseminated within broilers via vertical or horizontal transmission. Vertical contamination occurs when *Salmonella* is passed from the hen to the chick because of ovarian contamination of the hen (Guthrie, 1992). Horizontal transmission occurs when *Salmonella* is spread by direct contact between infected birds and uninfected birds, or by contaminated feed, water, or litter (Holt, 1995; Holt et al., 1998; Nakamura et al., 1997). The first opportunity for contamination comes from the breeder flock, with the opportunity for cross contamination occurring at the hatchery.

Breeder Flocks and Hatchery

The U.S. poultry industry produced over 12 billion broiler-hatching eggs in 2010 for use in commercial hatcheries (ERS, 2011). In an integrated poultry operation, the hatchery takes eggs from broiler-breeder flocks and distributes chicks to grow-out facilities. Thus, if one *Salmonella*-positive breeding flock exists, it could spread easily throughout the entire operation. Some studies have shown that *Salmonella* serotypes found on fully processed broiler carcasses originate predominately from hatcheries and breeder flocks (Bhatia and McNabb, 1980; Lahellec and Colin, 1985). Transmission of *Salmonella* has been reported through direct ovarian shedding of the organism into the egg before addition of the cell membrane (Mayes and Takeballi, 1983). Ovarian contamination occurs when *Salmonella* passes from the gastrointestinal tract to the ovaries via the bloodstream (Gordon and Tucker, 1965). Once *Salmonella* gets past the egg membranes, there are no effective means to eliminate or prevent further invasion of egg and developing embryo (Cason et al., 1994).

Salmonella can also penetrate the shell and membranes of a freshly laid egg and enter the interior of the egg via pores (Mayes and Takeballi, 1983). Conditions during incubation tend to favor the proliferation of these bacteria, and the *Salmonella* does not cause extensive decomposition of the fertile egg and so the chick hatches (Cason et al., 1994), resulting in the establishment of *Salmonella* reservoirs in commercial broiler operations (Cox et al., 1990, 1991; Blankenship et al., 1993). Bailey et al. (1992) demonstrated that a single egg contaminated with *Salmonella* may contaminate all eggs and newly hatched birds within a hatching cabinet. Even if the chicks are not contaminated by vertical transmission from the hen or horizontal transmission in the hatchery, there are a variety of means of contamination once the chicks reach the farm.

Feed

Feed is believed to be a major source of *Salmonella* contamination in poultry flocks (Snoeyenbos et al., 1970; Dougherty, 1976; Cox et al., 1983; Hoover et al., 1997; McIlroy, 1998). *Salmonella* sp. has been detected in poultry feed or feed ingredients in a number of studies (Williams, 1981; Stuart, 1984; Veldman et al., 1995). Meat and bone meal or animal by-product ingredients have been reported to have the highest incidence of *Salmonella*, with some estimates of contamination as high as 86% of the feeds sampled (Allred et al., 1967; Maciorowski et al., 2004; Williams et al., 1969). *Salmonella* has also been detected in plant protein sources including soybean meal and different protein sources have been examined for their potential to influence survival of *Salmonella* in feed as well as colonization and shedding (Alali et al., 2011; Grumbles and Flowers, 1961; Ha et al., 1998; Vanderwal, 1979). Recently, Petkar et al. (2011) did not detect differences in *Salmonella* survival after inoculation into organic and conventional broiler feeds when the two feed types were compared.

Inadequate time-temperature control of feed during pelleting, improper storage, and contamination during transportation can contribute to feed contamination with *Salmonella* before entering poultry houses (Maciorowski et al., 2004; McCapes and Riemann, 1998; Park et al., 2011). Feed moisture and conditioning time play crucial roles in the ability of the pelleting process to kill *Salmonella* (Himathongkham et al., 1996). Cox et al. (1983) reported that 92% of mash feed samples were positive for *Salmonella* but no pelleted samples were positive, indicating the importance of the pelleting process. Veldman et al. (1995) found that 21% of mash feeds but only 1.4% of pelleted feeds were positive for *Salmonella*, whereas Jones and Richardson (2004) found that 8.8% of mash feed samples and 4.2% of pelleted feed samples were contaminated with *Salmonella*.

Even though *Salmonella* is destroyed during heat treatments, the possibility of re-contamination still exists. Cross contamination can occur from raw feed ingredients to the plant environment and ultimately to the final feed product. Veldman et al. (1995) sampled raw ingredients and found that 130 samples of fish meal (31%), 83 samples of meat and bone meal (4%), 58 samples of tapioca (2%) and 15 samples of maize grits (27%) were positive for *Salmonella*. Jones and Richardson (2004) collected data that indicated that dust within a feed mill could serve as a major source of contamination to the final product, because vibrations of machinery and air currents around the pellet mill resulted in dust particles being dislodged and landing on the final pelleted feed. Cooling units have also been implicated in the spread of *Salmonella* within a mill (Davies and Wray, 1997).

Litter

Litter in broiler houses is a bedding material, such as wood shavings or rice hulls, which primarily acts to absorb moisture and facilitate the removal of feces at the end of the grow-out period (Roll et al., 2011). Since removal and disposal of used litter and replacing it with new material can be costly, multiple flocks of broilers are typically raised on the same litter. This litter can be a vector of *Salmonella* transmission in the grow-out facilities. Frequency and *Salmonella* serotype information for chicken carcasses can be assessed by examination of litter within poultry houses (Simmons and Byrnes, 1972). The infected birds shed *Salmonella* into the litter, which can harbor the organism from a few days to several weeks. Litter samples have been used as reliable indicators of flock contamination (Bhatia et al., 1979; Olesiuk et al., 1969; Snoeyenbos et al., 1967, 1969). Fanelli et al. (1970) reported that recycling of *Salmonella* between litter and birds appears to maintain intestinal colonization. However, reused litter eventually develops a *Salmonella* inhibitory effect (Bhatia et al., 1979; Tucker, 1967; Fanelli et al., 1970). Bactericidal activity of old litter has been associated with more rapid increases in pH and ammonia than in fresh litter (Dunkley et al., 2011; Opara et al., 1992; Snoeyenbos et al., 1967; Turnbull and Snoeyenbos, 1973,). Older litter may also assist young birds to develop a complex gut microflora that may help exclude *Salmonella* by competition (Fanelli et al., 1970; Hoover, 1996). Several serotypes, including *S.* Pullorum, *S.* Gallinarum, *S.* Typhimurium and *S.* Infantis, have been shown to be susceptible to the bactericidal effects of used litter (Botts et al., 1952; Snoeyenbos et al., 1967; Tucker, 1967; Fanelli et al., 1970; Olesiuk et al., 1971).

Water

Fecal contamination of drinking water by *Salmonella*-infected birds could result in rapid contamination of poultry houses (Bryan et al., 1968; Gauger and Greaves, 1946; Higgins et al., 1982; Morris et al., 1969; Stersky et al., 1981). Water can be initially contaminated with *Salmonella* by bird feces, litter, feed, and dust (Morgan-Jones, 1980; Poppe et al., 1986). High levels of *Salmonella* (10^4 CFU/mL) have been found in the drinking water of chicks less than 1 week of age (Poppe et al., 1986), and Lahellec and Colin (1985) found that 18% of drinker samples were contaminated with *Salmonella* in broiler flocks. Addition of chlorine and sanitizer to drinking water reduces *Salmonella* in broilers (Al-Chalaby et al., 1985; Poppe et al., 1986), but the type of drinkers influenced the level of available free chlorine in water and thus, the levels of *Salmonella* (Poppe et al., 1986). Other researchers have determined that *Salmonella* in water and water sources may actually become more virulent (Nutt et al., 2002, 2003).

Pests

Rodents, insects, birds, and wild animals have been implicated as vectors of *Salmonella* in poultry houses (Amick-Morris, 1998; Henzler and Opitz, 1992; Hoover, 1996; Jones and Twigg, 1976; Keymer et al., 1991; Nagaraja et al., 1991; Wray and Davies, 1998). Rats and mice are the major sources/vectors of *Salmonella*, and they can act as carriers after consuming infected chicken manure. Mice can transmit paratyphoid infections in poultry (Nagaraja et al., 1991). Mice usually stay within close proximity to feed and nesting places and can carry *Salmonella* within the poultry facility. Rats, on the other hand, travel long distances and may transmit *Salmonella* from farm to farm (Haynes and Smith, 1996).

Salmonella transmission may be amplified by mice or rats defecating in feed troughs or litter. Contamination can spread throughout the poultry house by automated feeding and manure removal equipment (Wray and Davies, 1998). Infected wild birds spread *Salmonella* on farms and pastures where domestic animals may acquire infections. Infected seagulls are able to transmit *Salmonella* to poultry houses (Reilly et al., 1981). Davies and Wray (1994) detected *Salmonella* in several species of wild birds near hatcheries and poultry processing units, and these birds could contaminate equipment left outside buildings. Darkling beetles, maggots, blowfly larvae, cockroaches, flies, and mealworm beetles have been implicated in mechanical transport of *Salmonella* in poultry houses (Amick-Morris, 1998; Baggessen et al., 1992; Bennett, 1993; Davies and Wray, 1995; Greenburg et al., 1970; Jones et al., 1991; Rivault et al., 1993; Wray and Davies, 1998).

Environmental Sources

Transmission of *Salmonella* within poultry houses may result from moving air and dust particles (Baskerville et al., 1992). Movement of personnel and birds, flapping of wings, and improper ventilation can spread *Salmonella* and other microorganisms in poultry houses (Jones et al., 1984). Wathes et al. (1988) reported that transmission occurs by inhalation and ingestion of contaminated airborne particles. *Salmonella* can be isolated from organs of chicks and adult birds after exposure to aerosols containing the organism (Clemmer et al., 1960; Baskerville et al., 1992; Wathes et al., 1988). Wray and Davies (1998) reported that dust particles within selected poultry houses were contaminated (8.5 to 220.4×10^2 CFU/L of air) with microorganisms including species of *Streptococcus*, *Staphylococcus*, and *Salmonella*.

Other Parameters

Management and husbandry practices, transportation, and uncontrollable environmental conditions such as temperature may stress poultry. This stress, in turn, could increase the potential for bird colonization (Bailey, 1988). Thaxton et al. (1971) found that day-old chicks reared at 29, 24, and 21°C suffered increased mortality by 0, 28, and 78%, respectively when infected with *S.* Paratyphi. Soerjadi et al. (1979) concluded that day-old chicks held at 18 to 22°C were more susceptible to low and moderate challenges of *S.* Typhimurium than chicks challenged and held at 32 to 36°C. Broilers withdrawn from feed for several hours before slaughter, crowded into transport coops, deprived of water, and subjected to hot and cold environmental temperatures during transportation could shed *Salmonella* and cross-contaminate birds before they enter the slaughter facility (Bailey, 1988).

CONTROL OF *SALMONELLA* DURING LIVE PRODUCTION

Controlling Feed Contamination

Salmonella contamination of poultry feed can be controlled by consistently and effectively decontaminating feed and preventing recontamination at the production facilities. Control measures would include purchasing *Salmonella*-free feed ingredients and implementing stringent sanitary measures during feed production and transportation (Hoover,

1996; Maciorowski et al., 2004). Organic acids are stable in feed and many of them occur naturally in living organisms, with the added advantage that they will leave no residues in food animals (Wales et al., 2010). Feeds may be treated with acids may be accomplished before or after production of the finished feed. Organic acids have been included in feeds at rates of 0.2 to 2% to inhibit *Salmonella* (Vahl, 1995), but the efficacy in feed varies widely. Activity of organic acids in feed is influenced by the level of contamination, the type of acid or blend of acids, the physical form, inclusion rate, the diet composition, moisture in the feed, and the chemical form of the product (i.e., free acid or acid salt) (European Food Safety Authority, 2008). The temperature of pelleting or extrusion may also affect the activity of organic acids, with higher temperatures resulting in greater efficacy (Garland, 1994; Rouse et al., 1988; Tabib et al., 1984). Killing *Salmonella* in feeds may require a high level of acid, but it may need several days to destroy existing bacteria (Vahl, 1995). In addition, using larger quantities of acid may be expensive, corrosive to equipment in the feed mill, affect feed palatability, and interfere with the availability of vitamins (European Food Safety Authority, 2008). Formaldehyde has been shown to be superior at decontaminating feed compared with acid products (Duncan and Adams, 1972; Smyser and Snoeyenbos, 1979). However, formaldehyde is quite volatile and evaporates in open systems (David et al., 1972; Khan et al., 2003), and workers must be protected from overexposure to this chemical because formaldehyde exposure has been associated with cancers of the lung, nasopharynx, oropharynx, and nasal passages in humans (Horvath et al., 1988). Early and sensitive detection of *Salmonella* in feeds would be helpful for implementing more effective control measures at critical areas of feed production where contamination is most likely to occur (Jarquin et al., 2009; Maciorowski et al., 1998; 2000; 2005, 2006; Park et al., 2011).

Biosecurity

The term biosecurity refers to preventive measures to reduce the risk of transmission of infectious diseases or zoonotic agents into a flock. Everything that enters a poultry house is potentially contaminated, so an effective control program needs to embrace several biosecurity measures. The starting point is to ensure that poultry breeding flocks, houses, feed, and litter are kept *Salmonella* free; there are published specific hygiene measures for equipment, animals, and people (European Food Safety Authority, 2004; Helm, 2005). However, these strategies are only partly effective for controlling pathogen colonization of the poultry house, and thus other methods are necessary to control *Salmonella* efficiently (Mead, 2004).

A comprehensive biosecurity program should consist of guidelines for location of farms and facilities (conceptual biosecurity), farm and fence layout (structural biosecurity), movement of personnel and equipment, manufacture and distribution of feed, water sanitation, rodent and pest control, cleaning and disinfection procedures, monitoring procedures and disease surveillance (operational biosecurity) (Rosales and Jensen, 1998). These guidelines should be simple, cost effective, and reviewed periodically. Protocols should include (1) procedures for poultry house cleaning and disinfection; (2) requirements for decontamination of buildings before and after placement of each flock; (3) requirements for employment and contract growing; (4) restrictions to avoid contact with avian and animal species; (5) requirements for personnel hygiene and health status; (6) disposal procedures for dead birds and manure; (7) source verification of litter suppliers; and (8) steps for decontamination of transport vehicles (Nayak, 2000).

An effective biosecurity program can never be "set in stone", and must it be continuously improved through revisions, updates, and periodic audits. Workshops on biosecurity and sanitation protocols should be organized to educate managers, flock supervisors, contract growers, farm employees, vaccination and monitoring crews, veterinarians, and others involved with poultry operations. A biosecurity program should be complemented by the use of competitive exclusion products, feed additives to prevent recontamination, litter and water treatments, and vaccination (Gast, 2010).

Vaccination

Prophylactic vaccination is another method of preventing vertical transmission of *Salmonella*. An understanding of host immunological responses to *Salmonella* is needed to develop effective vaccines. Unfortunately there is little known about the poultry immune response to virulent or attenuated *Salmonella* strains. Cell mediated immunity is important for tissue clearance (Barrow and Wallace, 2000; Nagaraja and Rajashekara, 1999) and systemic clearance (Farnell et al., 2001) of virulent *Salmonella* strains. Bacterins and live attenuated cultures have been used as vaccines in the prevention of avian salmonellosis (Nagaraja and Back, 1998). Components, such as ribosomes, outer membrane proteins, and polysaccharide-protein conjugates extracted from *Salmonella* have also been investigated as potential vaccines (Nagaraja et al., 1982, 1984, 1985, 1988). Killed vaccines do not induce sufficient protection to eliminate non-specific *Salmonella* serotypes colonizing chickens, likely because the killed pathogen primarily stimulates antibody production but is rapidly destroyed and eliminated from the host, and relevant antigens may be destroyed during the preparation of the vaccine (Barrow, 2007). Killed vaccines also do not induce cytotoxic T cells (Nagaraja and Rajashekara, 1999) or secretory IgA responses (Barrow and Wallace, 2000), both of which seem to be important for protecting mucosal surfaces. Vaccines prepared from live but attenuated *Salmonella* strains (Gallinarum, Typhimurium, Choleraesuis, and Enteritidis) have produced variable protection depending on delivery route and ability of the attenuated strain to survive the host (Pritchard et al., 1978; Barrow, 1990; Barrow et al., 1987, 1998, 1990a, 1990b, 1998; Hassan and Curtis, 1994). A few live vaccines are registered and commercially available for use in Europe only. For example, the rough strain *S.* Gallinarum 9R is registered for prevention of *S.* Enteritidis (Feberwee et al., 2001). A detailed review of vaccine types and effects can be found in Barrow (2007).

Feed or Water Additives

Klasing (1998) suggested that modifying the ingredients and/or nutrients in feed might reduce bird susceptibility to pathogens. More recently researchers have been investigating various feed or water additives, such as competitive exclusion, probiotics, prebiotics and synbiotics, for modulation of the gut flora.

Competitive Exclusion

Pivnic and Nurmi (1982) noted that newly hatched chicks may be colonized by a single cell of *Salmonella*, but older birds are more resistant to colonization because of a mature, complex gut microflora. Nurmi and Rantala (1973) had previously suggested that a suspension of the contents of the gastrointestinal (GI) tract of adult birds given orally to newly hatched chicks would establish an adult-type microflora in the chicks, which would protect them from *Salmonella* colonization. This process through which normal intestinal microflora protects the host against invading pathogens is called competitive exclusion (CE). This process is most often used to increase the resistance of young chicks to *Salmonella* (Mead, 2000), but has also been used after antibiotic therapy to restore the normal gut flora (Seo et al., 2000). The treatment is given as soon as possible after hatching, either by adding the culture to the first drinking water or by spraying in the hatchery or on the farm (Bailey et al., 2000; Palmu and Camelin, 1997; Schneitz, 2005). The spraying method was developed to overcome the reduced viability of anaerobic strains in water and the variable drinking water uptake in the first 24 h after hatching (Mead, 2000).

Two types of CE cultures, undefined (bacterial composition unknown) and defined (known bacterial composition) have been used (Stavric and D'Aoust, 1993; Mead, 1998). Studies have been carried out to determine the laboratory and field efficacy of undefined and defined CE cultures. Undefined CE cultures offer protection to chicks when challenged with a standard dose of *Salmonella* under laboratory conditions (Stavric and D'Aoust, 1993; Nisbet et al., 1994, 1996; Palmu and Camelin, 1997; Corrier et al., 1998; Fukata et al., 1999; Hume et al., 1998). However, field study results have been variable. Protective capacity of undefined cultures is influenced by source of microflora, culture conditions, method of administration, presence of feed additives, in-laboratory or natural environmental *Salmonella* challenge, and hygienic practices on the farm (Bailey, 1987; Savage, 1987). Formulation of undefined cultures has been difficult due to insufficient knowledge of microbial ecology, isolation/detection techniques, underlying protective mechanisms, and host (bird)-microbe and microbe-microbe interactions in the GI tract (Ricke and Pillai, 1999). Defined cultures are less effective than undefined cultures under laboratory conditions and afford little protection against *Salmonella* colonization (Stavric, 1987; Corrier et al., 1993; Stavric and D'Aoust, 1993). Commercial CE preparations such as Aviguard (Bayer AG, Leverkusen, Germany), Avi-Free (Alltech Ltd., Stamford, UK), Broilact (Orion Corporation, Espoo, Finland), CF3 (Milk Specialties Co., Dundee, IL), and Preempt (Milk Specialties Co., Dundee, IL) are currently available. All are mixed cultures derived from the cecal contents and/or gut wall of domestic birds (Schneitz, 2005).

Competitive exclusion cultures may exclude *Salmonella* by (1) competing for attachment sites and nutrients in the intestine; (2) excreting metabolic products such as bacteriocins, volatile fatty acids (VFAs), lactic acid, and hydrogen sulfide that are toxic to *Salmonella*; and/or (3) creating an intestinal environment conducive to the growth of obligate anaerobes. Effects of CE on *Salmonella* in the cecum appear to be bacteriostatic rather than bactericidal (Mead, 2000) and have been associated with production of VFAs by the bacteria (Schneitz, 2005). Hume et al. (1996) observed a significant increase in propionic acid in the ceca when chicks were challenged with *Salmonella* Typhimurium at 10^4 CFU at 4 h after treatment with a commercial CE treatment, CF-3, by oral gavage. Other proposed mechanisms are competition between pathogens and the CE flora for receptor sites in the intestinal tract, or competition for nutrients (Ewing, 2009; Mead, 2000). The exact mechanism(s) of action remains unknown.

Probiotics

A probiotic is defined as ''a live microbial feed supplement which beneficially affects the host animal by improving its intestinal microbial balance'' (Fuller, 1989). Jin et al (1998) found that feeding probiotic bacteria changed the community structure of the gut flora, stimulated the immune system, and had a growth-promoting effect. Several researchers have found that feeding of one or more probiotic strains to broilers may inhibit *Salmonella* colonization (Audisio et al., 2000; Higgins et al., 2007; Van Coillie et al., 2007). Proposed mechanisms of action of probiotics are competition for receptor sites, competition for limiting nutrients, and production of antimicrobial metabolites (e.g., bacteriocins, VFAs, and hydrogen peroxide) (Ewing, 2009; Ouwehandn et al., 1999; Servin, 2004).

Most probiotic organisms come from the genera *Lactobacillus*, *Enterococcus*, *Pediococcus*, and *Bacillus*, but the most extensive research focus has been on *Lactobacillus* species (Jin et al., 1996; Tsai et al., 2005; Van Coillie et al., 2007). Jin et al. (1996) examined the effect of *Lactobacillus fermentum* and *L. acidophilus* on attachment of *S.* Typhimurium and *S.* Pullorum, respectively and found a significant reduction in attachment of the pathogen to ileal epithelial cells. The mode of action in this study was concluded to be exclusion (lactobacilli prior to addition of salmonellae) and competition (lactobacilli versus salmonellae) (Jin et al., 1996). Another mode of action for *L. acidophilus* and *L. fermentum* against *S.* Typhimurium is production of lactic acid (Tsai et al., 2005). An *Enterococcus* spp. protected chickens against *Salmonella* challenge by the combined effects of lactic acid and bacteriocins (Audisio et al., 2000). In the previously described trials, the probiotic was given orally, but according to Jin et al. (1998) and Line et al. (1998) probiotics can be incorporated into the feed. Line et al. (1998) found that supplementing standard feed with live cells of *Saccharomyces boulardii* reduced cecal colonization from 1.64 to 0.15 log CFU/g in broiler chickens that had been co-challenged with *Salmonella* Typhimurium and *Campylobacter jejuni* at 4 days of age.

Prebiotics

Prebiotics are feed ingredients that are not digested or metabolized or are metabolized very little as they pass through the upper portion of the GI tract and thus are available to interact with the flora of the large intestine by serving as a substrate for beneficial bacteria (Grizard and Barthomeuf, 1999). Non-digestible fermentable feed carbohydrates and sugar alcohols are considered prebiotics (Suskovic et al., 2001); the non-digestible carbohydrates may be categorized according to their molecular weight. The most important prebiotics are the di- and oligosaccharides (Mussatto and Mancilha, 2007).

Prebiotics have beneficial health effects including inhibiting intestinal colonization by *Salmonella* (Grizard and Barthomeuf, 1999). One effect is directly binding to *Salmonella* in the GI tract, thus blocking adhesion to epithelial cells (Snijders and van Knapen, 2002). They may also have indirect effects by serving as specific nutrients for beneficial bacteria thus inhibiting pathogen colonization by CE, or by stimulating production of lactic acid, VFAs, or bacteriocins (Suskovic et al., 2001). Lactose, lactulose, and lactosucrose are natural disaccharides or trisaccharides that have been reported to have prebiotic effects in chickens (Tellez et al., 1993). Tellez et al. (1993) fed chicks lactose and found a significant reduction in the total number of organ invasions by *Salmonella* Enteritidis at 14 and 19 days after infection in chicks fed with lactose. Conversely, Barnhart et al. (1999) did not observe any reduction in *Salmonella* populations in the crop or cecum of broilers fed 2.5% lactose in the drinking water during the last 5 to 11 days of growth before slaughter. Fructooligosaccharides (FOS) and mannanoligosaccharides (MOS) have been studied extensively for prebiotic effects in chickens and activity against *Salmonella*. FOS reduce *Salmonella* colonization of chickens by means that differ with the mode of preparation of the FOS and at what point they are added to the experimental diet (Chambers et al., 1997). Donalson et al. (2007) discovered that FOS in combination with cecal contents acted in a synergistic manner to decrease *S.* Typhimurium growth when *S.* Typhimurium was introduced to 24 h cecal incubations. When laying hens were fed FOS-containing diets and compared to hens that were subjected to feed withdrawal it was observed that ovary and liver colonization by *S.* Enteritidis was reduced, and in some trials decreases of cecal counts of *S.* Enteritidis counts were also observed (Donalson et al., 2008). When 4000 ppm of MOS was incorporated into the diet of chicks that were subsequently inoculated with *S.* Dublin, the number of chicks with the pathogen in their ceca was 34% lower than in the control group without MOS (Spring et al., 2000).

Synbiotics

A logical extension is to create synbiotics, combinations of probiotics and prebiotics (Collins and Gibson, 1999; Schrezenmeir and de Vrese, 2001). Schrezenmeir and de Vrese (2001) reserve the term synbiotic for products in which the prebiotic selectively favors the probiotic. Kontula et al. (1998) found that three specific lactic acid bacteria were able to ferment β-glucooligosaccharides and xylooligosaccharides resulting in antimicrobial activity. Nisbet et al. (1993) studied a combination of lactose and CE for effects on *Salmonella* colonization in chicks and found that the combination was more effective than lactose alone or CE alone. However, Fasina et al. (2008) did not find any benefit from combining pectin and a commercial probiotic in reducing *Salmonella* in chicken ceca. Much research has been done on synbiotics in humans, but more work needs to be done using commercial probiotics and specific prebiotics for poultry (Vandeplas et al., 2010).

Litter Treatment

Roll et al. (2011) confirmed that reuse of litter actually inhibits *Salmonella* colonization. They determined that the decrease in samples positive for *Salmonella* was not due to chance, but was highly associated with reuse of the litter. They hypothesized that increases in moisture and denitrifying bacteria intensify degradation of urate from feces in the litter increasing ammonia production, and inhibiting *Salmonella*. Ricke et al (1997) also determined that *S.* Typhimurium was inhibited by ammonium salts, dependent on extracellular pH and type of ion forming the ammonium salt, but found that some adaptation occurred over time. High ammonium levels are known to not only be inhibitory to other bacteria but at lower concentrations can alter their metabolism (Ricke and Schaefer, 1991, 1996; Ricke et al., 1996). However, treatment of litter to decrease the pathogen load is often recommended.

Treating litter with organic acids formalin, sodium bisulfate, aluminum sulfate, and sulfuric acid to eliminate *Salmonella* and other pathogens has been described (Ivanov, 2001; Line, 2002; Pope and Cherry, 2000; Williams, 1980). Vicente et al. (2007) reported on the use of a product containing sulfuric acid that is used to control ammonia volatilization by converting litter ammonia to ammonium sulfate, consequently decreasing litter pH and leading to pathogen reduction in the litter, which might in turn lead to decreased *Salmonella* concentration in the cecum. However, Line (2002) found that aluminum sulfate and sodium bisulfate had no effect on *Salmonella* colonization in chickens raised on pine shavings. Stringfellow et al. (2010) studied steam pasteurization and/or the use of quicklime for reduction of *S.* Typhimurium in litter. They found that all steam treatments, with or without quicklime, significantly reduced *S.* Typhimurium by 3 logs, and significant reductions were also seen with quicklime alone.

CONTROL OF *SALMONELLA* DURING PROCESSING

Sources of Contamination

Although the frequency of *Salmonella*-positive birds entering a processing plant is generally low (National Advisory Committee on Microbiological Criteria in Foods, 1997), there are several opportunities for carcass cross-contamination during slaughter and subsequent processing (Bryan et al., 1968; Lillard, 1990; May, 1974; Morris et al., 1969).

The rate of *Salmonella* contamination, either from processing plants or retail markets, varies from 5 to 100% on broiler carcasses (Carraminana et al., 1997; Humphrey et al., 1988; Lammerding et al., 1988; National Advisory Committee on Microbiological Criteria in Foods, 1997; Todd, 1980). Possible sources of *Salmonella* contamination during poultry processing are summarized in Table 1 (Russell, 1998).

Table 1. Sources of Salmonella (and other microorganisms) contamination during poultry processing (abstracted from Russell, 1998)

Operation	Workers' hands	Equipment and tools	Bird to bird	Other environmental factors[1]
Stunning	-	-	-	*
Scalding	-	**	***	****
Picking	-	****	**	-
Washing	-	*	-	****
Rehanging	***	-	-	-
Eviseration	**	****	**	-
Inspection	****	-	-	-
Reprocessing	****	****	-	-
Washing	-	*	-	****
Chilling	-	-	**	****
Rehanging	****	-	-	-
Sizing	-	***	***	-
Boxing	****	*	*	-

[1] Processing parameters, water quality, and disinfectant level.

[*] Not a significant source of contamination to **** significant source of contamination.

Reviews on microbial contamination associated with individual processing steps have been published (Bryan and Doyle, 1995; National Advisory Committee on Microbiological Criteria in Foods, 1997; Russell, 1998).

INTERVENTION STRATEGIES IN THE PROCESSING PLANT

Although broiler slaughter operations do not include thermal processes that ensure elimination of *Salmonella*, a number of processing steps can be controlled to minimize and reduce microbiological hazards. Implementation of HACCP protocols in the slaughter facility and several chemical and physical treatments of broiler carcasses reduce/eliminate *Salmonella* associated with fresh poultry. The goals of HACCP for poultry slaughter operations are to prevent, eliminate, or reduce the incidence and level of pathogenic microorganisms such as *Salmonella* and to control bacterial recontamination and/or outgrowth (National Advisory Committee on Microbiological Criteria in Foods, 1997). In general, HACCP can be defined as a systematic, scientific approach used in food production to ensure food safety (National Advisory Committee on Microbiological Criteria in Foods, 1998).

In 1997, the Food Safety and Inspection Service (FSIS) of the United States Department of Agriculture (USDA) implemented mandatory HACCP regulations and switched from organoleptic to science-based inspection (Federal Register, 1996). This inspection includes microbiological testing and mandatory reporting of any incidence of pathogen recovery, and identification of actual sources of contamination and cross-contamination, as well as visual examination of carcasses for fecal contamination. To verify that HACCP systems are effective, the FSIS has set performance standards for *Salmonella* that slaughter plants must meet. Sampling and testing for *Salmonella* is carried out on an unannounced basis by federal inspectors. The original performance standards for broilers was set to be no more than 12 positives out of a 51 sample set (20%); in 2011 the standards were amended to no more than 5 positives out of the 51 sample set (7.5%) (Flynn, 2010). Failure to meet performance standards requires a plant to take immediate action to meet the guidelines, and results in web posting of establishments that fail.

In the slaughter facility, CCP's fall into two categories: (1) preventive measures to avoid contamination of carcasses with *Salmonella* and (2) risk minimization measures to limit spread of *Salmonella* from contaminated carcasses. Preventive measures include adequate live-bird surveillance on the farm, surveillance of personnel handling the birds, pest control, equipment sanitation, safe water supply, and good manufacturing practices in the processing units (McCapes et al., 1991). Risk minimization measures include chlorination of carcass rinse water, refrigeration, equipment cleaning and disinfection procedures, and personnel sanitation.

Several intervention strategies have been attempted to rid raw poultry carcasses of *Salmonella* and other poultry pathogens. Interventions can include physical, chemical or biological treatments (Bolder, 1997; Dincer and Baysal, 2004; Huffman, 2002; Koohmaraie et al., 2005; Ricke et al., 2005). Carcass decontamination in the United States and Canada frequently follows a multiple hurdle approach (Arthur et al., 2004; Bacon et al., 2000; Stopforth et al., 2007). In the European Union, carcass interventions using anything other than potable water are discouraged, although current legislation does not ban chemical decontamination but approval must be given by the European Food Safety Authority (European Food Safety Authority, 2010).

Water Based Interventions

Cold water has been shown to be effective for removing physical contaminants such as soil, feathers and other debris, but has little effect on bacterial numbers, because of the difficulty of removing attached bacteria from the carcass (Abu-Ruwaida et al., 1994; Firstenberg-Eden, 1981; Lillard, 1989). As might be expected, several researchers have had some success using either hot water sprays or immersion in hot water to reduce bacterial contamination (Avens and Miller, 1972; de Ledesma et al., 1996; Purnell et al., 2004; Whyte et al., 2003). In general researchers have found treatments to be more effective with higher temperatures or longer exposure times (Cox et al., 1974; Morrison and Fleet, 1985; Pickett and Miller, 1966). However, Northcutt et al. (2005) found that *Salmonella* inoculated onto broiler carcasses was lowered an average of 2 logs regardless of the temperature of the spray (21.1, 43.3, or 54.4°C) or whether or not the water contained chlorine.

Electrolyzed water, produced by electrolysis, is available for use as a sanitizer in processing plants. The electrolysis forms an acidic electrolyzed water (pH of 2 to 3, active chlorine content of 10 to 90 ppm), and a basic electrolyzed water that has a pH of 10 to 13. Acidic electrolyzed water was found to be more effective than chlorine in an immersion process, reducing total aerobic counts, coliforms and *S.* Typhimurium on poultry carcasses immediately after immersion and after 7 days of refrigerated storage (Fabrizio et al., 2002). However, when the electrolyzed water was applied by spray the acidic electrolyzed water was not significantly different from untreated carcasses either immediately after spray or during refrigerated storage (Fabrizio et al., 2002).

Chlorine Based Interventions

Presently, commercial processing plants in the U.S. use 20 to 50 ppm chlorine disinfectant (3-5 ppm residual chlorine) in immersion chillers (Thomson et al., 1979; Tamblyn et al., 1997). Chlorine has been widely used because it is relatively safe (GRAS status), readily available, and inexpensive (Tsai et al., 1991). Chlorine (20 ppm) has also been used by slaughter facilities to disinfect equipment surfaces, carcass rinse cabinets, and the inside-outside bird washer prior to the chiller. However, chlorinated immersion and spray methods for use on carcasses have been relatively ineffective against *Salmonella* due to the large amounts of organic matter (blood and feces) (Hargis et al., 1998). Another factor that affects bactericidal properties of chlorine is pH. In water, chlorine dissociates into hypochlorous acid (powerful disinfectant) and hypochlorite ion (weak disinfectant). Poultry chill water has a pH of 7.6 to 8.0. At this pH, less than 60% of the chlorine is available in the form of hypochlorous acid (Waldroup, 1998). However, if chill water pH is maintained between 6.0 and 6.5, about 95 to 98% of the chlorine would be available as hypochlorous acid. Hence, chill water tanks are injected with CO_2 that forms carbonic acid, thereby reducing the pH of the chill water (Waldroup, 1998). Alternative decontamination methods have been investigated as potential replacements for chlorine as the standard disinfectant.

Chlorine dioxide (1.5 to 3.0 ppm residual chlorine) has been permitted in U.S. poultry processing plants (Lillard, 1979, 1980; Waldroup, 1998). However, high cost and skin discoloration of raw carcasses have limited its use. Trisodium phosphate (8 to 12%) has also been approved for use in processing units to reduce *Salmonella* and other foodborne pathogens (Giese, 1993; Tamblyn et al., 1997).

Other Interventions

Several physical and chemical approaches such as air scrubbing (Dickson and Cox, 1992), heat (Davidson et al., 1985; Morrison and Fleet, 1985), irradiation (Mulder et al., 1977; Hanis et al., 1989; Thayer, 1995; Thayer et al., 1991; Abu-Tarboush et al., 1997), ozone (Yang and Chen, 1979, Sheldon and Brown, 1986; Waldroup, 1998), and several organic acids and chemicals have been used to reduce/eliminate *Salmonella* on carcasses and to minimize cross- contamination (Conner and Bilgili, 1994; Hwang and Beuchat, 1995; Tamblyn and Conner, 1997; Tamblyn et al., 1997; Xiong et al., 1998; Yang et al., 1998). The Food and Drug Administration (FDA) has approved irradiation of refrigerated or frozen uncooked meat, meat by products, and certain meat products to control foodborne pathogens and extend product shelf life (Food and Drug Administration, 1997). Organic acids such as lactic, acetic, citric, malic, propionic, and tartaric acid reduce *Salmonella* levels on poultry carcasses (Snijders et al., 1985; van der Marel et al., 1988; Hwang and Beuchat, 1995; Kolsarchi and Candogan, 1995; Tamblyn and Conner, 1997).

Among several chemical treatments, phosphates (Kim and Slavik, 1994; Lillard, 1994; Hwang and Beuchat, 1995; Salvat et al., 1997; Wang et al., 1997; Coppen et al., 1998), hydrogen peroxide (Lillard and Thomson, 1983), quaternary ammonium salts (Breen et al., 1995; Wang et al., 1997), glutaraldehyde (Thomson et al., 1977), sorbates (Robach and Sofos, 1982; Kolsarchi and Candogen, 1995), Tween 80 (Hwang and Beuchat, 1995), and a combination of lysozyme and EDTA (Samuelson et al., 1985) have been found to be effective in reducing *Salmonella* contamination on poultry carcasses. O'Bryan et al. (2008) found that some essential oils from citrus had activity against *Salmonella* spp. Multiple hurdle treatments using a combination of heat and acidified organic acids have also been successful in a laboratory environment (Milillo and Ricke, 2010; Milillo et al., 2011). For an excellent review of poultry carcass treatments see Loretz et al. (2010). Although these approaches reduce *Salmonella* on fresh poultry, they could adversely affect taste, color, flavor, texture, and/or appearance of the product (Breen et al., 1995; Hargis et al., 1998). Existing technologies reduce, but rarely eliminate, *Salmonella* on carcasses during processing because they are ineffective against bacterial cells that are attached to skin.

Salmonella Attachment to Poultry Skin/Carcasses

Salmonella incidence on broiler carcasses increases with successive stages of processing, possibly due to the ability of the pathogen to firmly attach to poultry tissues or skin (Lillard, 1986a, b; 1989a, b). According to Lillard (1989b), "attached" bacteria can be defined as bacteria that remain on the skin after exposure to a bacterial cell suspension for a predetermined time and following rinsing for one min under running water at 50 psi. Lillard (1989a) demonstrated that *Salmonella* cells are firmly attached to poultry skin before broilers arrive at the slaughter facility, and high levels are recovered after 40 consecutive whole carcass rinses of a single carcass. Salmonellae are not always recovered in the first whole carcass rinse, and so this sampling method could result in false negative reports. Attachment of *Salmonella* to poultry skin or the avian intestinal tract is complex and the mechanism(s) of action are not well understood.

The mechanism of bacterial attachment involves two steps (Kim and Doores, 1993). The first step involves retention of bacteria in a liquid film on the surface of skin and meat after the sample is immersed in the bacterial suspension (Thomas and McMeekin, 1981; Lillard, 1986a, 1986b; Thomas et al., 1987). Thomas and McMeekin (1984) demonstrated that, in the first 15 s of immersion, over 90% of *S.* Typhimurium cells were in the water film and less than 10% were recovered from the skin samples. However, after 30 and 60 min of immersion, 40 and 60% of cells were recovered from the skin, respectively, and fewer were found in the water film. These results indicate a transfer of cells from the water film to the skin as immersion time increases. Contamination of carcasses by *Salmonella* during immersion processes can be reduced by preventing formation of the surface film, and by altering the surface tension. Scanning electron micrographs have shown that *Salmonella* appears to be entrapped in deep crevices or ridges that become more prominent after poultry skin and muscle are immersed in water (Lillard, 1988). *Salmonella* cells lodged in these crevices or ridges of the skin are protected and not easily accessible. Certain chemical treatments used in chill water are effective in reducing salmonellae to non-detectable levels, but did not completely eliminate them from the carcasses (Lillard, 1979, 1980; Lillard and Thomson, 1983; Lillard et al., 1987). Nayak et al. (2001) have indicated that zinc ions ($ZnCl_2$) at 25 and 50 mM concentrations significantly reduced firmly attached *S.* Typhimurium cells by 82 and 91%, respectively, to chicken skin (model). The authors attributed the reduction in *Salmonella*, in part, to the bactericidal activity of $ZnCl_2$ in addition to bacterial cell detachment.

Firstenberg-Eden (1981) reported that bacteria are closely associated with each other and entrapped in certain inaccessible sites by physical forces. Attachment at this stage is reversible and balanced between attractive van der Waals and repulsive electrostatic forces (Gristina, 1987). Adhesion depends on characteristics of the bacterium, the surrounding medium, and the substrate surface to be colonized. Bacteria approach the binding site with flagella in motile organisms or through fluid flow or external propulsion in motile and non-motile organisms (Benedict, 1988). Although both surfaces (bacterial and meat tissue) possess a net negative surface charge favoring repulsion, variations in isoelectric points, through localized changes in the microenvironmental pH, may allow the two surfaces to approach within the minimum van der Waals forces, favoring attraction (Benedict, 1988).

The second step of attachment is characterized by a time-dependent, irreversible exopolymer formation. At this stage, bacteria multiply and form a microcolony, which can lead to the formation of a biofilm. Formation of these extracellular polysaccharides (glycocalyx) or attachment fibrils has been involved in the attachment process (Costerton et al., 1978; Butler et al., 1979, 1980; Schwach and Zottola, 1982).

The strongest form of *Salmonella* attachment involves high-affinity chemical attachment to specific receptor sites. Little is known about the mechanisms involved in the chemical attachment of *Salmonella* to avian intestinal tract or skin surfaces. Duguid et al. (1966) found that *S.* Typhimurium exhibited adhesive properties due to type 1 pili. Adhesive properties of type 1 pili were inhibited by D-mannose. However, Jones et al. (1980) found that type 1 pili were not involved in the attachment of *S.* Typhimurium to HeLa cells. Cell adhesin, which was released during homogenization of *S.* Typhimurium cells, inhibited attachment of the organisms to the HeLa cell receptor. A cell-bound, D- mannose resistant hemagglutinin that was responsible for attachment of *S.* Typhimurium to HeLa cells (Jones et al., 1980). Inhibition of *in vitro* attachment of *Salmonella* to inverted ceca (McHan et al 1989) and intestinal segments (Oyofo et al., 1989a) by D-mannose and inhibition of colonization in broilers by D-mannose (Oyofo et al., 1989b) indicated that mannose-sensitive adhesion (associated with type 1 fimbriae) plays a major role in the colonization of the avian intestinal tract by salmonellae (Craven and Williams, 1998). Lillard (1986b) also found that mannose-sensitive type 1 fimbriae were responsible for attachment of *S.* Typhimurium to chicken skin.

Attachment of bacteria depends on the presence and activity of flagella (Notermans and Kampelmacher, 1974; Butler et al., 1979; Farber and Idziak, 1984). Flagellated bacteria readily attach and non-flagellated bacteria rarely attach to poultry skin. Bouttier et al. (1997) observed a 90% reduction in *S.* Choleraesuis attachment to beef muscle tissues after mechanically removing the flagella or treating the bacteria with specific anti-flagella serum. The authors attributed this reduction to a loss of bacterial mobility leading to a reduction in the number of bacterial cells reaching the tissue during the period of contact. *Salmonella* attachment has also been associated with connective tissue, particularly collagen (Thomas and McMeekin, 1981; Benedict et al., 1991; Kim and Doores, 1993; Walls et al., 1993). Adhesion to hyaluronan has been identified as the likely explanation (Sanderson et al., 1991). Benedict (1988) demonstrated that *S.* Typhimurium attached to fresh meat surfaces by selectively binding to collagen fibers, particularly the reticulin type. Lipopolysaccharides and hydrophobic bonding have contributed to in vitro attachment of *S.* Typhimurium and *S.* California cells to chicken cecal mucus and enterocytes (Craven, 1994; Craven et al., 1992). The phenomenon of *Salmonella* attachment to poultry skin/tissue or the intestinal tract involves more than one mechanism. Water uptake and type of fimbriae, flagella, and cell wall components may, alone or in combination, influence *Salmonella* attachment to poultry skin. Reduction of *Salmonella* will depend on the extent of fecal contamination within the production facility.

CONCLUSIONS

Bacteria are naturally present in the environment and are found on all raw agricultural products. There are several means by which foodborne pathogens such as *Salmonella*, *Campylobacter*, *E. coli* O157:H7, and *Listeria*, can enter a food system. Factors such as temperature, stress, and unsanitary conditions in the facility may contribute to pre- and post-harvest contamination. *Salmonella* can survive minimal preservation treatment(s) and can continue to multiply if food products are abused.

Humans may introduce pathogens into food products during production, processing, distribution, storage, and preparation. Depending on individual susceptibility (old age, infants, or immunocompromised), foodborne pathogens can inflict mild to life-threatening diseases. The public health system in the U.S. needs to develop a more efficient early-warning network than the currently existing Foodborne Disease Active Surveillance Network (FoodNet) and pathogen DNA fingerprinting (PulseNet), to detect, control and/or prevent foodborne outbreaks. The 2011 Food Safety Modernization Act in the United States aims at strengthening the food safety system, thereby protecting public health. The key mandates and legislation included in this Act focuses on preventive controls, inspection and compliance, imported food safety, response to outbreaks, and enhanced partnerships.

Food safety research should involve more sensitive, rapid, and automated methods to accurately detect and characterize pathogens in food products. Food companies should strictly adhere to the food safety regulations and guidelines implemented by the federal agencies. Food safety educational training programs should be made mandatory for personnel working in the food companies. Food safety workshops can be held through extension services and universities to educate the public. Federal funding must be invested in educating school students and consumers through regular food-safety related programs on television, radio, and the social networking websites. Controlling the incidence of foodborne pathogens in food products from "The Farm to the Fork" must be a concerted effort on the part of all people involved in each segment of the food system – producers, integrators, shippers, retailers, processing companies, retailers, food service establishments, and consumers.

ACKNOWLEDGEMENTS

This manuscript was funded in part from a USDA Food Safety Consortium Grant and a USDA NIFSI grant #2008-51110-04339 to author Ricke.

REFERENCES

Abu-Ruwaida AS, Sawaya WN, Dashti BH, Murad M, Al-Othman HA. 1994. Microbiological quality of broilers during processing in a modern commercial slaughterhouse in Kuwait. *J. Food Prot.* 57: 887–892.

Abu-Tarboush H, Al-Kahtani H, Atai M, Abou-Arab A, Bajaber A, El-Mojaddidi M. 1997. Sensory and microbial quality of chicken as affected by irradiation and postirradiation storage at 4.0°C. *J. Food Prot.* 60:761-770.

Alali WQ, Hofacre CL, Mathis GF, Batal AB. 2011. Effect of plant-based protein meal use in poultry feed on colonization and shedding of *Salmonella* Heidelberg in broiler birds. Ag. *Food Analy. Bacteriol.* 1: 45-53.

Al-Chalaby ZAM, Hinton MH, Linton AH. 1985. Failure of drinking water sanitisation to reduce the incidence of natural *Salmonella* in broiler chickens. *Vet. Rec.* 116:364-365.

Allred JN, Walker JW, Beal VC, Germaine FS. 1967. A survey to determine the *Salmonella* contamination rate in livestock and poultry feeds. *JAVMA.* 151: 1857–1860.

Amick-Morris J. 1998. Insects' contribution to *Salmonella* transmission in turkey flocks. M.S. *Thesis.* West Virginia University, Morgantown.

Andrews WH, Hammack T. 2011. *Salmonella.* In *Bacteriological Analytical Manual.* Available at: http://www.fda.gov/Food/ScienceResearch/Laboratory Methods/ BacteriologicalAnalyticalManualBAM/ucm070149.htm Accessed 20 October 2011.

Arthur TM, Bosilevac JM, Nou XW, Shackelford SD, Wheeler TL, Kent MP, Jaroni D, Pauling B, Allen DM, Koohmaraie M. 2004. *Escherichia coli* O157 prevalence and enumeration of aerobic bacteria, *Enterobacteriaceae*, and *Escherichia coli* O157 at various steps in commercial beef processing plants. *J. Food Prot.* 67: 658-665.

Audisio MC, Oliver G, Apella MC. 2000. Protective effect of *Enterococcus faecium* J96, a potential probiotic strain, on chicks infected with *Salmonella* Pullorum. *J. Food Prot.* 63:1333–1337.

Avens JS, Miller BF. 1972. Pasteurisation of turkey carcasses. Poultry Sc. 51: 1781.

Bacon RT, Belk KE, Sofos JN, Clayton RP, Reagan JO, Smith GC. 2000. Microbial populations on animal hides and beef carcasses at different stages of slaughter in plants employing multiple-sequential interventions for decontamination. *J. Food Prot.* 63: 1080-1086.

Baggessen DC, Olsen JE, Bisgaard M. 1992. Plasmid profiles and phage types of *Salmonella typhimurium* isolated from successive flocks of chickens on three parent farms. *Avian Pathol.* 21:569-579.

Bailey JS. 1987. Factors affecting microbial competitive exclusion in poultry. *Food Technol.* 41:88-92.

Bailey JS. 1988. Integrated colonization control of *Salmonella* in poultry. *Poultry Sci.* 67:928-932.

Bailey JS. 1993. Control of *Salmonella* and *Campylobacter* in poultry production: A summary of work at Russell Research Center. *Poultry Sci.* 72:1169-1173.

Bailey JS, Cox NA, Blankenship LC, Stern NJ. 1992. Hatchery contamination reduces effectiveness of competitive exclusion treatments to control salmonellae colonization of broiler chicks. *Poultry Sci.* (Abstract) 71 (Suppl. 1):6.

Bailey JS, Stern NJ, Cox NA. 2000. Commercial field trial evaluation of mucosal starter culture to reduce *Salmonella* incidence in processed broiler carcasses. *J. Food Prot.* 63:867–870.

Barnhart ET, Caldwell DJ, Crouch MC, Byrd JA, Corrier DE, Hargis BM. 1999. Effect of lactose administration in drinking water prior to and during feed withdrawal on *Salmonella* recovery from broiler crops and ceca. *Poult. Sci.* 78:211–214.

Barrow PA. 1990. Immunity to experimental fowl typhoid in chickens induced by a virulence plasmid-cured derivative of *Salmonella gallinarum*. *Infect. Immun.* 58:2283-2288.

Barrow PA. 2007. *Salmonella* infections: *immune and nonimmune protection with vaccines.*

Barrow, P.A., Hassan, J.O. and Berchieri, A. 1990a. Reduction in faecal excretion of *Salmonella typhimurium* strain F98 in chickens vaccinated with live and killed *S. typhimurium* organisms. *Epidemiol. Infect.* 104:413-426.

Barrow, P.A., Huggins, M.B., Lovell, M.A. and Simpson, J.M. 1987. Observations on the pathogenesis of experimental *Salmonella typhimurium* infection in chickens. *Res. Vet. Sci.* 42:194-199.

Barrow PA, Lovell MA, Berchieri A. 1990b. Immunisation of laying hens against *Salmonella enteritidis* phage type 4 with live, attenuated vaccines. *Vet. Rec.* 126:241-242.

Barrow PA, Wallis TS. 2000. Vaccination against *Salmonella* infections in food animals: rationale, theoretical basis and practical application, p. 323–339. In A. Wray and C. Wray (ed.), *Salmonella in domestic animals.* Cab International, Oxford.

Barrow PA, Zhang-Barber L, Turner AK. 1998. Live vaccines for control of *Salmonella* in poultry. Proc. Intl. Symp. on Food-borne *Salmonella* in Poultry. pp. 201-211. Baltimore, Maryland. *Avian Pathol.* 36:1–13.

Baskerville A, Humphrey TJ, Fitzgeorge RB, Cook RW, Chart H, Rowe B, Whitehead A. 1992. Airborne infection of laying hens with *Salmonella enteritidis* phage type 4. *Vet. Rec.* 130:395-398.

Benedict RC. 1988. Microbial attachment to meat surfaces. *Recip. Meat Conf. Proc.* 41:1-6.

Benedict RC, Schultz FJ, Jones SB. 1991. Attachment and removal of *Salmonella* spp. on meat and poultry tissues. *J. Food Safety* 11:135-148.

Bennett G. 1993. Cockroaches as carriers of bacteria. *Lancet.* 341:732-735.

Berrang ME, Meinersmann RJ, Cox NA, Fedorka-Cray PJ. 2011. Application of chlorine dioxide to lessen bacterial contamination during broiler defeathering. *J. Appl. Poultry Res.* 20: 33-39.

Bhatia TRS, McNabb GD. 1980. Dissemination of *Salmonella* in broiler-chicken operations. *Avian Dis.* 24:616-624.

Bhatia TRS, McRobb GD, Wyman H, Rayer GPS. 1979. *Salmonella* isolation from litter as an indicator of flock infection and carcass contamination. *Avian Dis.* 23:838-847.

Blankenship LC, Bailey JS, Cox NA, Stern NJ, Brewer R, Williams O. 1993. Two step mucosal competitive exclusion flora treatment to diminish salmonellae in commercial broiler chickens. *Poultry Sci.* 72:1667-1672.

Bolder NM. 1997. Decontamination of meat and poultry carcasses. *Trends Food Sci. Technol.* 8: 221-227.

Botts CW, Ferguson LC, Birkeland JM, Winter AR. 1952. The influence of litter in the control of *Salmonella* infections in chicks. *Am. J. Vet. Res.* 13:562-566.

Bouttier S, Linxe C, Ntsama C, Morgant G, Bellon-Fontaine MN, Fourniat J. 1997. Attachment of *Salmonella choleraesuis* to beef muscle and adipose tissues. *J. Food Prot.* 60:16-22.

Breen PJ, Compadre CM, Kim Fifer E, Salari H, Serbus DC, Lattin DL. 1995. Quaternary ammonium salts inhibit and reduce the attachment of viable *Salmonella typhimurium* to poultry tissues. *J. Food Sci.* 60:1191-1196.

Bryan FL, Ayres JC, Kraft AA. 1968. Contributory sources of salmonellae on turkey products. *Am. J. Epidemiol.* 87:578-591.

Bryan FL, Doyle MP. 1995. Health risks and consequences of *Salmonella* and *Campylobacter jejuni* in raw poultry. *J. Food Prot.* 58:326-344.

Butler JL, Stewart JC, Vanderzant C, Carpenter ZL, Smith GC. 1979. Attachment of microorganisms to pork skin and surfaces of beef and lamb carcasses. *J. Food Prot.* 42:401-406.

Butler JL, Vanderzant C, Carpenter ZL, Smith GC, Lewis RE, Dutson TR. 1980. Influence of certain processing steps on attachment of microorganisms to pork skin. *J. Food Prot.* 43:699-705.

Carraminana JJ, Yanguela J, Blanco D, Rota C, Agustin AI, Arino A, Herrera A. 1997. *Salmonella* incidence and distribution of serotypes throughout processing in a Spanish poultry slaughterhouse. *J. Food Prot.* 60:1312-1317.

Cason JA, Cox NA, Bailey JS. 1994. Transmission of *Salmonella typhimurium* during hatching of broiler chicks. *Avian Dis.* 38:583-588.

CDC (Centers for Disease Control and Prevention). 2007. Three outbreaks of salmonellosis associated with baby poultry from three hatcheries— United States, 2006. *Morb. Mortal. Wkly. Rep.* 56:273–276.

CDC (Centers for Disease Control and Prevention). 2009a. Multistate outbreaks of *Salmonella* infections associated with live poultry—United States, 2007. *Morb. Mortal. Wkly. Rep.* 58:25–29.

CDC (Centers for Disease Control and Prevention). 2009b. Surveillance for foodborne disease outbreaks—United States, 2006. *Morb. Mortal. Wkly. Rep.* 58:609–615.

Chambers JR, Spencer JL, Modler HW. 1997. The influence of complex carbohydrates on *Salmonella typhimurium* colonization, pH, and density of broiler ceca. *Poult. Sci.* 76:445–451.

Chart H, Cheasty T, de Pinna E, Siorvanes L, Wain J, Alam D, Nizami Q, Bhutta Z, Threlfall EJ. 2007. Serodiagnosis of *Salmonella enterica* serovar Typhi and *S. enterica* serovars Paratyphi A, B and C human infections. *J. Med. Microbiol.* 56: 1161-1166.

Chittick P, Sulka A, Tauxe RV, Fry AM. 2006. A summary of national reports of foodborne outbreaks of *Salmonella* Heidelberg infections in the United States: Clues for disease prevention. *J Food Protect.* 69: 1150-1153.

Clemmer DI, Hickey JL, Bridges JF, Schliessmann DJ, Shaffer MF. 1960. Bacteriological studies of experimental air-borne salmonellosis in chicks. *J. Infect. Dis.* 106:197-210.

Collins DM, Gibson GR. 1999. Probiotics, prebiotics, and synbiotics: approaches for modulating the microbial ecology of the gut. *Am. J. Clin. Nutr.* 69:1052S1057S.

Conner DE, Bilgili SF 1994. Skin attachment model for improved laboratory evaluation of potential carcass disinfectants for their efficacy against *Salmonella* attached to broiler skin. *J. Food Prot.* 57:684-688.

Coppen P, Fenner S, Salvat G. 1998. Antimicrobial efficacy of AvGard™ carcass wash under industrial processing conditions. *Br. Poultry Sci.* 39:229-234.

Corrier DE, Hargis BM, Hinton A, Lindsey D, Caldwell DJ, Manning J, Deloach J. 1991. Effect of cecal colonization resistance of layer chicks to invasive *Salmonella enteritidis*. *Avian Dis.* 35:337-343.

Corrier DE, Nisbet DJ, Byrd II JA, Hargis BM, Keith NK, Peterson M, Deloach JR. 1998. Dosage titration of a characterized competitive exclusion culture to inhibit Salmonella colonization in broiler chickens during growout. *J. Food Prot.* 61:796-801.

Corrier DE, Nisbet DJ, Hollister AG, Scanlan CM, Hargis BM, Deloach JR. 1993. Development of defined cultures of indigenous cecal bacteria to control salmonellosis in broiler chicks. *Poultry Sci.* 72:1164-1168.

Costerton JW, Geesey GG, Cheng K-J. 1978. How bacteria stick. *Sci. Am.* 238:86-95.

Cox NA, Bailey JS, Mauldin JM, Blankenship LC. 1990. Presence and impact of salmonellae contamination in the commercial integrated broiler hatchery. *Poultry Sci.* 69:1606-1609.

Cox NA, Bailey JS, Mauldin JM, Blankenship LC, Wilson JL. 1991. Extend of salmonellae contamination in the breeder hatcheries. *Poultry Sci.* 70:416-418.

Cox NA, Bailey JS, Thomson JE, Juven BJ. 1983. *Salmonella* and other *Enterobacteriaceae* found in commercial poultry feed. *Poultry Sci.* 62:2169-2175.

Cox NA, Berrang ME, Cason JA. 2000. *Salmonella* penetration of egg shells and proliferation in broiler hatching eggs—a review. *Poult. Sci.* 79:1571–1574.

Cox NA, Mercuri AJ, Juven BJ, Thomson JE, Chow V. 1974. Evaluation of succinic acid and heat to improve the microbiological quality of poultry meat. *J. Food Sci.* 39: 985–987.

Craven SE. 1994. Altered colonizing ability for the ceca of broiler chicks by lipopolysaccharide-deficient mutants of *Salmonella typhimurium. Avian Dis.* 38:401-408.

Craven SE, Williams DD. 1998. In vitro attachment of *Salmonella tyhimurium* of chicken cecal mucus: Effect of cations and pretreatment with *Lactobacillus* spp. isolated from the intestinal tracts of chickens. *J. Food Prot.* 61:265-271.

D'Aoust J-Y, Maurer J. 2007. *Salmonella* species In Doyle MP and Beuchat LR, eds., *Food microbiology fundamentals and frontiers*, 3rd edition. Washington, DC: ASM Press. pp187-236.

D'Aoust J-Y, Purvis U. 1998. Isolation and identification of *Salmonella* from foods. MFHPB-20. *Health Protection Branch*. Health Canada, Ottawa, Ontario, Canada.

David WAL, Ellaby S, Taylor, G.1972. The fumigant action of formaldehyde incorporated in a semi-synthetic diet on the granulosis virus of *Pieris brassicae* and its evaporation from the diet. *J. Invertebr. Pathol.* 19:76–82.

Davidson CM, D'Aoust J-Y, Allwell, W. 1985. Steam decontamination of whole and cut-up raw chicken. *Poultry Sci.* 64:765-767.

Davies R, Wray C. 1997. Distribution of *Salmonella* contamination in ten animal feedmills. *Vet. Microbiol.* 57: 159-169.

de Ledesma AMR, Rieman HP, Farver TB. 1996. Short-time treatment with alkali and/or hot water to remove common pathogenic and spoilage bacteria from chicken wing skin. *J. Food Prot.*59: 746–750.

Dickson JA, Cox NA. 1992. The effect of air scrubbing on moisture pickup, aerobic plate counts, Enterobacteriaceae and the incidence of *Salmonella* on artificially inoculated broiler carcasses. *Poutlry Sci.* 71:560-564.

Dincer AH, Baysal T. 2004. Decontamination techniques of pathogen bacteria in meat and poultry. *Crit. Rev. Microbiol.* 30: 197-204.

Donalson LM, Kim WK, Chalova VI, Herrera P, Woodward CL, McReynolds JL, Kubena LF, Nisbet DJ, Ricke SC. 2007. *In vitro* anaerobic incubation of *Salmonella enterica* serotype Typhimurium and laying hen cecal bacteria in poultry feed substrates and a fructooligosaccharide prebiotic. *Anaerobe.* 13: 208-214.

Donalson LM, McReynolds JL, Kim WK, Chalova VI, Woodward CL, Kubena LF, Nisbet DJ, Ricke SC. 2008. The influence of a fructooligosaccharide prebiotic combined with alfalfa molt diets on the gastrointestinal tract fermentation, *Salmonella* Enteritidis infection, and intestinal shedding in laying hens. *Poultry Sci.* 87: 1253-1262.

Dougherty TJ. 1976. A study of *Salmonella* contamination in broiler flocks. *Poultry Sci.* 55:1811-1814.

Doyle MP, Erickson MC. 2006. Reducing the carriage of foodborne pathogens in livestock and poultry. *Poult. Sci.* 85:960–973.

Duguid JP, Anderson ES, Campbell I. 1966. Fimbriae and adhesive properties in salmonellae. *J. Pathol. Bacteriol.* 92:107-111.

Duncan MS, Adams AW. 1972. Effects of a chemical additive and of formaldehyde gas fumigation on *Salmonella* in poultry feeds. *Poult. Sci.* 51:797–802.

Dunkley CS, Cunningham DL, Ritz CW, Dunkley KD, Hinto A. 2011. Using mortality compost in vegetable production: A comparison between summer and winter composting and its use in cabbage production. *Ag. Food Analyt.* Bacteriol. 1: 6-14.

Dunkley KD, Callaway TR, Chalova VI, McReynolds JL, Hume ME, Dunkley CS, Kubena LF, Nisbet DJ, Ricke SC. 2009. Foodborne *Salmonella* ecology in the avian gastrointestinal tract. *Anaerobe.*15: 26-35.

ERS. 2011. Livestock, poultry and dairy outlook. Available at: http://www.ers.usda.gov/publications/ldp/2011/08Aug/LDPM206%20Text%20Only.pdf Accessed 25 October 2011.

European Food Safety Authority. 2004. Opinion of the Scientific Panel on Biological Hazards on the request from the Commission related to the use of antimicrobials for the control of *Salmonella* in poultry. *EFSA J.* 115:1–76.

European Food Safety Authority. 2008. Microbiological risk assessment in feedingstuffs for food-producing animals. Scientific opinion of the Panel on Biological Hazards. *EFSA J.* 720:1–84.

European Food Safety Authority. 2010. Decontamination of carcasses. Available at: http:// www. efsa.europa.eu/en/ahawtopics/topic/decontamination.htm Accessed November 2010.

Ewing WN. 2009. The living gut, 2nd ed. Nottingham University Press, Thrumpton, UK.

Fabrizio KA, Sharma RR, Demirci A, Cutter CN.2002. Comparison of electrolyzed oxidizing water with various antimicrobial interventions to reduce *Salmonella* species on poultry. *Poultry Sci.* 81: 1598-1605.

Fanelli MJ, Sadler WW, Brownell JR. 1970. Preliminary studies on persistence of salmonellae in poultry litter. *Avian Dis.* 14:131-141.

Fanelli MJ, Sadler WW, Franti CE, Brownell JR. 1971. Location of salmonellae within the intestinal tract of chickens. *Avian Dis.* 15:366-395.

Farber JM, Idziak ES. 1984. Attachment of psychrotrophic meat spoilage bacteria to muscle surfaces. *J. Food Prot.* 47:92-96.

Farnell MB, El Halawani M, You S, McElroy AP, Hargis BM, Caldwell DJ. 2001. *In vivo* biologic effects of recombinant-turkey interferon-gamma in neonatal leghorn chicks: protection against *Salmonella enteritidis* organ invasion. *Avian Dis.* 45:473–478.

Feberwee A, de Vries TS, Hartman EG, de Wit JJ, Elbers ARW, de Jong WA. 2001. Vaccination against *Salmonella enteritidis* in Dutch commercial layer flocks with a vaccine based on a live *Salmonella gallinarum* 9R strain: evaluation of efficacy, safety, and performance of serologic *Salmonella* tests. *Avian Dis.* 45:83–91.

Federal Register. 1996. Pathogen reduction: hazard analysis and critical control point (HACCP) systems. Available at: http://www.fsis.usda.gov/OPPDE/rdad/FRPubs/93-016F_Part_3.htm Accessed 08 November 2011

Firstenberg-Eden R. 1981 Attachment of bacteria to meat surfaces: a review. *J. Food Prot.* 44: 602–607.

Flynn D. Poultry industry gets new performance standards. Available at: http://www. foodsafetynews.com/2010/05/poultry-industry-gets-new-performance-standards/ Accessed 08 November 2011.

Food and Drug Administration. 1997. Irradiation in the reduction, processing, and handling of food. *Federal Register* 62:64107-64121.

Foley SL, Nayak R, Hanning IB, Johnson TJ, Han J, Ricke SC. 2011. Population dynamics of *Salmonella enterica* serotypes in commercial egg and poultry production. *Appl. Environ. Microbiol.* 77: 4273-4279.

Fukata T, Sasai K, Miyamoto T, Baba E. 1999. Inhibitory effects of competitive exclusion and fructooligosaccharides, singly and in combination, on *Salmonella* colonization of chicks. *J. Food Prot.* 62:229-233.

Fuller, R. 1989. Probiotics in man and animals. *J. Appl. Bacteriol.* 66:365–378.

Garland PW. 1994. In-feed *Salmonella* inhibitors. *Poult. Intern.* 33:40–42.

Gast RK. 2010. Preharvest control of *Salmonella*. Available at: http://wattagnet.com/Preharvest_control_of_salmonella.html Accessed 16 November 2011.

Gast RK, Stone HD, Holt PS. 1993. Evaluation of the efficacy of oil-emulsion bacterins for reducing fecal shedding of *Salmonella enteritidis* in laying hens. *Avian Dis.* 37:1085-1091.

Gauger HC, Greaves RE. 1946. Isolations of *Salmonella typhimurium* from drinking water in an infected environment. *Poultry Sci.* 25:476-478.

Geilhausen B, Mauff G, Vlaes L, Goossens H, Butzler JP. 1990. Restriction-fragment-length-polymorphism for the identification of Campylobacter jejuni isolates. Zbl. *Bakt-Int. J. Med. M.* 274: 366-371.

Genge NE. 2002. Working the scene: the evidence. *In The forensic casebook*. New York, New York: Randon House. Pp 21-135.

Giese J. 1993. *Salmonella* reduction process receives approval. *Food Technol.* 47:110-112.

Gordon RF, Tucker JF. 1965. The epizootology of *Salmonella menston* infection of fowls and the effect of feeding poultry food artificially infected with *Salmonella*. *Br. Poultry Sci.* 6:251-264.

Grimont F, Grimont PA. 1986. Ribosomal ribonucleic acid gene restriction patterns as potential taxonomic tools. *Ann. Inst. Pasteur Microbiol.* 137B:165-175.

Gristina AG. 1987. Biomaterial-centered infection: Microbial adhesion versus tissue integration. *Science* 237:1588-1595.

Grizard D, Barthomeuf C. 1999. Non-digestible oligosaccharides used as prebiotic agents: mode of production and beneficial effects on animal and human health. *Reprod. Nutr. Dev.* 39:563–588.

Greenburg B, Kowalski JA, Klowden MJ. 1970. Factors affecting the transmission of salmonellae by flies: Natural resistance to colonization and bacterial interference. *Infect. Immun.* 2:800-809.

Grumbles LC, Flowers AI. 1961. Epidemiology of paratyphoid infections in turkeys – Species encountered and possible sources of infection. *JAVMA.* 138: 261–262.

Guthrie RK. 1992. *Salmonella* enteritidis in eggs. In Guthrie RK, ed., *Salmonella.* Boca Raton, FL: CRC Press. pp 117-129.

Ha SD, Maciorowski KG, Kwon YM, Jones FT, Ricke SC. 1998. Indigenous feed microflora and *Salmonella typhimurium* marker strain survival in poultry feed with varying levels of protein. *Anim. Feed Sci. Technol.* 76: 23-33.

Hanis T, Jelen P, Klir P, Mnukova J, Perez B, Pesek M. 1989. Poultry meat irradiation – effect of temperature on chemical changes and inactivation of microorganisms. *J. Food Prot.* 52:26-29.

Harbottle H, White DG, McDermott PF, Walker RD, Zhao S. 2006. Comparison of multilocus sequence typing, pulsed-field gel electrophoresis, and antimicrobial susceptibility typing for characterization of *Salmonella enterica* serotype Newport isolates. *J. Clin. Microbiol.* 44: 2449-2457.

Hargis BM, Caldwell DJ, Brewer RL, Corrier DE, DeLoach JR. 1995. Evaluation of the chicken crop as a source of *Salmonella* contamination for broiler carcasses. *Poultry Sci.* 74:1548-1552.

Hargis BM, Caldwell DJ, Byrd JA, Corrier DE, Stanker LH. 1998. Preharvest crop contamination and *Salmonella* recovery from broiler carcasses at processing. Proc. Intl. Symp. on Food-borne *Salmonella* in Poultry. pp. 220-231. Baltimore, MD.

Harvey PC, Watson M, Hulme S, Jones MA, Lovell M, Berchieri A, Young J, Bumstead N, Barrow P. 2011. *Salmonella enterica* serovar Typhimurium colonizing the lumen of the chicken intestine grows slowly and upregulates a unique set of virulence and metabolism genes. *Infect. Immun.* 79: 4105-4121.

Hassan JO, Curtis R. 1994. Development and evaluation of experimental vaccination program using a live-avirulent *Salmonella typhimurium* strain to protect immunized chickens against challenge with homologous and heterologous *Salmonella* serotypes. *Infect. Immun.* 62:5519-5527.

Haynes RL, Smith TW. 1996. Control of commensal rodents in poultry houses. Available at: http://www.poultry.msstate.edu/extension/pdf/rodent_control.pdf Accessed 16 November 2011.

Helm, J. D. 2005. Practical disease prevention, biosecurity on poultry farms. Available at: http://www.clemson.edu/public/lph/ahp/disease_links/images/poultrybiosecurity.pdf Accessed 2 November 2011.

Henzler DJ, Opitz HM. 1992. The role of mice in the epizootiology of *Salmonella enteritidis* infection in chicken layer farms. *Avian Dis.* 36:625-631.

Higgins JP, Higgins SE, Vicente JL, Wolfenden AD,Tellez G, Hargis BM. 2007. Temporal effects of lactic acid bacteria probiotic culture on Salmonella in neonatal broilers. *Poult. Sci.* 86:1662–1666.

Higgins R, Malo R, Rene-Roberge E, Gauthier R. 1982. Studies on the dissemination of *Salmonella* in nine broiler-chicken flocks. *Avian Dis.* 26:26-33.

Himanthonkham S, das Gracas Periera M, Riemann H. 1996. Heat destruction of *Salmonella* in poultry feeds. *Avian Dis.* 40: 72-77.

Holder GT. 1998. Meat-type poultry industry initiatives to control *Salmonella*. Proc. Intl. Symp. on Food-borne *Salmonella* in Poultry. pp. 70-74. Baltimore, MD.

Holt PS. 1995. Horizontal transmission of *Salmonella enteritidis* in molted and unmolted layint chickens. *Avian Dis.* 39: 239-249.

Holt PS, Mitchell BW, Gast RK. 1998. Airborne horizontal transmission of *Salmonella enteritidis* in chickens. *Avian Dis.* 42: 45-52.

Hoorfar J, Ahrens P, Rådström P. 2000. Automated 5′ Nuclease PCR assay for identification of *Salmonella enterica. J. Clin. Microbiol.* 38: 3429-3435.

Hoorfar J, Baggesen DL, Porting PH. 1999. A PCR-based strategy for simple and rapid identification of rough presumptive *Salmonella* isolates. *J. Microbiol. Methods* 35: 77-84.

Hoover NJ. 1996. Sources of *Salmonella* colonization in turkey production. M.S. Thesis. West Virginia University, Morgantown.

Hoover NJ, Kenney PB, Amick J-A, Hypes WA. 1997. Preharvest sources of *Salmonella* colonization in turkey production. *Poultry Sci.* 76:1232-1238.

Horvath EP, Anderson H, Pierce WE, Hanrahan L, Wendlick JD. 1988. Effects of formaldehyde on the mucous membranes and lungs. J. *Am. Med. Assoc.* 259: 701-707.

Howard ZR, O'Bryan CA, Crandall PG, Ricke SC. *Salmonella* Enteritidis in shell eggs: current issues and prospects for control. *Food Res. Int.* http://dx.doi.org/10.1016/j.foodres.2011.04.030.

Huffman RD. 2002. Current and future technologies for the decontamination of carcasses and fresh meat. *Meat Sci.* 62 (SI): 285-294.

Hume ME, Corrier DE, Nisbet DJ, DeLoach JR. 1996. Reduction of *Salmonella* crop and cecal colonization by a characterized competitive exclusion culture in broilers during grow-out. *J. Food Prot.* 59:688–693.

Hume ME, Corrier DE, Nisbet DJ, Deloach JR. 1998. Early *Salmonella* challenge time and reduction in chick cecal colonization following treatment with a characterized competitive exclusion culture. *J. Food Prot.* 61:673-676.

Humphrey TJ, Mead GC, Rowe B. 1988. Poultry meat as a source of human salmonellosis in England and Wales. *Epidem. Infect.* 100:175-184.

Hwang C-A, Beuchat LR. 1995. Efficacy of selected chemicals for killing pathogenic and spoilage microorganisms on chicken skin. *J. Food Prot.* 58:19-23.

Ivanov IE. 2001. Treatment of broiler litter with organic acid. *Res. Vet. Sci.* 70:169–173.

Jarquin R, Hanning I, Ahn S, Ricke SC. 2009. Development of rapid detection and genetic characterization of *Salmonella* in poultry breeder feeds. *Sensors* 9: 5308-5323.

Jin LZ, Ho YW, Abdullah N, Ali MA, Jalaludin S. 1998. Effects of adherent *Lactobacillus* cultures on growth, weight of organs and intestinal microflora and volatile fatty acids in broilers. *Anim. Feed Sci. Technol.* 70:197–209.

Jin LZ, Ho YW, Ali MA, Abdullah N, Jalaludin S. 1996. Effect of adherent *Lactobacillus* spp. on in vitro adherence of salmonellae to the intestinal epithelial cells of chicken. *J. Appl. Bacteriol.* 81:201–206.

Jones FT, Axtell RC, Rives RV, Scheideler SE, Tarver Jr FR, Walker RL, Wineland MJ. 1991. A survey of *Salmonella* contamination in modern broiler production. *J. Food Prot.* 54:502-507.

Jones FT, Richardson KE. 2004. *Salmonella* in commercially manufactured feeds. *Poult. Sci.* 83, 384-391.

Jones GW, Richardson LA, Vanden Bosch JL. 1980. Phases in the interaction between bacteria and animal cells. In. *Microbial Adhesion to Surfaces*. pp 211. Ellis Harwood Ltd., Chichester, England.

Jones PW, Twigg GI. 1976. Salmonellosis in wild animals. J. Hyg. 77:51-54.

Jones W, Morring K, Olenchock SA, Williams T, Hickey J. 1984. Environmental study of poultry confinement buildings. *Am. Ind. Hyg. Assoc. J.* 45:760.

Kaldhone P, Nayak R, Lynne AM, White DG, Logue CM, Foley SL. 2008. Characterization of *Salmonella enterica* serotype Heidelberg from turkey-associated sources. *Appl. Environ. Microbiol.* 74:5038-5046.

Keymer I, Gibson EA, Reynolds DJ. 1991. Zoonoses and other findings in hedgehogs (*Erinacaeus europaeus*) – a survey of mortality and review of the literature. *Vet. Rec.* 128:245-249.

Khan MZ, Ali Z, Muhammad G, Khan A, Mahmood F. 2003. Pathological effects of formalin (37% formaldehyde) mixed in feed or administered into the crops of White Leghorn cockerels. *J. Vet. Med. A Physiol. Pathol. Clin. Med.* 50:354–358.

Kim J-W, Doores S. 1993. Attachment of *Salmonella typhimurium* to skins of turkey that had been defeathered through three different systems: Scanning electron microscopic examination. *J. Food Prot.* 56:395-400.

Kim J-W, Slavik MF. 1994. Removal of *Salmonella typhimurium* attached to chicken skin by rinsing with trisodium phosphate solution: Scanning electron microscopic examination. *J. Food Safety* 14:77-84.

Klasing KC. 1998. Nutritional modulation of resistance to infectious diseases. *Poult. Sci.* 77:1119–1125.

Kolsarchi N, Candogan K. 1995. The effect of potassium sorbate and lactic acid on the shelf life of vacuum-packed chicken meats. *Poultry Sci.* 74:1884-1893.

Kontula P, von Wright A, Mattila-Sandholm T. 1998. Oat bran β-gluco- and xylo-oligosaccharides as fermentative substrates for lactic acid bacteria. *Int. J. Food Microbiol.* 45:163–169.

Koohmaraie M, Arthur TM, Bosilevac JM, Guerini M, Shackelford SD, Wheeler TL. 2005. Post-harvest interventions to reduce/eliminate pathogens in beef. *Meat Sci.* 71: 79-91.

Kotetishvili M, Stine OC, Kreger A, Morris JG, Sulakvelidze A. 2002. Multilocus sequence typing for characterization of clinical and environmental *Salmonella* strains, *J. Clin. Micro.* 40: 1626-1635.

Lahellec C, Colin P. 1985. Relationship between serotypes of *Salmonella* from hatcheries and rearing farms and those from processed poultry carcasses. *Br. Poultry Sci.* 26:179-186.

Lammerding AM, Garcia MM, Mann ED, Robinson Y, Dorward WJ, Truscott RB, Tittiger, F. 1988. Prevalence of *Salmonella* and thermophilic *Campylobacter* in fresh pork, beef, veal and poultry in Canada. *J. Food Prot.* 51:47-52.

Landeras E, Gonzalez-Hevia MA, Alzugaray R, Mendoza MC. 1996. Epidemiological differentiation of pathogenic strains of *Salmonella enteritidis* by ribotyping, *J. Clin. Microbiol.* 34: 2294-2296.

Lillard HS. 1979. Levels of chlorine and chlorine dioxide of equivalent bactericidal effect in poultry processing water. *J. Food Sci.* 44:1594-1597.

Lillard HS. 1980. Effect on broiler carcasses and water of treating chiller water with chlorine or chlorine dioxide. *Poultry Sci.* 59:1761-1766.

Lillard HS. 1986a. Distribution of "attached" *Salmonella typhimurium* cells between poultry skin and a surface film following water immersion. *J. Food Prot.* 49:449-454.

Lillard HS. 1986b. Role of fimbriae and flagella in the attachment of *Salmonella typhimurium* to poultry skin. *J. Food Sci.* 51:54-56, 65.

Lillard HS. 1988. Effect of surfactant or changes in ionic strength on the attachment of *Salmonella typhimurium* to poultry skin and muscle. *J. Food Sci.* 53:727-730.

Lillard HS. 1989a. Factors affecting the persistence of *Salmonella* during the processing of poultry. *J. Food Prot.* 52: 829–832.

Lillard HS. 1989b. Incidence and recovery of salmonellae and other bacteria from commercially processed poultry carcasses at selected pre- and post-evisceration steps. *J. Food Prot.* 52:88-91.

Lillard HS. 1990. The impact of commercial processing procedures on the bacterial contamination and cross-contamination of broiler carcasses. *J. Food Prot.* 53:202-204.

Lillard HS. 1994. Effect of trisodium phosphate on salmonellae attached to chicken skin. *J. Food Prot.* 57:465-469.

Lillard HS, Blankenship LC, Dickens JA, Craven SE, Shackelford AD. 1987. Effect of acetic acid on the microbiological quality of scalded picked and unpicked boiler carcasses. *J. Food Prot.* 50:112-114.

Lillard HS, Thomson JE. 1983. Efficacy of hydrogen peroxide as a bactericide in poultry chiller water. *J. Food Sci.* 48:125-126.

Line JE. 2002. *Campylobacter* and *Salmonella* populations associated with chickens raised on acidified litter. *Poult. Sci.* 81: 1473–1477.

Line JE, Bailey JS, Cox NA, Stern NJ, Tompkins T. 1998. Effect of yeast-supplemented feed on *Salmonella* and *Campylobacter* populations in broilers. *Poult. Sci.* 77:405–410.

Loretz M, Stephan R, Zweifel C. Antimicrobial activity of decontamination treatments for poultry carcasses: A literature survey. *Food Control* 21: 791-804.

Maciorowski KG, Herrera P, Jones FT, Pillai SD, Ricke SC. 2006. Cultural and immunological detection methods for *Salmonella* spp. in animal feeds- A review. *Vet. Res. Comm.* 30: 127-137.

Maciorowski KG, Jones FT, Pillai SD, Ricke SC. 2004. Incidence, sources, and control of food-borne *Salmonella* spp. in poultry feeds. *Worlds Poultry Sci. J.* 60: 446-457.

Maciorowski KG, Pillai SD, Jones FT, Ricke SC. 2005. Polymerase chain reaction detection of foodborne *Salmonella* spp. in animal feeds. *Crit. Rev. Microbiol.* 31: 45-53.

Maciorowski KG, Peña J, Pillai SD, Ricke SC. 1998. Application of gene amplification in conjunction with a hybridization sensor for rapid detection of *Salmonella* spp. and fecal indicators in animal feeds. *J. Rapid. Meth. Automation Microbiol.* 6: 225-238.

Maciorowski KG, Pillai SD, Ricke SC. 2000. Efficacy of a commercial polymerase chain reaction-based assay for detection of *Salmonella* spp. in animal feeds. *J. Appl. Microbiol.* 89: 710-718.

Maiden MC, Bygraves JA, Feil E, Morelli G, Russell JE, Urwin R, Zhang Q, Zhou J, Zurth K, Caugant DA, Feavers IM, Achtman M, Spratt BG. 1998. Multilocus sequence typing: a portable approach to the identification of clones within populations of pathogenic microorganisms. *Proc. Natl. Acad. Sci. USA* 95: 3140-3145.

Matsui T, Matsuda M, Murayama O, Millar BC, Moore JE. 2001. *recA* genotyping of *Salmonella enteritidis* phage type 4 isolates by restriction fragment length polymorphism analysis. *Lett. Appl. Microbiol.* 32: 424-427.

May KN. 1974. Changes in microbial numbers during final washing and chilling of commercially slaughtered broilers. Poultry Sci. 53:1282-1285.

Mayes FJ, Takeballi MA. 1983. Microbial contamination of the hen's egg: A review. *J. Food Prot.* 46:1092-1098.

McCapes RH, Riemann HP. 1998. Obstacles to control of *Salmonella* in foods of avian origin. In Proceedings of the International Symposium on Food-Borne Salmonella in Poultry. *American Association of Avian Pathologists*, Baltimore, Maryland. Pages 23-42.

McHan F, Cox NA, Blankenship LC, Bailey JS. 1989. *In vitro* attachment of *Salmonella typhimurium* to chick ceca exposed to selected carbohydrates. *Avian Dis.* 33:340-344.

McIlroy SG. 1998. Control of *Salmonella* contamination of poultry feeds. Proc. Intl. Symp. on Food-borne *Salmonella* in Poultry. pp. 88-92. Baltimore, MD.

McMeekin TA, Thomas CJ, Pennington PI. 1984. Contamination and decontamination of poultry carcass neck tissue. *J. Food Safety*. 6:79-88.

Mead GC. 1998. Prospects for "competitive exclusion" treatment in controlling *Salmonella* and other pathogens in poultry. Proc. Intl. Symp. on Food-borne *Salmonella* in Poultry. pp. 176-193. Baltimore, Maryland.

Mead GC. 2000. Prospects for competitive exclusion treatment to control *Salmonella* and other foodborne pathogens in poultry. *Vet. J.* 159:111–123.

Mead GC. 2004. Current trends in the microbiological safety of poultry meat. *World Poult. Sci. J.* 60:112–118.

Mendoza MC, Landeras E. 1999. Molecular epidemiological methods for differentiation of *Salmonella enterica* serovar Enteritidis strains. In Saeed AM, Gast RE, Potter ME, Wall PG, eds,*Salmonella enterica serovar Enteritidis in humans and animals: epidemiology, pathogenesis, and control*. Ames, IA: Iowa University Press, pp. 125-140.

Milillo SR, Martin E, Muthaiyan A, Ricke SC. 2011. Immediate reduction of *Salmonella enterica* serotype Typhimurium viability via membrane destabilization following exposure to multiple-hurdle treatments with heated, acidified organic acid salt solutions. *Appl. Environ. Microbiol.* 77: 3765-3772.

Milillo SR, Ricke SC. 2010. Synergistic reduction of *Salmonella* in a model raw chicken media using a combined thermal and acidified organic acid salt intervention treatment. *J. Food Sci.* 75: M121-M125.

Morgan-Jones SC. 1980. The occurrence of *Salmonella* during the rearing of broiler birds. *Br. Poultry Sci.* 21:463-470.

Morris GK, McMurray BL, Galton MM, Wells JG. 1969. A study of the dissemination of salmonellosis in a commercial boiler chicken operation. *Am. J. Vet. Res.* 30:1413-1421.

Morrison GJ, Fleet GH. 1985. Reduction of *Salmonella* on chicken carcasses by immersion treatments. *J. Food Prot.* 48: 939–943.

Mulder RW, Notermans S, Kampelmacher, E.H. 1977. Inactivation of salmonellae on chilled and deep frozen broiler carcasses by irradiation. *J. Appl. Bacteriol.* 42:179-185.

Mussatto SI, Mancilha IM. 2007. Non-digestible oligosaccharides: a review. *Carbohydr. Polym.* 68:587–597.

Nagaraja KV, Back, A. 1998. Vaccination against *Salmonella* infection: Killed and subunit vaccines. Proc. Intl. Symp. on Food-borne *Salmonella* in Poultry. pp. 194-200. Baltimore, Maryland.

Nagaraja KV, Kim CJ, Pomeroy BS. 1988. Outer membrane proteins in prophylactic vaccines for *Salmonella*. *J. Am. Vet. Med. Assoc.* 192:1784.

Nagaraja KV, Kumar MC, Newman JA, Pomeroy BS. 1985. Control of *Salmonella arizonae* infection in turkey breeding flocks by immunization. *J. Am. Vet. Med. Assoc.* 187:309.

Nagaraja KV, Newman JA, Pomeroy BS. 1984. Use of oil adjuvant vaccines for the control of *Salmonella* infections in turkeys. *Proc. Intl. Symp. on Salmonella.* 90:84-87.

Nagaraja KV, Pomeroy BS, Newman JA, Peterson I. 1982. Vaccination of turkeys with killed oil adjuvant *Salmonella san-diego* vaccine. *J. Am. Vet. Med. Assoc.* 181:284.

Nagaraja KV, Pomeroy BS, Williams JE. 1991. Paratyphoid infections. In: *Diseases of Poultry*, 9th Ed. Eds. B.W. Calnek, H.J. Barnes, C.W. Beard, W.M. Reid and H.W. Yoder, Jr. pp 99-130. Iowa State University Press, Ames, Iowa.

Nagaraja KV, Rajashekara G. 1999. Vaccination against *Salmonella enterica* serovar Enteritidis infection: dilemma and realities, p. 397–404. In A. M. Saeed (ed.), *Salmonella enterica* serovar Enteritidis in humans and animals: epidemiology, pathogenesis, and control. Iowa State University Press, Ames.

Nakamura M, Takagi M, Takahashi T, Suzuki S, Sato S, Takehara K. 1997. The effect of the flow of air on horizontal transmission of *Salmonella enteritidis* in chickens. *Avian Dis.* 41:354-360

National Advisory Committee on Microbiological Criteria in Foods. 1997. Generic HACCP application in broiler slaughter and processing. *J. Food Prot.* 60:579-604.

National Advisory Committee on Microbiological Criteria for Foods. 1998. Hazard analysis and critical control point principles and application guidelines. *J. Food Prot.* 61:762-775.

Nayak R. 2000. Foodborne pathogens in poultry production and post-harvest control. Ph.D. dissertation, West Virginia University, Morgantown, WV.

Nayak R, Kenney PB, Bissonnette GK. 2001. Inhibition and reversal of *Salmonella* Typhimurium attachment to poultry skin using zinc chloride, *J. Food Prot.* 64:456-461.

Nayak R, Kenney PB, Keswani J, Ritz C. 2003. Isolation and characterisation of *Salmonella* in a turkey production facility. *Br. Poultry Sci.* 44:192-202.

Nayak R, Stewart T, Rong-Fu W, Lin J, Cerniglia C. 2004. Genetic diversity and virulent gene determinants of antibiotic-resistant *Salmonella* isolated from preharvest turkey production sources. *Int. J. Microbiol.* 91:51-62.

Nayak R, Stewart-King T. 2008. Molecular epidemiological analysis and bacterial source tracking of antimicrobial-resistant *Salmonella enterica* serovars in turkey production environment. *Foodborne Path. Dis.* 5:115-126.

Nisbet DJ, Corrier DE, DeLoach JR. 1993. Effect of mixed cecal microflora maintained in continuous culture and of dietary lactose on *Salmonella typhimurium* colonization in broiler chicks. *Avian Dis.* 37:528–535.

Nisbet DJ, Corrier DE, Ricke SC, Hume ME, Byrd II JA, Deloach JR. 1996. Maintenance of biological efficacy in chicks of a cecal competitive-exclusion culture against *Salmonella* by continuous-flow fermentation. *J. Food Prot.* 59:1279-1283.

Nisbet DJ, Ricke SC, Scanlan CM, Corrier DE, Hollister AG, DeLoach JR. 1994. Inoculation of broiler chicks with a continuous-flow derived bacterial culture facilitates early native cecal bacterial colonization and increases resistance to *Salmonella typhimurium*. *J. Food Prot.* 57: 12-15.

Northcutt JK, Smith DP, Musgrove MT, Ingram KD, Hinton A. 2005. Microbiological impact of spray washing broiler carcasses using different chlorine concentrations and water temperatures. *Poultry Sci.* 84: 1648-1652.

Notermans S, Kampelmacher EH. 1974. Attachment of some bacterial strains to the skin of broiler chickens. *Br. Poultry Sci.* 15:573-585.

Nurmi E, Rantala H. 1973. New aspects of *Salmonella* infection in broiler production. *Nature* 241:210-211.

Nutt JD, Kubena LF, Nisbet DJ, Ricke SC. 2002. Virulence response of a *Salmonella* Typhimurium *hilA*: *lacZY* fusion strain to spent media from pure cultures of selected bacteria and poultry cecal mixed culture. *J. Food Safety.* 22: 169-181.

Nutt JD, Pillai SD, Woodward CL, Sternes KL, Zabala-Diaz IB, Kwon YM, Ricke SC. 2003. Use of a *Salmonella* Typhimurium *hilA* fusion strain to assess effects of environmental fresh water sources on virulence gene expression. *Water Res.* 37: 3319-3326.

O'Bryan CA, Crandall PG, Chalova VI, Ricke SC. 2008. Orange essential oils antimicrobial activities against *Salmonella* spp. J. Food Sci. 73: M264-M267.

Olesiuk O, Carlson V, Snoeyenbos G, Smyser C. 1969. Experimental *Salmonella typhimurium* infection in two chicken flocks. Avian Dis. 13:500-508.

Olive DM, Bean P. 1999. Principles and applications of methods for DNA-Based typing of microbial organisms. *J. Clin. Microbiol.* 37: 1661-1669.

Olsen JE, Skov MN, Threlfall EJ, Brown DJ. 1994. Clonal lines of *Salmonella enterica* serotype Enteritidis documented by IS200-, ribo-, pulsed-field gel electrophoresis and RFLP typing. *J. Med. Microbiol.* 40: 15-22.

Opara OO, Carr LE, Russek-Cohen E, Tate CR, Mallinson ET, Miller RG, Steward LE, Johnston RW, Joseph SW. 1992. Correlation of water activity and other environmental conditions with repeated detection of *Salmonella* contamination on poultry farms. *Avian Dis.* 36:664-671.

Ouwehand AC, Kirjavainen PV, Shortt C, Salminen S. 1999. Probiotics: mechanisms and established effects. *Int. Dairy J.* 9:43–52.

Oyofo BA, Droleskey RE, Norman JO, Mollenhauer HH, Ziprin RL, Corrier DE, DeLoach JR. 1989a. Inhibition by mannose of *in vitro* colonization of chicken small intestine by *Salmonella typhimurium*. *Poultry Sci.* 68:1351-1356.

Oyofo BA, DeLoach JR, Corrier DE, Norman JO, Ziprin RL, Mollenhauer HH. 1989b. Prevention of *Salmonella typhimurium* colonization of broilers with D-mannose. *Poultry Sci.* 68:1357-1360.

Palmu L, Camelin I. 1997. The use of competitive exclusion in broilers to reduce the level of *Salmonella* contamination on the farm and at the processing plant. *Poult. Sci.* 76:1501–1505.

Park H, Hung Y-C, Brackett RE. 2002. Antimicrobial effect of electrolyzed water for inactivating *Campylobacter jejuni* during poultry washing. *Int. J. Food Microbiol.* 72: 77-83.

Park SH, Jarquin R, Hanning I, Almeida G, Ricke SC. 2011. Detection of *Salmonella* spp. survival and virulence by targeting the *hilA* gene. *J. Appl. Microbiol.* 111: 426-432.

Park SY, Woodward CL, Kubena LF, Nisbet DJ, Birkhold SG, Ricke SC. 2008. Environmental dissemination of foodborne *Salmonella* in preharvest poultry production: Reservoirs, critical factors, and research strategies. *Crit. Rev. Environ. Sci. Technol.* 38: 73-111.

Petkar A, Alali WQ, Harrison MA, Beuchat LR. 2011. Survival of *Salmonella* in organic and conventional broiler feed as affected by temperature and water activity. *Agric. Food Anal. Bacteriol.* (In press).

Pickett LD, Miller BF. 1966. The effect of high temperature immersion on the microbial population of whole turkey carcasses. *Poultry Sci.* 45: 1116.

Pivnick H, Nurmi E. 1982. The Nurmi concept and its role in the control of *Salmonella* in poultry. In. Developments in Food Microbiology. Ed. R. Davis. pp 41-70. *Applied Science Publisher Ltd.*, Essex, England.

Pope MJ, Cherry TE. 2000. An evaluation of the presence of pathogens on broilers raised on Poultry Litter Treatment®–treated litter. *Poult. Sci.* 79:1351–1355.

Poppe C, Barnum DA, Mitchell WR. 1986. Effect of chlorination of drinking water on experimental *Salmonella* infection in poultry. *Avian Dis.* 30:362-369.

Pritchard DG, Nivas SC, York MD, Pomeroy BS. 1978. Effect of Gal-E mutant of *Salmonella typhimurium* on experimental salmonellosis in chickens. *Avian Dis.* 22:562-575.

Purnell G, Mattick K, Humphrey T. 2004. The use of 'hot wash' treatments to reduce the number of pathogenic and spoilage bacteria on raw retail poultry. *J. Food Eng.* 62: 29–36.

Reilly WJ, Forbes GI, Patterson GM, Sharp JCM. 1981. Human and animal salmonellosis in Scotland associated with environmental contamination. *Vet. Rec.* 108:553-555.

Ribot EM, Fair Ma, Gautom R, Cameron DN, Hunter SB, Swaminathan B, Barrett TJ. 2006. Standardization of Pulsed-Field Gel Electrophoresis protocols for the subtyping of *Escherichia coli* O157:H7, *Salmonella*, and *Shigella* for PulseNet. *Foodborne Path. Dis.* 3: 59-67.

Ricke SC. 2003. The gastrointestinal tract ecology of *Salmonella* Enteritidis colonization in molting hens. *Poultry Sci.* 82: 1003-1007.

Ricke SC, Kundinger MM, Miller DR, Keeton JT. 2005. Alternatives to antibiotics: Chemical and physical antimicrobial interventions and foodborne pathogen response. *Poultry Sci.* 84: 667-675.

Ricke SC, Martin SA, Nisbet DJ. 1996. Ecology, metabolism, and genetics of ruminal selenomonads. *Crit. Reviews Microbiol.* 22: 27-65.

Ricke SC, Nisbet DJ, Maciorowski KG. 1997. Batch culture growth response of a poultry *Salmonella typhimurium* isolate to ammonium salts. *Bioresource Technol.* 60: 107-111.

Ricke SC, Pillai, SD. 1999. Conventional and molecular methods for understanding probiotic bacteria functionality in gastrointestinal tracts. *Crit. Rev. Microbiol.* 25: 19-38.

Ricke SC, Schaefer DM. 1991. Growth inhibition of the rumen bacterium *Selenomonas ruminantium* by ammonium salts. *Appl. Microbiol. Biotechnol.* 36: 394-399.

Ricke SC, Schaefer DM. 1996. Growth and fermentation responses of *Selenomonas ruminantium* to limiting and non-limiting concentrations of ammonium chloride. *Appl. Microbiol. Biotechnol.* 46: 169-175.

Rivault C, Cloarec A, Leguyader A. 1993. Bacterial load of cockroaches in relation to urban environment. *Epidemiol. Infect.* 110:317-321.

Robach MC, Sofos JH. 1982. Use of sorbates in meat products, fresh poultry and poultry products: *A review. J. Food Prot.* 45:374-383.

Roll VFB, Pra MAD, Roll AP. 2011. Research on *Salmonella* in broiler litter reused for up to 14 consecutive flocks. *Poultry Sci.* 90: 2257-2262.

Rosales AG, Jensen EL. 1998. Biosecurity and disinfection for *Salmonella* control. Proc. Intl. Symp. on Food-borne *Salmonella* in Poultry. pp. 105-117. Baltimore, Maryland.

Rouse J, Rolow A, Nelson C E. 1988. Effect of chemical treatment of poultry feed on survival of *Salmonella*. *Poult. Sci.* 67:1225–1228.

Russell SM. 1998. The effect of poultry processing steps on populations of bacteria on fresh broiler chicken carcasses. Proc. Intl. Symp. on Food-borne *Salmonella* in Poultry. pp. 232-236. Baltimore, MD.

Salvat G, Poppen P, Allo JC, Fenner S, Laisney MJ, Toquin MT, Humbert F, Colin P. 1997. Effects of AvGard^{TM} treatment on the microbiological flora of poultry carcases. *Br. Poultry Sci.* 38:489-498.

Samuelson KJ, Rupnow JH, Frowning GW. 1985. The effect of lysozyme and ethylenediaminetetraacetic acid and *Salmonella* on broiler parts. *Poultry Sci.* 64:1488-1490.

Sanderson K, Thomas CJ, McMeekin TA. 1991. Molecular basis of the adhesion of *Salmonella* serotypes to chicken muscle fascia. *Biofouling* 5:89-101.

Savage DC. 1987. Factors influencing biocontrol of bacterial pathogens in the intestine. *Food Technol.* 41:82-87.

Scallan E, Hoekstra RM, Angulo FJ, Tauxe RV, Widdowson M-A, Roy SL, Jones JL, Griffen PM. 2011. Foodborne illness acquired in the United States—major pathogens. *Emerg. Infect. Dis.* 17: 7-15.

Scharff RL. 2010. Health-related costs from foodborne illness in the United States. http://www.producesafetyproject.org/admin/assets/files/Health-Related-Foodborne-Illness-Costs-Report.pdf-1.pdf Accessed 18 October 2011.

Schneitz C. 2005. Competitive exclusion in poultry—30 years of research. *Food Control* 16:657–667.

Schrezenmeir J, de Vrese M. 2001. Probiotics, prebiotics, and synbiotics—approaching a definition. *Am. J. Clin. Nutr.* 73(Suppl. 2):361S–364S.

Schwach RS, Zottola EA. 1982. Use of scanning electron microscopy to demonstrate microbial attachment to beef and beef contact surfaces. *J. Food Sci.* 47:1401-1405.

Schwartz DC, Cantor CR. 1984. Separation of yeast chromosome-sized DNAs by pulsed-field gradient gel electrophoresis. *Cell* 37:67-75.

Seo KH, Holt PS, Gast RK, Hofacre CL. 2000. Elimination of early *Salmonella enteritidis* infection after treatment with competitive-exclusion culture and enrofloxacin in experimentally infected chicks. *Poult. Sci.* 79:1408–1413.

Servin AL. 2004. Antagonistic activities of lactobacilli and bifidobacteria against microbial pathogens. *FEMS Microbiol. Rev.* 28:405–440.

Sheldon BW, Brake J. 1991. Hydrogen peroxide as an alternative hatching egg disinfectant. *Poult. Sci.* 70:1092–1098.

Sheldon BW, Brown AL. 1986. Efficacy of ozone as a disinfectant for poultry carcasses and chill water. J. Food Sci. 51:305-309.

Simmons GC, Byrnes RV. 1972. The origin of *Salmonella* in chickens and chicken carcasses. *Aust. Vet. J.* 48:186-189.

Smith CL, Cantor CR. 1987. Purification, specific fragmentation, and separation of large DNA molecules. *Methods Enzymol.* 155:449-467.

Smith CL, KIco SR, Cantor CR. 1988. Pulsed field gel electrophoresis and the technology of large DNA molecules. In Davies K ed., *Genome analysis: a practical approach.* Oxford, UK:IRL Press pp. 41-72.

Smyser CF, Snoeyenbos GH. 1979. Evaluation of organic acids and other compounds as *Salmonella* antagonists in meat and bone meal. *Poult. Sci.* 58:50–54.

Snijders JMA, van Knapen F. 2002. Prevention of human diseases by an integrated quality control system. *Livest. Prod. Sci.* 76:203–206.

Snijders JMA, van Logtestijn JG, Mossel DAA, Smulders FJM. 1985. Lactic acid decontaminant in slaughter and processing procedures. *Vet. Q.* 7:277-282.

Snoeyenbos GH, Carlson VL, McKie BA, Smyser CF. 1967. An epidemiological study of salmonellosis of chickens. *Avian Dis.* 11:653-667.

Snoeyenbos GH, Carlson VL, Smyse CF, Olesuik OM. 1969. Dynamics of *Salmonella* infection in chicks reared on litter. *Avian Dis.* 13:72-83.

Snoeyenbos GH, McKie BA, Smyser CF, Weston CR. 1970. Progress in identifying and maintaining *Salmonella*-free commercial chicken breeding flocks. *Avian Dis.* 14:683-696

Snoeyenbos GH, Soerjadi AS, Weinack OM. 1982. Gastrointestinal colonization by *Salmonella* and pathogenic *Escherichia coli* in monozenic and holoxenic chicks and poults. *Avian Dis.* 26:566-575.

Soerjadi AS, Druitt JH, Llyod AB, Cumming RB. 1979. Effect of environmental temperature on susceptibility of young chickens to *Salmonella typhimurium*. *Aust. Vet. J.* 55:413-417.

Spring P, Wenk C, Dawson KA, Newman KE. 2000. The effects of dietary mannanoligosaccharides on cecal parameters and the concentrations of enteric bacteria in the ceca of *Salmonella* challenged broiler chicks. *Poult. Sci.* 79:205–211.

Stavric S. 1987. Microbial colonization control of chicken intestine using defined cultures. *Food Technol.* 41:93-98.

Stavric S, D'Aoust, J–Y. 1993. Undefined and defined bacterial preparations for the competitive exclusion of *Salmonella* in poultry – A review. *J. Food Prot.* 56:173-180.

Stersky A, Blanchfield B, Thacker C, Pivnick H. 1981. Reduction of *Salmonella* excretion into drinking water following treatment of chicks with Nurmi culture. *J. Food Prot.* 44:917-920.

Stopforth JD, O'Connor R, Lopes M, Kottapalli B, Hill WE, Samadpour M. 2007. Validation of individual and multiple-sequential interventions for reduction of microbial populations during processing of poultry carcasses and parts. *J. Food Prot.* 70: 1393-1401.

Stringfellow K, Caldwell D, Lee J, Byrd A, Carey J, Kessler K, McReynolds J, Bell A, Stipanovic R, Farnell M. 2010. Pasteurization of chicken litter with steam and quicklime to reduce *Salmonella* Typhimurium. *J. Appl. Poultry Res.*19: 380-386.

Stuart JC. 1984. The introduction of *Salmonella* into poultry flocks. *J. Sci. Food Agric.* 35: 632–633.

Sukhnanand S, Alcaine S, Warnick LD, Su WL, Hof J, Craver MP, McDonough P, Boor KJ, Wiedmann M. 2005. DNA sequence-based subtyping and evolutionary analysis of selected *Salmonella enterica* serotypes. *J. Clin. Microbiol.* 43: 3688-3698.

Suskovic J, Kos B, Goreta J, Matosic S. 2001. Role of lactic acid bacteria and bifidobacteria in symbiotic effect. *Food Technol. Biotechnol.* 39:227–235.

Tabib Z, Jones FT, Hamilton PB. 1984. Effect of pelleting of poultry feed on the activity of molds and mold inhibitors. *Poult. Sci.* 63:70–75.

Tamblyn KC, Conner DE. 1997. Bactericidal activity of organic acids against *Salmonella typhimurium* attached to broiler chicken skin. *J. Food Prot.* 60:629-633.

Tamblyn KC, Conner DE, Bilgili SF. 1997. Utilization of skin attachment model to determine the antibacterial efficacy of potential carcass treatments. *Poultry Sci.* 76:1318-1323.

Tankouo-Sandjong B, Sessitsch A, Liebana E, Kornschober C, Allerberger F, Hachler H, Bodrossy L. 2007. MLST-v, multilocus sequence typing based on virulence genes, for molecular typing of *Salmonella enterica* subsp. *enterica* serovars. *J. Microbiol. Methods* 69: 23-36.

Tellez G, Petrone VM, Escorcia M, Morishita TY, Cobb CW, Villasenor L. 2001. Evaluation of avian-specific probiotic and *Salmonella* Enteritidis–, *Salmonella* Typhimurium–, and *Salmonella* Heidelberg–specific antibodies on cecal colonization and organ invasion of *Salmonella* Enteritidis in broilers. *J. Food Prot.* 64:287–291

Thayer D. 1995. Use of irradiation to kill enteric pathogens in meat and poultry. *J. Food Safety* 15:181-192.

Thayer D, Songprasertchai S, Boyd G. 1991. Effects of heat and ionizing radiation on *Salmonella typhimurium* in mechanically deboned chicken meat. *J. Food Prot.* 54:718-724.

Thaxton P, Wyatt RD, Hamilton PB. 1971. Cold stress and *Salmonella* as a cause of early mortality in chickens. *Poultry Sci.* 50:1636 (Abstr.).

Thomas CJ, McMeekin TA. 1984. Effect of water uptake by poultry tissues on contamination by bacteria during immersion in bacterial suspensions. *J. Food Prot.* 47:398-402.

Thomas CJ, McMeekin TA, Patterson JT. 1987. Prevention of microbial contamination in the poultry processing plant. In. *Elimination of Pathogenic Organisms from Meat and Poultry.* (Ed.) F.J.M. Smulders, pp 163-179. Elsiever, Amsterdam.

Thomson JE, Bailey JS, Cox NA, Posey DA, Carson MO. 1979. Salmonella on broiler carcasses as affected by fresh water input rate and chlorination of chiller water. *J. Food Prot.* 42:954-955.

Thomson JE, Cox NA, Bailey JS. 1977. Control of *Salmonella* and extension of shelf life of broiler carcasses with a glutaraldehyde product. *J. Food Sci.* 42:1353-1355.

Thong KL, Ngeow YF, Altwegg M, Navaratnam P, Pang T. 1995. Molecular analysis of Salmonella enteritidis by pulsed-field gel electrophoresis and ribotyping. *J. Clin. Microbiol.* 33: 1070-1074.

Todd ECD. 1980. Poultry-associated foodborne disease – its occurrence, cost, sources and prevention. *J. Food Prot.* 43:129-139.

Tompkins LS, Troup N, Labigne-Rousel A, Cohen M. 1986. Cloned random chromosomal sequences as probes to identify *Salmonella* species. *J. Infect. Dis.* 154:156-162.

Torpdahl M, Skov MN, Sandvang D, Baggesen DL. 2005. Genotypic characterization of *Salmonella* by multilocus sequence typing, pulsed-field gel electrophoresis and amplified fragment length polymorphism. *J. Microbiol. Methods* 63: 173-184.

Tsai, C-C, Hsih H-Y, Chiu H-H, Lai Y-Y, Liu J-H, Yu B, Tsen H-Y. 2005. Antagonistic activity against *Salmonella* infection in vitro and in vivo for two *Lactobacillus* strains from swine and poultry. *Int. J. Food Microbiol.* 102:185–194.

Tsai LS, Schade JE, Molyneux BT. 1991. Chlorination of poultry chill water: chlorine demand and disinfection efficacy. Poultry Sci. 71:188-196.

Tucker JF. 1967. Survival of salmonellae in built-up litter for housing of rearing and laying fowl. *Br. Vet. J.* 123:92-103.

Turnbull PCB, Snoeyenbos GH. 1973. The roles of ammonia, water activity, and pH in the salmonellacidal effect of long-used poultry litter. *Avian Dis.* 17:72-86.

Urwin R, Maiden MCJ. 2003. Multi-locus sequence typing: a tool for global epidemiology. *Trends Microbiol.* 11: 479-487.

Vahl IJ. 1995. Breaking the *Salmonella* chain at the feed mill. *Feed Mix* 3:14–17.

Van Coillie E, Goris J, Cleenwerck I, Grijspeerdt K, Botteldoorn N, Van Immerseel F, De Buck J, Vancanneyt M,Swings J, Herman L, Heyndrickx M. 2007. Identification of lactobacilli isolated from the cloaca and vagina of laying hens and characterization for potential use as probiotics to control *Salmonella* Enteritidis. *J. Appl. Microbiol.* 102:1095–1106.

van der Marel GM, van Logtestijn JG, Mossel DAA. 1988. Bacteriological quality of broiler carcasses as affected by inplant lactic acid decontamination. *Int. J. Food Microbiol.* 6:31-42.

Vandeplas S, Dauphin RD, Beckers Y, Thonart P, Thewis A. 2010. *Salmonella* in chicken: current and developing strategies to reduce contamination at farm level. *J. Food Prot.* 73: 774-785.

Vanderwal P. 1979. *Salmonella* control of feedstuffs by pelleting or acid treatment. *World's Poultry Sci. J.* 35: 70-78.

Vareltzis K, Soultos N, Koidis P, Ambrosiadis J, Genigeorgis C. 1997. Antimicrobial effects of sodium tripolyphosphate against attached to the surface of chicken carcasses. *Lebensm.-Wiss. Technol.* 30, 665–669.

Veldman A, Vahl HA, Borggreve GJ, Fuller DC. 1995. A survey of the incidence of *Salmonella* species and Enterobacteriaceae in poultry feeds and feed components. *Vet. Rec.* 136: 169–172.

Vicente JL, Higgins SE, Hargis BM, Tellez G. 2007. Effect of poultry guard litter amendment on horizontal transmission of *Salmonella enteritidis* in broiler chicks. *Int. J. Poult. Sci.* 6:314–317.

Waldroup AL. 1998. Chemical control of microorganisms on raw poultry. *Proc. Intl. Symp.* On Food-borne *Salmonella* in Poultry. pp. 237-241. Baltimore, MD.

Wang W-C, Li Y, Slavik MF, Xiong H. 1997. Trisodium phosphate and cetylpyridinium chloride spraying on chicken skin to reduce attached *Salmonella typhimurium. J. Food Prot.* 60:992-994.

Wales AD, Allen VM, Davies RH. 2010. Chemical treatment of animal feed and water for the control of *Salmonella. Foodborne Path. Dis.* 7: 3-15.

Walls I, Cooke PH, Benedict RC, Buchanan RL. 1993. Sausage casing as a model for attachment of *Salmonella* to meat. *J. Food Prot.* 56:390-394.

Wathes CM, Zaiden WAR, Pearson GR, Hinton M, Todd N. 1988. Aerosol infection in calves and mice with *Salmonella typhimurium. Vet. Rec.* 123:590-594.

White PL, Baker AR, James WO. 1997. Strategies to control *Salmonella* and *Campylobacter* in raw poultry products. *Rev. Sci. Tech.* 16:525–541.

Whyte P, McGill K, Collins JD. 2003. An assessment of steam pasteurization and hot water immersion treatments for the microbiological decontamination of broiler carcasses. *Food Microbiol.* 20: 111–117.

Williams JE. 1980. Formalin destruction of *Salmonella* in poultry litter. *Poult. Sci.* 59:2717–2724.

Williams JE. 1981. Salmonellas in poultry feeds – A worldwide review. Part I. Introduction and Part II. Methods in isolation and identification. *World's Poultry Sci. J.* 37: 6–25.

Winokur PL. 2003. Molecular epidemiological techniques for *Salmonella* strain discrimination. *Frontiers in Biosci.* 8: 14-24.

Wray C, Davies RH. 1998. Environmental problems in poultry production: Dust and pests. Proc. Intl. Symp. on Food-borne Salmonella in Poultry. pp. 93-104. Baltimore, Maryland.

Xiong H, Li Y, Slavik MF, Walker JT. 1998. Spraying chicken skin with selected chemicals to reduce attached *Salmonella typhimurium. J. Food Prot.* 61:272-275.

Yang PPW, Chen TC. 1979. Stability of ozone and its germicidal properties on poultry meat microorganisms in liquid phase. *J. Food Sci.* 44:501-504.

Yang Z, Li Y, Slavik M. 1998. Use of antimicrobial spray applied with an inside-outside birdwasher to reduce bacterial contamination of prechilled chicken carcasses. *J. Food Prot.* 61:829-832.

In: Salmonella: Classification, Genetics and Disease Outbreaks ISBN: 978-1-61942-928-4
Editors: Adelaide S. Monte, Paulo Eduardo De Santos © 2012 Nova Science Publishers, Inc.

Chapter 2

THE *SALMONELLA* PATHOGENICITY ISLAND ENCODED TYPE III SECRETION SYSTEMS AND THEIR ROLE IN INFECTION OF POULTRY

Taseen Desin, Amanda Wisner, Aaron White, Andrew Potter and Wolfgang Köster
Vaccine and Infectious Disease Organization, University of Saskatchewan, Canada

Many strains of *Salmonella enterica* represent oonotic pathogens which are capable of causing disease in humans. One major source of food poisoning is *Salmonella enterica* serovar Enteritidis which is often found associated with chicken meat, meat products and eggs. A number of virulence factors enable this bacterium to colonize and systemically infect poultry. In this review we will concentrate on the *S.* Enteritidis Type III Secretion System (T3SS) located on *Salmonella* Pathogenicity Island-1 and highlight its role in invasion of chickens. The structural components of the complex secretion apparatus and the secreted effector proteins will be introduced. Aspects of T3SS assembly, its expression regulation under different conditions as well as its involvement in colonization and invasion of poultry will be discussed in the context of the recent findings.

1. INTRODUCTION

1.1. Nomenclature

The bacterial genus *Salmonella* was named following the discovery of this pathogen by the United States Department of Agriculture (USDA) veterinary bacteriologist Dr. Daniel E. Salmon (1850-1914) [1]. *Salmonella* is a Gram negative, facultative intracellular, rod-shaped (0.7-1.5 μm wide x 2-5 μm long) and non-spore forming member of the enterobacteriacae family. Most *Salmonella* species have peritrichous flagella and are motile and have an optimal growth temperature of 37° Celsius [2]. The genus *Salmonella* is divided into two species, *Salmonella bongori* and *Salmonella enterica*. *S. enterica* consists of six subspecies:

enterica, *salamae*, *arizonae*, *diarizonae*, *indica*, and *houtenae* [3]. *S. enterica* subspecies *enterica* is mainly associated with infection of warm blooded animals, while the other subspecies and *Salmonella bongori* rarely cause infection in these animals [4-5]. *S. enterica* subspecies *enterica* consists of more than 2000 serovars [6] which are classified based on the O factor (O antigen) of the lipopolysaccharide (LPS) and the H antigens of the flagella [7].

1.2. *Salmonella* Enteritidis

S. enterica subspecies *enterica* serovar Enteritidis (*S.* Enteritidis) has a genome size of approximately 4.69 Mbp [8] and is one of the most prevalent serovars with respect to human *Salmonella* infections world wide [9]. The consumption of contaminated meat (mainly poultry) and eggs are major sources of *S.* Enteritidis human infections [10]. Typically human infections result in a localized gastrointestinal disease which is characterized by a massive influx of neutrophils (hallmark of these infections) in the terminal ileum and colon (enterocolitis) resulting in nausea, vomiting and diarrohea [11]. These infections are usually self-limiting and clear within 3-5 days. However, *S.* Enteritidis infections can also lead to systemic disease, requiring antibiotic treatment and hospitalization. On rare occasions, *S.* Enteritidis infections can also lead to the development of pain in the joints, eye irritation and painful urination (referred to as Reiter's Syndrome) [12]. It is estimated that there are approximately 1.4 million cases of human salmonellosis in the United States annually [12], while in Canada the number of cases has been estimated to be close to 0.5 million every year [13]. The economic impact of these infections is massive in the U.S. and Canada due to medical care, loss of work and death [14].

1.3. Virulence Factors

1.3.1. Flagella

The primary role of *Salmonella* flagella is for cell propulsion [15]. Rotation of the flagellar filament propels the bacterial cell either in a forward motion or random reorientation, depending on the chemical stimulus in the environment (chemotaxis). In addition to their primary role, under certain conditions, flagella have been shown to secrete SPI-1 T3SS effector proteins, SptP and SopE [16].

The major components of the flagellum that are exposed on the surface consist of the proteins FliD (cap), FliC (filament – about 5 to 10 μm in length) and FlgE (hook – about 55 nm in length). The basal structure of the flagellum consists of an outer membrane anchored L ring (FlgH), a periplasmic rod, a periplasmic P ring (FlgI), an inner membrane MS ring (FliF), Mot proteins that constitute the stator element of the motor (Mot A and MotB), C ring (FliM and FliN) and a type 3 flagellar protein export apparatus (FlhA, FlhB, FliO, FliP, FliQ, FliR) [17]. The motility of the bacterial flagellum is powered by the proton motive force [16], while the assembly of the flagellar apparatus is powered by an ATPase known as FliI. The components of the basal structure of the flagellum share sequence homology to inner membrane components of T3SS, while components of the surface structure share little or no homology to T3SS components [17].

Salmonella flagella have been shown to be important for adherence to and invasion of epithelial cells in vitro. Studies with mouse and bovine models of infection have shown that flagella are not required, but are important for virulence. In the bovine model of infection, flagellar mutants were found to cause less inflammation [18]. This is most likely due to the fact that flagellin, the major monomeric subunit of the filament, is a powerful inducer of host innate immunity via toll-like receptor 5 (TLR5) [19].

1.3.2. Fimbriae

Fimbriae are found on the surface of most, if not all, *Salmonella* strains. These hair-like structures are protein polymers, typically comprised of one or two repeated subunits. Fimbriae play an important role in adhesion of the bacterium to the intestinal epithelium and hence are important virulence factors [20]. To date, 13 fimbrial loci have been identified [6], four of which are well defined in *S.* Enteritidis. These operons correspond to Type I fimbriae (*fimAICDHF*), SEF 14 (*sefABCD*), curli (*csgDEFG* and *csgBAC*) and plasmid encoded fimbriae (*pefABCD*) [21]. Type 1 fimbriae are about 7-8 nm in diameter and up to 100 nm long; FimA is the major structural monomer. Type 1 fimbriae are peritrichously distributed and bind α-D-mannose receptors on eukaryotic cells. SEF14 fimbriae are less than 3 nm in diameter; SefA is the major structural component. These fimbriae have an important role in serological tests used for the detection of *S.* Enteritidis. Curli (also known as thin aggregative fimbriae or SEF 17) are approximately 3-4 nm wide; AgfA is the major structural unit. Plasmid-encoded fimbriae (PEF) are encoded from the *Salmonella* virulence plasmid (described below). PEF are thought to play an important role in attachment to intestinal epithelial cells in vivo. However, the tissue specificity of type I fimbriae, SEF14 and curli during *Salmonella* infection has not been determined [20-21].

1.3.3. Plasmid Encoded Virulence Genes

S. Enteritidis strains carry a 59 kb virulence plasmid which is also present in other serovars (although the sizes may differ). The main virulence-associated genes include *spvRABCD* (*Salmonella* plasmid virulence) genes, *rck* (resistance to complement killing), *pef* (plasmid-encoded fimbriae), *srgA* (SdiA-regulated gene, putative disulphide bond oxireductase) and *mig-5* (macrophage-inducible gene encoding for putative carbonic anhydrase). The *spv* genes play an important role in macrophage survival and hence are important in causing systemic disease. The *rck* gene products increase the resistance of *S.* Enteritidis to complement mediated killing while the *pef* genes encode for a class of fimbriae described above. The roles of the *srgA* and *mig-5* genes in virulence are not very well known [22]. Certain *Salmonella* species also carry other plasmids which confer antibiotic resistance [22] and the presence of such plasmids makes these strains difficult to treat in human infections.

1.3.4. Type III Secretion Systems and Pathogenicity Islands

S. Enteritidis uses a complex syringe-like secretion pathway known as the Type III Secretion System (T3SS) to inject virulence factors directly into host cells. T3SSs are found in many other gram negative pathogens. The *Salmonella* T3SS apparatus is composed of more than 20 proteins and spans the inner membrane, periplasmic space including peptidoglycan layer, outer membrane, and extracellular space. Bacterial virulence factors (known as effector proteins) are secreted and translocated through the T3SS into eukaryotic cells in a contact dependent manner, which results in the manipulation of host cellular architecture [23]. *S.* Enteritidis has two distinct T3SSs, both of which are important during the infection process. These molecular syringes are encoded by regions of the chromosome known as *Salmonella* Pathogenicity Islands (SPI) which are hypothesized to have been acquired via horizontal gene transfer. One T3SS is encoded on *Salmonella* Pathogenicity Island 1 (SPI-1), while the other T3SS is located on SPI-2. The SPI-1 T3SS plays a very important role in invasion and inflammation during the initial stages of infection. On the other hand, the SPI-2 T3SS is crucial for intracellular survival and systemic spread of *Salmonella* after the invasion of host cells [24-26].

To date, twelve SPI's have been identified, of which SPI-1 to SPI-5 are well characterized [27]. SPI-3, SPI-4 and SPI-5 are mainly involved in growth and survival of the bacteria in the host species. The SPI's are characterized by a lower GC content (i.e., 37 - 47 %) relative to the rest of the *Salmonella* chromosome (~ 52 %), are flanked by direct repeats or insertion sequences (IS) and are generally conserved between the different *Salmonella* serovars [26].

2. *Salmonella* Pathogenicity Island-1 Type III Secretion System

The SPI-1 T3SS is about 40 kb in size (Figure 1) [25]. This T3SS is important for invasion of intestinal epithelial cells. During the process of infection, *S.* Enteritidis injects several effector proteins into the host cell which results in actin polymerization and membrane ruffling. This ultimately leads to uptake of the bacterium. Hence *S.* Enteritidis is able to breach the intestinal surface to gain access to underlying tissue and spread systemically [24, 26, 28].

2.1. Structure

The SPI-1 T3SS apparatus (Figure 2) belongs to an injectisome family which includes T3SS structures from *Shigella flexneri*, *Bordetella pseudomallei* and *Yersinia enterocolitica* [17]. The surface structure of this apparatus consists of a needle and a translocon which is involved in pore formation. The SPI-1 needle is formed by PrgI, while the translocon consists of SipB, SipC, and SipD. The basal structure of this apparatus consists of outer membrane and inner membrane proteins that are connected by a periplasmic protein. InvG is the outer membrane protein and forms a pair of rings [29].

This protein is a member of the secretin family of transporters which are also found in other secretion systems [17, 29-30]. The InvG secretin is connected by PrgJ, a periplasmic protein, to the inner membrane structure that mainly consists of PrgH and PrgK [31]. InvA, SpaP, SpaQ, SpaR and SpaS form part of the export machinery that is connected to PrgH and PrgK [32]. The SPI-1 apparatus also contains a motor-like energy source known as the "ATPase" (InvC) that provides the energy required for the secretion of proteins through this channel [33].

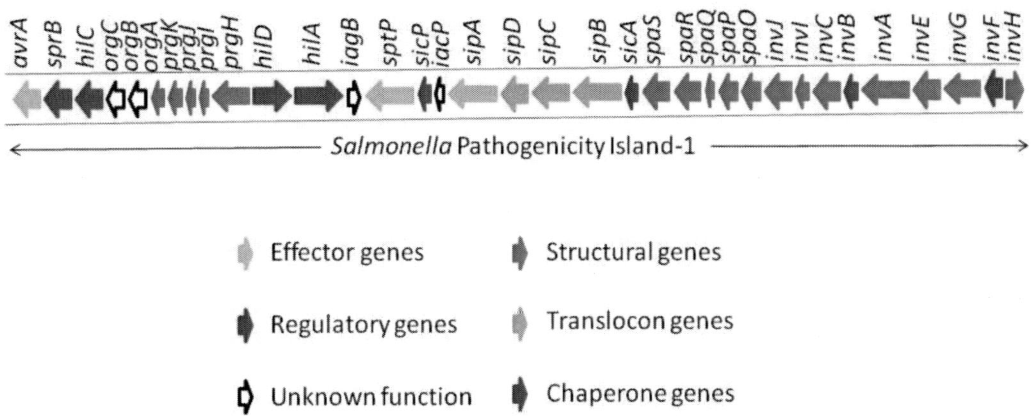

Figure 1. Schematic representation of *Salmonella* Pathogenicity Island-1 genes. The *sitABCD* operon downstream of *avrA* is not shown since it does not play a part in invasion[34].

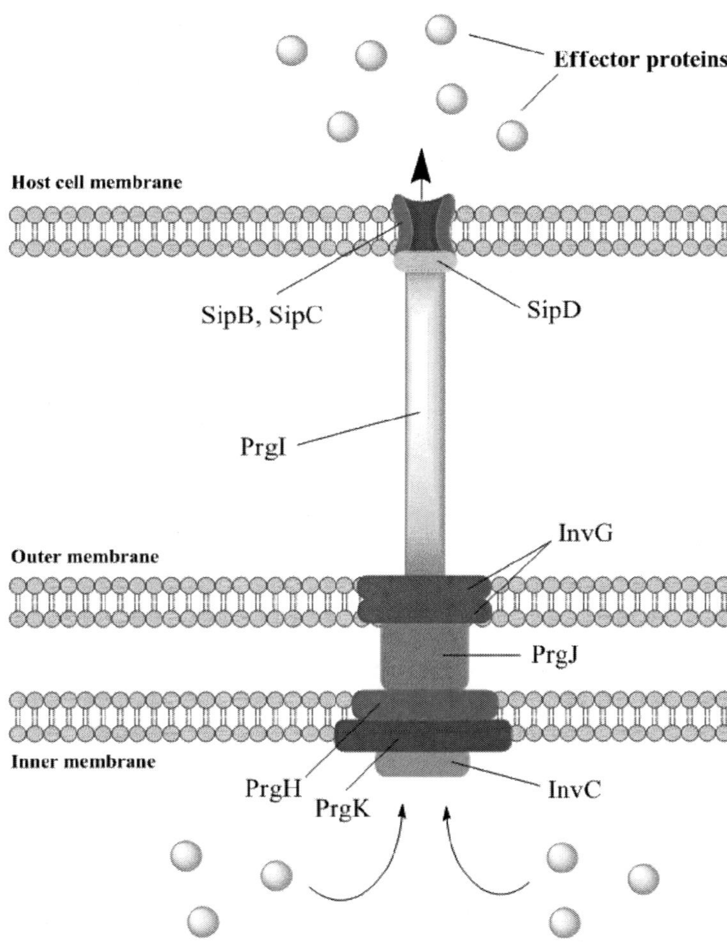

Figure 2. Structure of the *S*. Enteritidis SPI-1 Type III Secretion System. Diagram was modified from [17].

2.2. Assembly

The first step in assembly of the SPI-1 T3SS is the export of the inner membrane proteins PrgH and PrgK, and the outer membrane secretin InvG (which requires the help of a secretin specific protein InvH), by the general secretory (sec) pathway. This step is thought to occur in a sec-dependent fashion since each of these proteins contain N-terminal sec-dependent signal sequences [29, 35]. Once the assembly of PrgH, PrgK and InvG is completed, the export apparatus (InvA, SpaP, SpaQ, SpaR and SpaS) and the ATPase (InvC and SpaL) are formed. This completes the formation of the basal structure and is followed by the secretion of PrgI (needle) and PrgJ (inner rod) through the newly formed export apparatus [29]. As the needle reaches approximately 80 nm in length the export of PrgI is stopped by InvJ [29, 36]. The SipD protein is secreted through this system, forms the tip of the PrgI needle and plays an important role in mediating *Salmonella* species attachment to host cells in order to secrete effector proteins. SipD is present at the tip of the needle complex prior to contact with host cells, while the other members of the translocase (SipB and SipC) are exposed after contact with host cells [37].

2.3. Secretion

Salmonella species secrete many effector proteins through the SPI-1 T3SS, most of which are translocated into host cells. Contact with host cells [38] and the presence of cholesterol (host cell membrane) [39] are the main triggers of effector protein secretion. It has recently been proposed that the needle acts as a sensor via a structural change once in contact with host cells, leading to the secretion of effector proteins [40]. To date, at least 15 effectors have been identified that are secreted using the SPI-1 T3SS (Table 1).

After the secretion of effector proteins into host cells by *Salmonella*, the host cellular architecture is modulated; leading to the formation of membrane ruffles and lamellipodial extensions, which triggers bacterial internalization. *Salmonella* species employ the concerted action of 7 effector proteins to directly (SipA and SipC) or indirectly (SipB, SopB, SopD, SopE and SopE2) modulate the dynamics of actin filaments [28], which are the most dominant structural components in the lamellipodium [41].

The assembly of actin filaments is not a favourable process due to the instability of actin dimers and trimers [41]. Therefore, SipA promotes actin polymerization by binding to actin filaments and reducing the critical concentration for actin assembly as well as stabilizing the filaments [72]. In addition, SipA also enhances the activity of T-plastin (a host cell actin bundling protein) and prevents the binding of ADF/cofilin (actin depolymerising proteins) to actin filaments [45-46]. SipC on the other hand, forms part of the SPI-1 translocon and enhances the formation of actin trimers and bundles actin filaments [54]. Another SPI-1 effector protein, SipB, forms part of the SPI-1 apparatus translocon and has not been implicated with actin polymerization. However, SipB binds to cholesterol in the plasma membrane and it is thought that this may also represent one of the steps in triggering the secretion of SPI-1 effector proteins [53].

Table 1. List of effector proteins secreted by the *S.* Enteritidis SPI-1 T3SS. Table was adapted and modified from [28]

Effector protein	Gene location	Function	Reference
AvrA	SPI-1	Inhibits inflammation and apoptosis, stabilizes epithelial cell tight junctions.	[42-44]
SipA	SPI-1	Promotes actin polymerization by binding to actin filaments, induces infiltration of PMN across the intestinal epithelial layer, maintains perinuclear position of SCV, stimulates intracellular replication.	[45-49]
SipB	SPI-1	Forms part of translocon, binds to cholesterol and is involved in triggering secretion of effector proteins, contributes to inflammation and macrophage cell death.	[50-53]
SipC	SPI-1	Forms part of translocon, enhances actin polymerization	[54]
SipD	SPI-1	Forms part of translocon structure and the tip of the secretion system, is involved in mediating attachment to epithelial cells.	[28, 37]
SopA	outside SPI-1	Induces migration of PMN's across the intestinal epithelial layer, allows *Salmonella* to escape from the SCV.	[55-56]
SopB	SPI-5	Promotes actin polymerization, enhances membrane fission, induces expression of pro-inflammatory cytokines like IL-8, plays a role in SCV maturation.	[28, 57-62]
SopD	outside SPI-1	Enhances membrane fission	[59]
SopE	Bacteriophage	Promotes actin polymerization through GEF activity, induces inflammation, enhances SCV maturation.	[28, 60-61, 63]
SopE2	Bacteriophage	Promotes actin polymerization through GEF activity, induces inflammation.	[60-61, 63]
SptP	SPI-1	Allows cell to regain its original architecture following invasion, down regulates inflammatory response.	[64-67]
SlrP	Outside SPI-1	Causes cell death *in vitro*.	[68]
SspH1	Bacteriophage Gifsy-3	Inhibits NF-κB expression resulting in reduced inflammation.	[69-70]
SteA	outside SPI-1	Localizes to the Golgi network in infected cells.	[71]
SteB	outside SPI-1	Unknown.	[71]

Salmonella also causes the polymerization of actin filaments indirectly through other pathways. This involves the activation of Cdc42 and Rac-1, which are members of the Rho subfamily of actin-organizing small guanine binding proteins. These proteins are active when they are bound to guanosine triphosphate (GTP) and inactive when guanosine diphosphate (GDP) is bound to them. The activities of Cdc42 and Rac-1 are controlled by two classes of regulatory proteins: guanine nucleotide exchange factors (GEFs) and GTPase activating proteins (GAPs). GEFs catalyze GTP loading to Cdc42 and Rac-1, while the latter (GAPs) enhance GTP hydrolysis to GDP [65, 73]. The SPI-1 effector protein SopE acts as a GEF through activation of Cdc42 and Rac1, while SopE2 performs a similar function mainly in association with Cdc42 [63]. *Salmonella* also activates Cdc42 and Rac-1 indirectly through the activity of SopB. SopB hydrolyzes phosphatidyl inositol phosphate and inositol phosphate compounds, generating secondary messengers (such as phosphatidyl inositol-4,5-diphosphate), which in turn also activate Cdc42 and Rac-1 [57-58]. Once activated, Cdc42 and Rac-1 activate members of the Wiskott-Aldrich Syndrome protein (WASP) family.

WASP family proteins recruit and activate the actin-related protein-2/3 (Arp2/3) complex, which plays a very important role in actin nucleation, as well as branching and cross-linking of actin filaments [41, 61, 74]. Another SPI-1 effector protein, SopD, enhances membrane fission and macropinosome formation, along with SopB, at the site of bacterial invasion. However, the exact mechanisms by which SopD performs its role are not known [59]. Following *Salmonella* invasion, another effector protein, SptP, hydrolyzes GTP to GDP on Cdc42 and Rac1, thus deactivating these proteins. Hence, this counteracts the effects of SopB, SopE and SopE2 allowing the host cell to regain its original architecture [64-65].

The secretion of effector proteins by the SPI-1 T3SS also results in the modulation of host signaling pathways, leading to inflammation. SopB-, SopE- and SopE2-mediated activation of Cdc42 results in the stimulation of different mitogen activated protein kinase (MAPK) cascades (i.e., Erk, Jnk and p38 pathways) which in turn activate transcription factors activator protein-1 (AP-1) and nuclear factor kappa B (NF-κB). This entire process induces the expression of pro-inflammatory cytokines, such as IL-8, causing an influx of polymorphonuclear leukocytes (PMN), and eventually leading to diarrhoea [60-61]. The SPI-1 effector protein SipA, also induces signaling pathways that activate protein kinase Cα, resulting in the secretion of PMN chemoattractant hepoxillin A3 which enhances the infiltration of PMN across the intestinal epithelial layer [47-48]. The influx of neutrophils in the intestine is accompanied by fluid secretion from intestinal epithelial cells, which is regulated by chloride secretion. Increased levels of intracellular inositol phosphate (Ins[1,4,5,6]P4), as a result of SopB activity, leads to an influx of chloride ions. Hence, this process also contributes to the diarroheal response in the host [47]. Another SPI-1 effector protein, SipB, also contributes to the inflammatory response by inducing rapid macrophage cell death. This occurs when SipB binds to and activates caspase-1 in macrophages [50]. Activated caspase-1 causes the activation and release of pro-inflammatory cytokines IL-1β and IL-18, which stimulate the recruitment of immune cells and enhance the inflammatory response. Further, activated caspase-1, through other downstream processes, causes the formation of membrane pores leading to the release of cellular contents and cell lysis [51-52]. The recruitment of PMNs across the intestinal epithelium is also promoted by the SPI-1 effector protein SopA, through its E3 ubiquitin ligase activity. Ubiquitination is the process of attaching ubiquitin (regulatory protein) to proteins, so that the proteins are either labeled for degradation or directed to different cellular compartments. It controls a variety of cellular processes and involves a cascade of enzymes including E1 (ubiquitin-activating enzyme), E2 (ubiquitin-conjugating enzyme) and E3 (ubiquitin protein ligase). SopA mimics host E3 enzymes by binding host E2 enzymes and catalyzing the transfer of ubiquitin to itself. Thereafter, ubiquitinated SopA induces migration of PMNs across the intestinal epithelial layer [55-56, 75].

The aforementioned inflammatory responses are suppressed by the SPI-1 effector proteins AvrA, SptP and SspH1. AvrA is a cysteine protease that possesses deubiquitinase and acetyltransferase activity. This effector removes ubiquitin (deubiquitinates) from IκBα and β–catenin (inhibitors of NF-κB signalling), preventing them from proteasomal degradation. Hence, IκBα and β–catenin are able to suppress NF-κB signalling, leading to reduced inflammation and apoptosis [42]. In addition, AvrA also acetylates certain residues of upstream activators of MAPKs (MAPK Kinase MKK4/7) preventing their subsequent phosphorylation. This leads to the inhibition of MAPK pathways resulting in reduced inflammation [43]. Moreover, AvrA has also been associated with stabilizing epithelial cell tight junction structure, which is disrupted during *Salmonella* invasion [44]. Similarly, the SPI-1 effector SptP employs its tyrosine phosphatase activity to dampen inflammatory responses. Tyrosine kinases play an important role in the activation of MAPK pathways during *Salmonella* infection, which leads to the secretion of pro-inflammatory cytokines. SptP dephosphorylates proteins involved in the extracellular-regulated kinase (ERK) MAPK pathway, resulting in an inhibition of the pathways. Hence, this process lowers the inflammatory response [66-67]. Likewise, SspH1 reverses the host inflammatory reaction to *Salmonella* infection through its E3 ubiquitin ligase activity by ubiquitinating protein kinase N1 (PKN1). Ubiquitinated PKN1 inhibits NF-κB dependent gene expression [69-70].

SPI-1 effector proteins also play a role in processes following invasion (where SPI-2 effector proteins are the major players) including maturation and positioning of the *Salmonella* containing vacuole (SCV) and intracellular replication [6, 28]. SopB and SopE play important roles in maturation of the SCV, by recruiting cellular markers associated with early endosomes such as Rab5 (member of the Rab GTPase family). This in turn leads to the recruitment of other proteins (Vps34 and endosomal antigen-1) that results in the accumulation of phosphatidyl inositol 3 phosphate at the SCV membrane (important for SCV membrane maturation). SopB also prevents the SCV from entering the endosomal maturation pathway [28, 62]. As well, SopB mediated activation of a host kinase protein (Akt) prevents SCV phagosome-lysosomal fusion, thus allowing *Salmonella* to persist and replicate in the SCV [76]. The positioning of the SCV in close proximity to the nucleus (perinuclear position) is mediated in part by the SPI-1 effector, SipA, along with other SPI-2 effector proteins. SipA also plays a role in stimulating the replication of intracellular *Salmonella* [28, 49]. Another mechanism by which SPI-1 effector proteins are involved in late stages of infection deals with *Salmonella* escaping from the SCV. SopA has been implicated in allowing *Salmonella* to escape from the SCV through interaction with another host E3 ligase known as the RING finger protein with membrane anchor (HsRMA-1) [55].

In addition to the SPI-1 effector proteins described above, recently other effector proteins have been discovered that are also secreted using this system. This includes, SlrP, SteA and SteB. However, these proteins are also secreted by the SPI-2 T3SS. SlrP ubiquitinates mammalian thioredoxin (regulatory protein) which ultimately causes cell death in vitro [68]. Despite being secreted by both SPI-1 and SPI-2 systems, the expression of SlrP is induced by a SPI-1 regulator [77]. SteA and SteB are secreted by both the SPI-1 and SPI-2 T3SS. SteA localizes to the Golgi network in infected cells and is required for colonization of mouse spleens, while SteB does not appear to play a role in the colonization of mice. The regulation of SteA and SteB is not known [71].

In summary, SPI-1 effector proteins have diverse functions including mediating invasion, positively and negatively regulating the inflammatory response and SCV maturation and positioning.

2.4. Regulation

Regulation of the SPI-1 T3SS locus is complex and involves the actions of both local and global regulatory proteins, in response to specific environmental factors. The HilA protein (encoded on SPI-1) is one of the main local regulators of SPI-1 gene expression. HilA binds directly to promoters on the *inv-spa* and *prg-org* operons (Figure 3), which results in transcriptional activation. Read-through from the *inv-spa* operon also leads to the activation of InvF, which subsequently activates transcription of the *sic-sip* operon. In addition, InvF, along with SicA (chaperone), induces the expression of several non-SPI-1 effectors. Transcription of *hilA* is controlled by HilC, HilD and RtsA. Once HilD is expressed, it activates the transcription of *hilC* and *rtsA*. HilC and RtsA further enhance the expression of each other and themselves. Along with HilD, HilC and RtsA activate the transcription of *hilA*, which ultimately leads to the expression of SPI-1 genes [34].

Many global regulators affect the expression of SPI-1 genes through the transcriptional activator HilD. One such system is the EnvZ/OmpR two-component regulatory system. This system controls the expression of two major outer membrane proteins, OmpC and OmpF, primarily in response to changes in osmolarity. OmpC and OmpF form aqueous channels allowing passive diffusion of small molecules across the outer membrane. EnvZ acts as a sensor, monitoring conditions in the external environment and transfers this information to OmpR through phosphorylation [78]. Once phosphorylated, OmpR induces the expression of *hilD* (along with the regulation of several other bacterial genes) which ultimately leads to the expression of SPI-1 genes [79]. A second global regulator of SPI-1 genes is the BarA/SirA two component regulatory system which regulates genes involved in metabolism, motility, biofilm formation and invasion [34]. BarA is the sensor kinase which phosphorylates SirA in response to environmental signals, which are currently unknown. Phosphorylated SirA activates expression of two small RNA molecules *csrB* and *csrC*, which in turn prevent CsrA action; CsrA is a repressor of *hilD*. Hence, HilD expression is increased leading to increased SPI-1 gene expression [34, 80]. The ferric uptake regulator (Fur) is one of the most important iron dependent regulators in *Salmonella* and is another global regulator of SPI-1 gene expression. In response to high iron levels (as in the intestinal lumen), Fur binds Fe^{2+} and represses the expression of several genes involved in the uptake of iron and other metals. Fur affects *hilA* activity (SPI-1 gene expression) by regulating HilD at the post-transcriptional level either by repressing a negative regulator of HilD or controlling the level of HilD required to activate the *hilD* promoter and thus the expression of SPI-1 genes [81]. The PhoP/PhoQ two-component system is yet another global regulator of SPI-1 gene expression. PhoQ (sensor) activates PhoP in response to low levels of Mg^{2+} and Ca^{2+} (as in the intracellular and phagosomal environment) [25, 82]. This results in the activation of hilE expression, which represses HilD leading to the repression of SPI-1 gene expression [34]. This regulation is an important mechanism of switching off or lowering the expression of the SPI-1 T3SS genes, since they are not major players in intracellular survival and replication (summarized in Figure 3).

Environmental signals that affect the expression of SPI-1 T3SS genes include pH, osmolarity, and the levels of oxygen and magnesium. Since the main site of invasion by *Salmonella* is the small intestine, the environmental conditions associated with it lead to increased expression of SPI-1 virulence genes. The pH level of the small intestine is near neutral and has been shown to increase expression of genes associated with the SPI-1 locus. Similarly, the osmolarity of the small intestine is high which increases expression of SPI-1 genes, possibly signaling through OmpR and EnvZ. The intestinal lumen is anaerobic, while the brush border is microaerophilic.

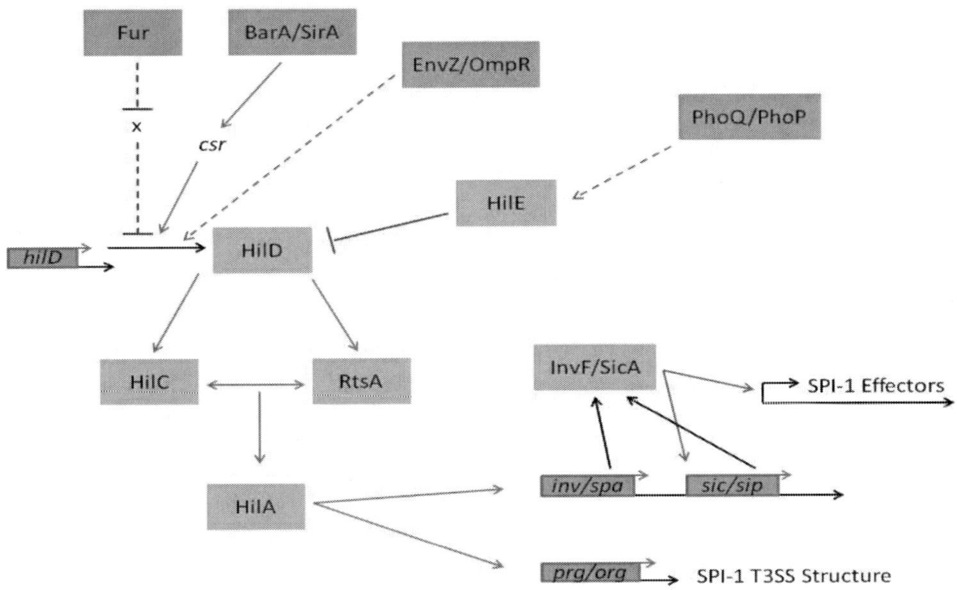

Figure 3. Regulation of the *S.* Enteritidis SPI-1 T3SS by local and global regulators. Lines with blunt ends represent repression. Lines with dashes indicate that the exact mechanism of regulation is not known. Diagram was modified from [34].

Low oxygen conditions have been shown to elevate the expression of SPI-1 genes. Finally, high levels of magnesium in the extracellular environment of the small intestine and elsewhere in the host result in repression of the PhoP/PhoQ system which normally represses SPI-1 gene expression. Taken together, this demonstrates that SPI-1 regulation is fairly complex and involves several parameters that include local, global and environmental regulators [83-84].

2.5. Role in Virulence

The role of the SPI-1 T3SS has been extensively studied in the bovine and murine (streptomycin-treated mice) models of infection [47]. These studies have been mainly performed with *Salmonella enterica* serovar Typhimurium (*S.* Typhimurium) which causes a similar non-typhoidal disease in humans and animal models. Oral infection of streptomycin treated mice and calves results in a massive neutrophil influx in the gastro-intestinal tract causing inflammation, which is analogous to the clinical and histological manifestations of the disease in humans. As well, in susceptible mice, the infection spreads to internal organs causing systemic disease [11]. *Salmonella* SPI-1 mutants have been shown to cause reduced inflammation and fluid influx in the animal models described above, demonstrating that SPI-1 is critical for the intestinal form of the disease [47]. Moreover, recently it has been demonstrated that SPI-1 effector proteins are also synthesized during later stages of infection in mice, suggesting that SPI-1 may play a role in systemic disease [85]. In chickens, the function of SPI-1 is not as well characterized and has mostly been observed using S. Typhimurium. Studies have revealed that SPI-1 mutants affect the colonization of chicken ceca [86-87], while one report suggests that this effect is age dependent [88]. Further, it has been shown that the absence of SPI-1 can affect levels of *Salmonella* in internal organs [88-89].

In order to examine the role of *S.* Enteritidis SPI-1 in chickens, we first tested the invasiveness of deletion mutants in SPI-1 (Δ SPI-1) relative to the wild type strain in both polarized human intestinal epithelial cells and chicken intestinal tissue explants. Our results confirmed that the absence of *S.* Enteritidis SPI-1 reduced the invasiveness of the mutant strains as compared to the wild type strain [90]. In chickens, we observed that oral challenge of two-week-old birds by a Δ SPI-1 mutant strain did not affect the colonization of the cecal contents on days 1-4 post challenge. However, the levels of *S.* Enteritidis were lower in the livers and spleens of the Δ SPI-1 challenged group relative to the wild type challenged group on the first two days post challenge. These findings suggest that *S.* Enteritidis SPI-1 plays a role in systemic infection of chickens but does not affect colonization of the cecal contents.

3. *Salmonella* Pathogenicity Island-2 Type III Secretion System

The SPI-2 T3SS is located between centisome 30 and 31 of the *Salmonella* chromosome and is 40 kb in size. It encodes approximately 31 genes that are organized in two operons.

Table 2. List of effector proteins secreted by the *S.* Enteritidis SPI-2 T3SS. Table was adapted and modified from [28]

Effector protein	Gene location	Function	Reference
GogB	Bacteriophage Gifsy-1	Unknown	[102]
PipB	SPI-5	Associates with the SCV and sifs but is not required for intracellular survival or virulence in mice	[103]
PipB2	Outside SPI-2	Enhances growth of sifs	[101]
SifA	Outside SPI-2	SCV positioning, sif formation and re-directing traffic to SCV	[28, 100]
SifB	Outside SPI-2	Localizes with SCV and travels away from SCV along sifs	[104]
SopD2	Outside SPI-2	Localizes to the SCV membrane, involved in sif formation and is important for replication in macrophage and mice	[105-106]
SpiC	SPI-2	Prevents fusion of late endosomes with SCV, required for translocation of SPI-2 proteins, important for survival in macrophages and virulence in mice	[95, 107]
SseF	SPI-2	Plays a role in Sif formation, re-directs traffic to SCV and maintains perinuclear position	[28, 100, 108]
SseG	SPI-2	Similar to SseF	
SseI	Bacteriophage Gifsy-1	Involved in the formation of actin surrounding the SCV	[98]
SseJ	Outside SPI-2	Maintains the integrity of the SCV membrane	[61, 97]
SseK1	Outside SPI-2	Localize to the host cytoplasm and has not been associated with virulence in mice	[109]
SseK2	Outside SPI-2	Similar to SseK1	[109]
SseK3	Bacteriophage	Unknown	[109]
SseL	Outside SPI-2	Suppresses NF-κB activity and causes cell death	[110-111]
SspH2	Bacteriophage	Involved in the formation of actin surrounding the SCV	[98]
SteC	Outside SPI-2	Involved in the formation of actin surrounding the SCV	[99]
SpvB	*spv* plasmid	Inhibits SCV associated actin polymerization	[98]
SpvC	*spv* plasmid	Down regulates the inflammatory response	[112-113]

One operon encodes genes of the secretion system apparatus (*ssa*), secretion system effectors (*sse*) and secretion system chaperones (*ssc*), while the other operon encodes the SsrAB two-component secretion system regulator (*ssr*) [91]. The SPI-2 secretion system plays a major role in intracellular survival and replication [92].

3.1. Structure

The surface structure of the SPI-2 apparatus consists of a translocon, filament and needle. SseC and SseD form the translocon at the tip of the T3SS apparatus, while SseB forms a filament-like structure that connects the translocon to the needle protein, SsaG. The basal structure is composed of SsaC (outer membrane protein), SsaJ (periplasmic protein) and a complex of proteins that consist of the inner membrane and the export apparatus (SsaD, SsaR, SsaS, SsaT, SsaU and SsaV). The SPI-2 apparatus also contains an "ATPase" that provides the energy required for the secretion of effector proteins through this structure. The major candidates for this function are SsaN, SsaK and SsaQ [91].

3.2. Secretion

Salmonella species secrete many effector proteins across the vacuolar membrane of the SCV. The secretion of these proteins is mainly triggered in response to the intracellular phagosomal environment encountered by *Salmonella* inside host cells [93]. However, expression of SPI-2 genes has recently been reported in the intestinal lumen of mice, suggesting that expression of these genes may occur prior to invasion of host cells [94]. To date, at least 19 effector proteins have been identified that are secreted through the SPI-2 T3SS (Table 2), some of which are located on SPI-2, while others are located outside this pathogenicity island. These virulence factors are involved in SCV maturation, trafficking and positioning. In addition, the SPI-2 T3SS effector proteins also modulate the inflammatory response associated with *Salmonella* infection [28].

The SPI-2 effector proteins SpiC, SseJ, SteC, SseI and SspH2 are involved in SCV maturation and trafficking. SpiC prevents the fusion of late endosomes with the SCV, which assists in delaying fusion of the SCV and lysosomes, allowing *Salmonella* to persist and replicate [95-96]. SseJ, has deacylase activity and is involved in maintaining the integrity of the SCV membrane [61, 97]. SteC, SseI and SspH2 all play a role in the formation of a filamentous-actin (F-actin) meshwork surrounding the SCV [98-99].

As the SCV continues to mature, it moves towards the nucleus (perinuclear position). The SPI-2 effector, SifA, is involved in maintaining the position of the SCV. SifA, as well as SseF and SseG, are important for the formation of *Salmonella* induced filaments (sifs) [28], which are tube-like membranes that contain aggregates of lysosomal glycoproteins [100]. The growth of the Sifs are enhanced by the SPI-2 effector protein, PipB2 [101]. In addition, SifA, along with SseF and SseG, re-directs transport of exocytic vesicles to the SCV, a process which allows *Salmonella* to gain access to nutrients for bacterial replication and for the growing SCV [100].

Effector proteins secreted by the SPI-2 secretion system also play a role in down-regulating the inflammatory response associated with *Salmonella* infections and have been linked with causing cell death. The SPI-2 effector, SseL, suppresses NF-κB activation by inhibiting IκBα ubiquitination, as a result of its deubiquitinase activity. This prevents IκBα degradation and consequently, IκBα suppresses NF-κB activity leading to lower levels of inflammation [110]. SseL has also been shown to cause cell death. *Salmonella* Typhimurium sseL- mutant strains cause significantly less cytotoxicity in macrophages and have been shown to be attenuated for virulence in mice, relative to the wild type strain [111].

In summary, the main functions of SPI-2 effector proteins are SCV maturation and positioning, re-directing SCV traffic and modulating the inflammatory response.

3.3. Regulation

The SsrA/SsrB two-component system is the master regulator of SPI-2 T3SS expression. SsrA is a sensor kinase that, in response to environmental stimuli, phosphorylates the response regulator SsrB, which activates the expression of SPI-2 T3SS genes encoded on SPI-2 as well as outside this pathogenicity island [114-116].

The SsrA/SsrB two-component system is regulated by the OmpR/EnvZ (described earlier in section 2.4) and PhoP/PhoQ two-component systems [116]. When *Salmonella* is grown under SPI-2 inducing conditions, EnvZ phosphorylates OmpR which in turn binds to the promoters of the SsrA/SsrB two component system, leading to activation of SPI-2 gene expression [117-118]. Similarly, in conditions of low magnesium and low pH (conditions resembling the SCV), the PhoQ sensor kinase phosphorylates PhoP which then activates the expression of the SsrA/SsrB system [119-120].

The transcription of SPI-2 T3SS genes is also controlled by a family of proteins known as nucleoid associated proteins (NAPs) [116]. These proteins bind to bacterial chromosomal DNA and play an important role in the organization and compaction of bacterial chromatin. Hence, the NAPs are able to repress or activate the transcription of certain genes depending on different cellular requirements [121]. H-NS, YgdT and Hha are three NAPs that repress the transcription of SPI-2 genes [116]. On the other hand, integration host factor (IHF) and inversion stimulation (Fis) are two NAPs that are required for complete expression of SPI-2 genes. IHF is important for DNA bending and compaction, while Fis directly activates the transcription of SPI-2 genes by binding to the promoters of *spiR* and *ssaG* genes [122-124].

3.4. Role in Virulence

The role of the SPI-2 T3SS has been studied extensively in mice, since *Salmonella* infections lead to systemic disease (explained in section 2.5). S. Typhimurium SPI-2 mutants are highly attenuated in mice relative to wild type strains. Lower bacterial loads were detected in the internal organs of infected mice, suggesting that SPI-2 mutant strains were impaired in their ability to survive and replicate in host organs [125-126]. Moreover, recent experiments have illustrated that the SPI-2 T3SS contributes to the intestinal form of disease in the murine and bovine models of infection [127-128]. This finding implies that the role of this secretion system may not be exclusive to systemic disease during non-host adapted *Salmonella* pathogenesis. The role of the SPI-2 secretion system has also been evaluated in chickens, but this has not been extensively studied relative to the studies in the mouse and bovine models.

Three studies performed in chickens indicated that lower levels of SPI-2 mutants (non-host adapted Salmonella species) were recovered from the internal organs of chickens relative to the wild type strain, implying that the SPI-2 T3SS is an important virulence factor in chickens [88, 129-130].

4. *Salmonella* Enteritidis Infections in Poultry

4.1. Sources of Infection

Poultry flocks become infected with *S.* Enteritidis from a variety of sources. Incubation of *Salmonella* contaminated eggs with *Salmonella* free eggs at the hatchery results in high numbers of *Salmonella* positive chicks, suggesting that the hatchery is an important source of *Salmonella* infection. Similarly, poultry can also become infected by the transmission of this pathogen via aerosols from infected birds. The litter in poultry barns is another source of contamination since chicks contaminate the litter with fecal content containing *Salmonella*. Hence, other chickens easily become infected with *Salmonella* when they pick on fecal droppings from their littermates. Poultry flocks can also become contaminated with *Salmonella* after consumption of water. This happens when the chicks are young and their drinkers are located close to the ground. The chicks often defecate in the drinkers resulting in the contamination of the water and spread of the organism to the rest of the flock. Rodents also form a major source of *Salmonella* infection in poultry houses. They often shed high levels of *Salmonella* species in their feces [131]. In addition to the sources mentioned above, the presence of insects on poultry houses can significantly contribute to the dissemination of *Salmonella* species in poultry flocks. These insects include cockroaches, lesser mealworms, flies and darkling beetles [132-135].

4.2. Pathogenesis

Chickens that come in contact with *S.* Enteritidis mostly develop gastrointestinal colonization, which results in shedding of the bacterium through the fecal contents. The bacteria may also cause a systemic infection leading to the spread of the organism to the internal organs (liver and spleen) [1, 131]. This occurs when *S.* Enteritidis breaches the intestinal epithelial surface via enterocytes, M cells or dendritic cells [136]. Once the bacteria reach the lamina propria they are internalized by macrophages and rapidly disseminate to the liver, spleen and other parts of the body through the thoracic duct [1, 6]. Systemic infection may also lead to infection of chicken ovaries resulting in the production of contaminated eggs. Young chicks (first few days of life) are more susceptible to colonization by *S.* Enteritidis relative to older birds and younger birds are more likely to develop a systemic infection. On rare occasions, young chicks can develop clinical signs that include progressive somnolence, drooping wings, ruffled feathers, anorexia, and diarrohea. In addition, chickens infected with other infectious agents like *Eimeria tenella* or immunosuppressive pathogens become more susceptible to infection by *Salmonella* species. The detection of *S.* Enteritidis in poultry flocks is often difficult because *S.* Enteritidis colonization is mainly asymptomatic [1, 131].

4.3. Immune Response to *S.* Enteritidis

4.3.1. Innate Immune Response

The innate immune system is the first line of defense encountered by *S.* Enteritidis during the process of infection. The innate system is comprised of several components including physical barriers (e.g. epithelial surfaces), antimicrobial chemical components, complement system and specialized cells, such as natural killer cells, macrophages, dendritic cells and heterophils [137].

Investigation of the dynamics of immune cell filtration in day old chicks infected with *S.* Enteritidis has revealed that heterophils were the first group of cells that infiltrated the cecal lamina propria at 12 hours post infection, followed by macrophages and T-lymphocytes at 20 hours post infection, and B cells at 24 hours post infection [138-139]. This suggested that the chicken innate immune system was important for resisting against *Salmonella* infection. This notion was supported by a study in which heterophil-depleted chickens were more susceptible to *S.* Enteritidis organ invasion [140-141]. Recently it was demonstrated that chicken heterophils release Cathelicidin-2, an antimicrobial peptide with potent bactericidal activity [142], upon contact with *Salmonella*. Cathelicidin-2 also has the capacity to bind to LPS and block LPS-mediated proinflammatory gene expression [137].

Another important component of the chicken innate immune system are toll-like receptors (TLRs). TLRs are transmembrane sensor proteins that recognize pathogen associated molecular patterns (PAMPs) leading to the induction of innate immunity [143]. In chickens, TLR-4 plays an important role in the host response to *Salmonella* infection. This receptor recognises *Salmonella* LPS leading to the activation of heterophils and an increase in the secretion of pro-inflammatory cytokines IL-1β, IL-6 and IL-18 [144-145]. In the same way, chicken TLR-5 recognizes *Salmonella* flagella leading to an upregulation of IL-1β, which causes local inflammation. Interestingly, flagella-deficient strains of *S.* Typhimurium do not upregulate IL-1β, and are isolated at higher levels from the internal organs of chickens. This suggests that the absence of the flagella allows *S.* Typhimurium to evade recognition by the host immune system [143, 146].

Similarly, other experiments have revealed that oral inoculation of chickens with non-host adapted *Salmonella* species (*S.* Enteritidis or *S.* Typhimurium) resulted in the up-regulation of IL-1β, IL-18 and TGF-β4 mRNA levels (as determined by real-time reverse transcription (RT)-PCR) in the spleens of infected birds, while the level of IL-4 was down-regulated [147-150]. In the ceca of infected chickens, it has been observed that the mRNA levels of IL-1β, IL-6, IL-8, IL-12, IL-18 and TGF-β4 have been upregulated relative to non-infected control birds [149-152]. The cytokines IL-1β, IL-6 and IL-8 are pro-inflammatory cytokines that lead to the recruitment of immune cells leading to inflammation in the host tissue. On the other hand, the increase in the levels of IL-12 and IL-18, in response to *Salmonella* infection, is indicative of a cellular immune response [153].

4.3.2. Adaptive Immune Response

Chickens infected orally with *S.* Typhimurium have been associated with higher levels of interferon-gamma (IFNγ) in splenocytes relative to control birds. In addition, levels of IFNγ gradually declined as the infection started to clear, suggesting that IFNγ (a strong indicator of cell mediated immunity) played an important role in clearance of *S.* Typhimurium infection [147]. As well, it has been demonstrated that intraperitoneal administration of IFNγ to chickens results in lower organ colonization following *S.* Typhimurium challenge [154]. Similarly, another group has shown that chickens infected with *S.* Typhimurium developed strong T cell responses (as measured by proliferation assays) relative to control birds and this also correlated with clearance of the infection [150]. In a more detailed study, the authors characterized the T cell composition of lymphocytes in the blood as well as in different organs following *S.* Typhimurium infection. CD8+ T cells were upregulated in the blood, ceca, bursa of fabricius and the spleen relative to the non-infected birds [155]. This provided further support to imply that cell mediated immunity was an important component in the defense against *S.* Typhimurium infections.

Infection of chickens with *S.* Typhimurium has often been associated with significant serum IgM, IgG (IgY) and IgA antibody titers 5-7 days post-infection. However, high antibody titers do not appear to correlate with lower levels of *Salmonella* or clearance of the organism [156]. To examine the role of antibodies in *Salmonella* infections, B cell depleted chickens have been tested. Chickens that were chemically bursectomized (using cyclophosphamide or testosterone proprionate) had higher levels of *S.* Enteritidis in cecal contents relative to healthy chickens, but this difference was not observed in internal organs. The authors hypothesized that secretory IgA plays a role in clearance of *Salmonella* infections from the chicken gut [157]. However, recently, it has been demonstrated that surgically bursectomized chickens had levels of *Salmonella* that were identical to healthy chickens in cecal contents as well as in internal organs. Moreover, the chickens were able to clear the infection at the same rate as healthy chickens [158]. This study suggests that the humoral response may not be critical for defense against *Salmonella* infections in chickens. Additionally, a recent report has indicated that using chemical methods to deplete B cells in chickens also affects other cells [156], adding further support to the findings in the study which used surgically bursectomized chickens [158]. Taken together, these studies imply that the humoral response to *Salmonella* infection may not be crucial in the clearance of infection. However, the importance of antibodies for chicken immunity to *Salmonella* infection can not be ruled out until further work is done to investigate the dynamics of the immune response [156].

5. CONTROL OF *SALMONELLA* ENTERITIDIS

5.1. Management Practices

Good flock management and sanitation practices are important since *S.* Enteritidis can be introduced into poultry houses from many different sources as discussed in section 4.1. One of the most important aspects of poultry house management is to ensure that eggs or chicks coming into the facility are from a breeding flock that has been extensively tested for

Salmonella species and is proven to be *Salmonella* free. Secondly, eggs that are set for hatching should be properly disinfected and hatched under strict conditions to minimize the chances of *Salmonella* contamination. In addition, between flocks, the poultry house should be cleaned and disinfected using an effective method since not all methods are effective in eliminating *S.* Enteritidis [159-160]. Formaldehyde fumigation has been shown to highly effective and should be used to disinfect poultry facilities [161]. Fourthly, since rodents and insects are important vectors of *Salmonella* transmission in poultry houses (discussed in section 4.1), strict control measures should be in place, especially given that a single mouse dropping can contain 10^5 *S.* Enteritidis cells [162]. Moreover, a study has shown that the levels of *S.* Enteritidis in mice from a poultry house positive for this pathogen were four times higher than in mice from a facility negative for *S.* Enteritidis [163]. Biosecurity is also an important component of good management practices at poultry houses. This includes ensuring that all personnel entering the facility either change their footware or use the boot dip disinfection method. In addition, equipment and machinery that is in use at the facility should be cleaned and disinfected [160, 164]. The feed that is used for chickens at the poultry houses should not contain any animal proteins and should be *Salmonella* free [160]. This can be achieved by the addition of antimicrobials in the feed, or by using heat or irradiation [164]. Another important component of good management practices includes a *Salmonella*-free water supply; water contaminated with *S.* Enteritidis has been associated with contamination of a laying flock [165]. Other factors that involve good management at facilities housing poultry flocks are controlling moisture levels and ensuring that there is adequate ventilation [160].

5.2. Bacteriophages

Bacteriophage therapy in chickens involves the use of phages that are orally administered to chickens a few days after oral challenge with non-host specific *Salmonella* species (e.g. *S.* Enteritidis and *S.* Typhimurium). These phages target specific receptors on the *Salmonella* surface prior to injection of DNA into the bacterial cell, followed by phage replication and cell lysis [166].

A recent study evaluated the efficacy of broad host range phages against *S.* Enteritidis. Chickens were treated orally with either 10^9 plaque forming units (pfu) or 10^{11} pfu of phages two days after oral challenge with *S.* Enteritidis. At the higher dose, the levels of *S.* Enteritidis were significantly lower in the cecal contents (about 2 to 4 log units lower) relative to the control group. However, the study did not examine the effect of phage therapy on systemic levels of *S.* Enteritidis [167]. On the other hand, results from other studies have given variable results suggesting that phage therapy may have potential as a pre-harvest intervention measure and that more research needs to be performed to investigate the effects of phage therapy on *S.* Enteritidis colonization in chickens [166].

5.3. Competitive Exclusion

Competitive exclusion, in the context of poultry, refers to the administration and redistribution of normal bacterial flora from the gastrointestinal tract of poultry to reduce colonization by enteric pathogens [168]. The inhibitory effect is thought to occur by either interference with the attachment of the enteric pathogen to the host intestinal wall or inhibition of the growth of the pathogen due to a change in the intestinal environment. In the case of *Salmonella* species, competitive exclusion products from older chickens have been given orally to younger birds leading to reduced *Salmonella* levels in the gastrointestinal tract of these pathogens [160, 168]. Reduction in the levels of this pathogen has also been associated with lower numbers of carcass contamination [169]. Hence, the use of competitive exclusion products is an attractive strategy that can be used as one of the components to form part of a comprehensive *Salmonella* control program. However, the use of this approach also has certain limitations. First of all, many of these "probiotics" are composed of undefined cultures. Thus, this involves introducing undefined live organisms into chickens and the poultry houses. Additionally, it may also lead to the introduction of antibiotic resistant bacteria and possibly result in the transfer of antibiotic resistance to other non-resistant bacterial strains. Nonetheless, attempts have been made to define competitive exclusion cultures; possible candidates responsible for protective effects have been suggested to include *Lactobacillus* species, *Bifidobacterium* species, *Escherichia coli*, *Bacillus subtilis* and *Streptococcus cristatus*. Secondly, the protective effect of these cultures has been observed in younger birds that have not yet developed a mature intestinal microflora. Thus, the use of these products may not be a reliable option for older birds. Thirdly, this treatment is not very effective in chickens that have an altered microflora due to antibiotic treatment or chickens that have been subject to feed or water withdrawal [160].

5.4. Vaccination

Vaccination of chickens for protection against non-host specific *Salmonella* serotypes has been widely used as an intervention strategy to reduce the prevalence of *Salmonella* in poultry flocks in order to protect consumers from food-borne disease transmission [160, 164, 170-171]. This strategy aims to utilize the chicken's immune system to decrease the levels of the pathogen that are associated with the animal upon infection. In the United Kingdom, extensive vaccination of chickens since 1997 has successfully reduced the incidence of human *S.* Enteritidis infections [10]. In the same way, vaccination along with other intervention strategies has drastically lowered the number of human *S.* Enteritidis infections in Belgium [172]. The *Salmonella* vaccines that have been used to date are generally classified into three categories: Live attenuated strains, killed *Salmonella* and subunit vaccines.

5.4.1. Live Attenuated Vaccines

Live attenuated strains of *Salmonella* are constructed mainly by the mutation or deletion of genes that are important for virulence, metabolism or survival. These vaccine strains have several advantages; they can be administered orally and to young chicks, they induce rapid protection, and can activate both humoral and cell-mediated responses. However, the main concern with live attenuated strains is that they consist of a living organism which may persist for extended periods in the chickens as well as their environment, posing a threat to human health [170].

S. Enteritidis *aroA* mutants, which are impaired in the ability to synthesize aromatic compounds, have been tested as live vaccines in chickens. Oral vaccination with aroA strains resulted in reduction of the levels of *S.* Enteritidis in the livers, spleens, cecal contents and ovaries relative to the non-vaccinated group [173]. Similarly, oral vaccination of 1 or 14 day old chicks with a *cya-crp S.* Typhimurium double mutant (deletion in the genes encoding adenylate cyclase and cyclic adenosine monophosphate receptor protein) significantly reduced the levels of the challenge strain in the ceca (approximately 6 log units) relative to the unvaccinated control group. As well, the levels of the challenge strain in the spleen were not detectable in the vaccinated group. However, when the same vaccine was used for protection against *S.* Enteritidis oral challenge, the levels of the challenge strain in the ceca were only slightly lower relative to the control group, while the levels in the spleen were not detectable in the vaccinated group [174]. A temperature sensitive *S.* Enteritidis mutant (able to grow at 28°C and not at 37°C) has also been evaluated as a live attenuated vaccine strain in chickens. Chickens were immunized at 1 and 14 days of age orally or intra-peritoneally with 10^{10} cfu of the mutant strain and were challenged (orally) at 28 days of age with 10^{8} cfu of virulent *S.* Enteritidis. All vaccinated groups demonstrated lower levels (several log units lower) of the challenge strain in the ceca and spleens compared to the control group [175].

The *Salmonella enterica* subspecies *enterica* serovar Gallinarum (*S.* Gallinarum) 9R strain (modification in the LPS) is another live attenuated strain that has been widely used in chickens for protection against *S.* Enteritidis. This strain has been tested under field conditions where chickens were vaccinated subcutaneously at 6 weeks, followed by a booster injection at 14-16 weeks of age as per the recommendation of the commercial vaccine (Nobilis SG 9R). Chickens were monitored for *S.* Enteritidis shedding prior to the 1st vaccination and up to 6 weeks after the 1st vaccination. The results indicated that 2.5 % of the flocks were positive for *S.* Enteritidis in the vaccinated groups relative to the control group (11.5 %) [176]. TAD *Salmonella* vac® E is a *S.* Enteritidis live vaccine constructed by chemical mutagenesis which has prolonged generation times and as a result is less virulent. To evaluate the efficacy of this strain, chickens were vaccinated orally with 10^{8} cfu of TAD *Salmonella* vac® E at 1 day of age, followed by two boosters at 6 and 16 weeks of age. The chickens were intravenously challenged at 24 weeks of age with 10^{7} cfu of *S.* Enteritidis. Vaccinated chickens had significantly lower numbers of positive livers (12/28) and oviducts (6/28) relative to the non-vaccinated chickens (23/30 livers and 15/29 oviducts). Similarly, eggs obtained from vaccinated chickens had fewer positive samples (9/35) compared to the control group (15/35) at 22 weeks of age [177].

In the studies described above, live attenuated *Salmonella* strains were tested for their ability to confer protection against *Salmonella* challenge. In most of the experiments, oral challenge was conducted shortly after immunization with the vaccine strain, therefore, it is possible that the vaccination strain may have colonization-inhibition effects that lead to reduced colonization and systemic spread of the challenge strain [170]. Moreover, not all the live attenuated strains (described above) have been tested under field conditions. In addition, these vaccine strains have not been very effective in inducing cross-protection against other non-host adapted serovars [160].

5.4.2. Killed Vaccines

Killed *Salmonella* vaccines consist of whole cell bacteria that have been inactivated using either heat, formalin or acetone. Most of these strains are delivered subcutaneously and require at least two injections. A major advantage conferred by this class of vaccines is that they do not contain a live organism that could potentially survive in the environment and affect human health. However, the use of these vaccines has been mainly associated with strong antibody responses [160, 170], which do not always correlate with protection.

Salenvac® is a commercially available killed vaccine licensed for use in the United Kingdom. It consists of an inactivated *S.* Enteritidis strain grown under iron limiting conditions (growth under iron limiting conditions is thought to stimulate the production of virulence factors in order to mimic the host environment). The efficacy of Salenvac® was evaluated in a study in which laying chickens were vaccinated subcutaneously at day 1 and 4 weeks of age (group 1), while the second group followed the same regime with a third immunization at 8 weeks of age (group 2). The chickens were challenged intravenously at different ages (8, 17, 23, 30 or 59 weeks) with 10^7 cfu of *S.* Enteritidis. Vaccinated birds had significantly lower *S.* Enteritidis fecal shedding, organ colonization and egg contamination (shells and internal contents) relative to the control birds [178]. It is obvious that the Salenvac® vaccine is highly effective in protecting laying chickens against a high dose of S. Enteritidis challenge. However, this study would have been more relevant if an oral challenge had been given since that would be closer to the real situation.

Layermune SE® is a killed *S.* Enteritidis vaccine that is commercially available. It is composed of multiple strains of *S.* Enteritidis formulated in an oil based adjuvant. This vaccine was tested in a study in which layers and broilers were vaccinated subcutaneously at five and nine weeks of age. The chickens were orally challenged at ten weeks of age with 10^8 cfu of *S.* Enteritidis. The vaccine reduced the levels of *S.* Enteritidis in the ceca, livers and spleens of the vaccinated group by several log units relative to the control group in layers but was not very effective in broiler chickens [179].

Similarly, Poulvac SE®, a commercially available killed *S.* Enteritidis vaccine, has been evaluated for protection in progeny derived from broiler breeders vaccinated with this strain. Broilers were vaccinated subcutaneously at twelve and twenty weeks of age. Progeny derived from these hens were orally challenged at 1 day or two weeks of age with 10^5 cfu or 10^9 cfu of *S.* Enteritidis, respectively. The results indicated that the number of birds positive for *S.* Enteritidis were much lower in the progeny derived from the vaccinated group (7/25) challenged at 1 day of age compared to the control group (25/25). However, the vaccine was not very effective in progeny challenged at two weeks of age relative to the control group. The vaccine did not cause a significant drop in the levels of *S.* Enteritidis in the livers, spleens and ceca of progeny obtained from the vaccinated chickens that were challenged at 1 day or at two weeks of age [180]. Another study evaluated the efficacy of a *S.* Enteritidis killed strain. In this study killed *S.* Enteritidis was formulated with microspheres and used to vaccinate chickens orally or intramuscularly at two weeks of age. The chickens were orally challenged at six weeks of age with 10^9 cfu of *S.* Enteritidis. Vaccination reduced the number of organs (ceca, liver and spleen) that were positive for *S.* Enteritidis (18-26 %) relative to the control group (44 %) [181].

5.4.3. Subunit Vaccines

Subunit vaccines consist of a single protein or a mixture of proteins that are usually expressed on the surface of the cell and are considered to be important in virulence. Such proteins are mainly delivered subcutaneously, unless they are formulated appropriately for oral delivery.

A vaccine containing an extract of *S.* Enteritidis outer membrane proteins was evaluated in chickens. The chickens were immunized orally or subcutaneously at 8 weeks of age, followed by a booster at 11 weeks of age. At thirteen weeks of age, the chickens were orally challenged with 10^7 cfu of *S.* Enteritidis. The numbers of chickens positive for *S.* Enteritidis, as determined by cloacal swabbing, were mostly negative in the vaccinated group relative to the control group (100% positive). However, this study did not examine the levels of *S.* Enteritidis present in the liver, spleen or ceca [182]. In the same way, another group evaluated the effect of immunizing chickens with *S.* Enteritidis outer membrane proteins. The chickens were immunized subcutaneously at nine and eleven weeks of age. At twelve weeks of age, the chickens were orally challenged with 10^8 cfu of *S.* Enteritidis. Vaccinated chickens had lower levels of *S.* Enteritidis (2-3 log units) in the ceca and small intestine relative to the control group. However, the levels of the challenge strain were not determined in the internal organs [183].

S. Enteritidis type 1 fimbriae have been evaluated as potential subunit vaccine candidates. Chickens were vaccinated subcutaneously at 18 weeks of age with purified type 1 fimbriae, followed by a booster injection at 21 weeks of age. At 24 weeks of age, the birds were challenged intravenously with 10^7 cfu of *S.* Enteritidis. The results suggested that the vaccine did not have an effect on the levels of *S.* Enteritidis in the ceca, livers or spleens. However, there was a mild reduction in the number of egg shells and oviducts contaminated with S. Enteritidis in the vaccinated group compared to the non-vaccinated control [184]. In another study, a peptide containing part of the FliC protein (forms the flagellar filament) was used to immunize chickens subcutaneously at 3 and 5 week of age, with an oral challenge of 10^7 cfu of S. Enteritidis at 7 weeks of age. The FliC based vaccine significantly reduced (2 log units) the levels of the challenge strain at 3 weeks post challenge in the cecal contents based on direct plating relative to the control group. The vaccine did not affect the levels of the challenge strain in the livers and spleens of the vaccinated birds [185].

Similarly, our group was interested in determining if *S.* Enteritidis SPI-1 T3SS proteins could be used for protection against *S.* Enteritidis oral challenge in chickens. Prior to testing the efficacy of the SPI-1 T3SS proteins in protection, we used sera against these proteins in a functional assay using polarized Caco-2 cells to determine if the sera could block invasion by *S.* Enteritidis. Interestingly, our results demonstrated that anti-SipD serum blocked *S.* Enteritids entry, while sera against InvG, PrgI, SipA, SipC, SopB, SopE and SopE2 did not [186]. Vaccination of chickens subcutaneously with SPI-1 T3SS proteins induced a significant antigen specific serum IgG response and resulted in lower levels of the *S.* Enteritidis challenge strain in the livers and spleens of vaccinated birds. However, the levels of *S.* Enteritidis in the cecal contents of vaccinates were not affected as compared to the control group [187]. These results suggest that *S.* Enteritidis SPI-1 T3SS proteins may have some potential as vaccine candidates and that further research needs to be performed.

Taken together, it can be concluded that vaccination of chickens with either live attenuated, killed or subunit vaccines has resulted in lowering the levels of *S.* Enteritidis (summarized in Table 3). Based on the data presented from different vaccine efficacy studies, it is difficult to infer that one class of vaccines confers greater protection than the other, although few studies have examined the efficacy of subunit vaccines. Recently, one study examined the efficacy of four commercially available *Salmonella* vaccines (3 live attenuated strains and 1 killed strain) in the U.K. in reducing *S.* Enteritidis colonization of laying hens.

Table 3. Summary of major studies carried out to evaluate the efficacy of *Salmonella* vaccines in protection against *S*. Enteritidis challenge (for details please see text)

Vaccine (type)	Route of delivery	Frequency of vaccination	Bacterial challenge	Results of vaccinated group
S. Enteritidis Δ*aroA* (live)	Oral 10^5 or 10^9 cfu	1 day of age	10^8 cfu *S*. Enteritidis (oral) at 8 wks	Levels of challenge strain were 1-2 log units lower in the liver and spleen and much lower in the ceca at 1 and 4 days postchallenge.
S. Typhimurium Δ*cya-crp* (live)	Oral 10^8 cfu	1 and 14 days of age	10^6 cfu *S*. Enteritidis (oral) at 4 wks	Challenge strain was not detectable in the spleen and levels in the ceca were similar to the control at 2 weeks postchallenge.
Ts *S*. Enteritidis mutant (live)	Oral 10^{10} cfu and/or intraperitoneal 10^8 cfu	1 and 14 days of age	10^9 cfu *S*. Enteritidis (oral) at 4 wks	Challenge strain was 2-5 log units lower in the spleen and 5 log units lower in the ceca upto 21 days postchallenge in orally vaccinated group.
S. Gallinarum 9R Nobilis® (live)	Subcutaneous	6 weeks and 14-16 weeks	Field conditions	2.5 % of the vaccinated flocks were positive for *Salmonella* relative to the control group (11.5%) as determined by fecal swabs.
TAD *Salmonella* vac® E (live)	Oral 10^8 cfu	1 day of age, 6 weeks and 16 weeks	10^7 cfu *S*. Enteritidis (i.v.) at 24 weeks	12/28 livers and 6/28 oviducts were positive for *Salmonella* relative to the control, 23/30 and 15/29, respectively, at 3 weeks postchallenge.
Salenvac® (killed)	Subcutaneous	Day 1 and 4 weeks	10^7 cfu *S*. Enteritidis (i.v.) at 17, 23, 30 and 59 wks	22.6% of cloacal swabs and 12.5% internal organs were positive for *Salmonella* over 21 days postchallenge compared to the control (48.0% and 28.0%, respectively).
Vaccine (type)	Route of delivery	Frequency of vaccination	Bacterial challenge	Results of vaccinated group
Layermune SE® (killed)	Subcutaneous	5 and 9 weeks	10^8 cfu *S*. Enteritidis (oral)	Levels of challenge strain were 1-2 log units lower in liver, spleen and ceca of vaccinated layers but not broilers.
Poulvac SE® (killed)	Subcutaneous	12 and 20 weeks	10^5 cfu *S*. Enteritidis (oral) for day old progeny 10^9 cfu *S*. Enteritidis for two week old progeny	7/25 birds were positive for *Salmonella* relative to the control (25/25) in day old progeny, while 2/25 birds were positive relative to the control (9/25).
S. Enteritidis outer membrane protein extract	Oral or subcutaneous	8 and 11 weeks	10^7 cfu *S*. Enteritidis (oral) at 13 weeks	Very few chickens shed the challenge strain compared to the control (100%) up to 4 weeks postchallenge.
75.6 and 82.3 kDa *S*. Enteritidis outer membrane proteins	Subcutaneous	9 and 11 weeks	10^8 cfu *S*. Enteritidis (oral) at 12 weeks	Levels of the challenge strain were 2-3 log units lower in the ceca relative to the control.

Table 3. (Continued)

Vaccine (type)	Route of delivery	Frequency of vaccination	Bacterial challenge	Results of vaccinated group
S. Enteritidis Type I fimbriae	Subcutaneous	18 and 21 weeks	10^7 cfu *S.* Enteritidis (i.v.) at 24 weeks	Levels of the challenge strain were similar in the liver, spleen and ceca relative to the control upto 3 weeks postchallenge.
S. Enteritidis FliC protein	Subcutaneous	3 and 5 weeks	10^7 cfu *S.* Enteritidis (oral) at 7 weeks	Levels of the challenge strain were 3 log units lower in the cecal contents at 3 weeks postchallenge relative to the control.

Chickens vaccinated with the killed strain had significantly lower levels of *S.* Enteritidis relative to the other groups, suggesting that killed *Salmonella* strains may be more effective in controlling the prevalence of *Salmonella* in poultry [188]. Moreover, killed *Salmonella* strains and subunit vaccines have an advantage over live attenuated strains since the latter are composed of a living organism. With the continued prevalence of *S.* Enteritidis human infections, there is still a need for improved and well defined vaccines to control the spread of this bacterium along with other intervention strategies [170].

5.5. Consumer Education

Since the aim of *Salmonella* control programs is to ultimately reduce the number of human *Salmonella* infections, it is crucial that consumers are also informed about strategies that can be applied in their daily lives to lower their chances of becoming infected with this pathogen. Consumption of undercooked poultry meat and eggs is a significant pathway for human exposure not only to *Salmonella* species, but also to other pathogens such as *Campylobacter* species. Therefore, informing consumers (through different educational tools) to thoroughly cook all foods that contain poultry meat or eggs is an important step in risk reduction. As well, labeling poultry meat and eggs or products containing the aforementioned will remind consumers to be cautious and follow procedures.

Similarly, it has been determined that cross-contamination of food products with *Salmonella* species while handling poultry meat or eggs is also a major source of human exposure to this pathogen. Hence, consumers must be advised to use either separate cutting boards and utensils in the kitchen when handling poultry products or to properly wash and clean them before handling other food products [189].

5.6. Testing

In order to ensure that the above mentioned intervention strategies are successful in reducing the levels of *S.* Enteritidis, it is crucial that regular microbiological testing is carried out. This should include testing of chicken fecal shedding, internal organs, eggs and poultry facilities for the presence of *S.* Enteritidis [160]. As well, it is important that other post-slaughter intervention strategies are put in place that include microbiological testing for *Salmonella* species at slaughter houses and meat processing plants. This would be greatly enhanced by the adoption of Hazard Analysis Critical Control Point (HACCP) programs that have been developed by several government agencies like the Canadian Food Inspection Agency and the Food Safety and Inspection Service in the U.S. Department of Agriculture. These programs are specially designed to monitor, control and prevent food safety risks.

CONCLUSION

Human infections with *S.* Enteritidis are still a concern in the U.K., North America, Europe and other parts of the world. This is largely the result of the consumption of contaminated poultry meat and eggs. Therefore, reducing the levels of *S.* Enteritidis in chickens is a critical component of any given *Salmonella* control program. In order to achieve this, it is important that we thoroughly understand *S.* Enteritidis pathogenesis. The SPI-1 T3SS has been extensively studied in the mouse and bovine models of infection, where it has been shown to be a significant virulence factor. Our results demonstrate that the *S.* Enteritidis SPI-1 T3SS is an important virulence factor in vitro, ex vivo and in chickens. In addition, vaccination of chickens with proteins encoded by this system suggests that these components, along with other vaccine candidates, may form an efficacious subunit vaccine against *S.* Enteritidis. However, further research still needs to be performed to study *S.* Enteritidis pathogenesis in chickens in order to design a vaccine that is safe, effective and well defined.

REFERENCES

[1] R.K. Gast, Salmonella infections, p. 567. In Y. M. Saif, H. J. Barnes, J. R. Glisson, A. M. Fadly, and L. R. McDougald (ed.), Diseases of Poultry, 11th ed., Iowa State Press, (2003).

[2] J.G. Holt, N.R. Krieg, P.H.A. Sneath, J.T. Staley, S.T. Williams, Part 5, p. 186. In J. G. Holt, N. R. Krieg, P. H. A. Sneath, J. T. Staley, and S. T. Williams (ed.), Bergey's Manual of Determinative Bacteriology, 9th ed., Williams and Wilkins, USA, (1994).

[3] B.J. Tindall, P.A. Grimont, G.M. Garrity, J.P. Euzeby, Nomenclature and taxonomy of the genus Salmonella, *Int J Syst Evol Microbiol* 55 (2005) 521-524.

[4] R.A. Kingsley, A.D. Humphries, E.H. Weening, M.R. de Zoete, S. Winter, A. Papaconstantinopoulou, G. Dougan, A.J. Baumler, Molecular and phenotypic analysis of the CS54 island of Salmonella enterica Serotype Typhimurium: identification of intestinal colonization and persistence determinants, Infect. *Immun.* 71 (2003) 629-640.

[5] S. Porwollik, F. Boyd, C. Choy, P. Cheng, L. Florea, E. Proctor, M. McClelland, Characterization of Salmonella enterica subspecies I genovars by use of microarrays, *J. Bacteriol.* 186 (2004) 5883-5898.

[6] J.A. Ibarra, O. Steele-Mortimer, Salmonella- the ultimate insider. Salmonella virulence factors that modulate intracellular survival, Cell Microbiol (2009).

[7] P.A. Grimont, F. Grimont, P. Bouvet, Taxonomy of the genus Salmonella, p. 5. In C. Wray and A. Wray (ed.), Salmonella in domestic animals, CABI Publishing., (2000).

[8] N.R. Thomson, D.J. Clayton, D. Windhorst, G. Vernikos, S. Davidson, C. Churcher, M.A. Quail, M. Stevens, M.A. Jones, M. Watson, A. Barron, A. Layton, D. Pickard,

R.A. Kingsley, A. Bignell, L. Clark, B. Harris, D. Ormond, Z. Abdellah, K. Brooks, I. Cherevach, T. Chillingworth, J. Woodward, H. Norberczak, A. Lord, C. Arrowsmith, K. Jagels, S. Moule, K. Mungall, M. Sanders, S. Whitehead, J.A. Chabalgoity, D. Maskell, T. Humphrey, M. Roberts, P.A. Barrow, G. Dougan, J. Parkhill, Comparative genome analysis of Salmonella Enteritidis PT4 and Salmonella Gallinarum 287/91 provides insights into evolutionary and host adaptation pathways, *Genome Res* 18 (2008) 1624-1637.

[9] WHO, World Health Organization Global Salm-Surv Country Databank (CDB), 2009.

[10] T.A. Cogan, T.J. Humphrey, The rise and fall of Salmonella Enteritidis in the UK, *J Appl Microbiol 94 Suppl* (2003) 114S-119S.

[11] R.L. Santos, Animal models of Salmonella infections: enteritis versus typhoid fever, *Microbes Infect.* 3 (2001) 1335-1344.

[12] S.L. Foley, A.M. Lynne, Food animal-associated Salmonella challenges: pathogenicity and antimicrobial resistance, *J Anim Sci* 86 (2008) E173-187.

[13] L.J. Martin, M. Fyfe, K. Dore, J.A. Buxton, F. Pollari, B. Henry, D. Middleton, R. Ahmed, F. Jamieson, B. Ciebin, S.A. McEwen, J.B. Wilson, Increased burden of illness associated with antimicrobial-resistant Salmonella enterica serotype typhimurium infections, *J Infect Dis* 189 (2004) 377-384.

[14] A.C. Voetsch, T.J. Van Gilder, F.J. Angulo, M.M. Farley, S. Shallow, R. Marcus, P.R. Cieslak, V.C. Deneen, R.V. Tauxe, FoodNet estimate of the burden of illness caused by nontyphoidal Salmonella infections in the United States, *Clin Infect Dis 38 Suppl 3* (2004) S127-134.

[15] R.M. Macnab, Type III flagellar protein export and flagellar assembly, *Biochim Biophys Acta.* 1694 (2004) 207-217.

[16] L. Journet, K.T. Hughes, G.R. Cornelis, Type III secretion: a secretory pathway serving both motility and virulence, *Mol. Membr. Biol.* 22 (2005) 41-50.

[17] G.R. Cornelis, The type III secretion injectisome, Nat. *Rev. Microbiol.* 4 (2006) 811-825.

[18] C.K. Schmitt, J.S. Ikeda, S.C. Darnell, P.R. Watson, J. Bispham, T.S. Wallis, D.L. Weinstein, E.S. Metcalf, A.D. O'Brien, Absence of all components of the flagellar export and synthesis machinery differentially alters virulence of Salmonella enterica serovar Typhimurium in models of typhoid fever, survival in macrophages, tissue culture invasiveness, and calf enterocolitis, *Infect Immun* 69 (2001) 5619-5625.

[19] A.T. Gewirtz, T.A. Navas, S. Lyons, P.J. Godowski, J.L. Madara, Cutting edge: bacterial flagellin activates basolaterally expressed TLR5 to induce epithelial proinflammatory gene expression, *J Immunol* 167 (2001) 1882-1885.

[20] K.H. Darwin, V.L. Miller, Molecular basis of the interaction of Salmonella with the intestinal mucosa, *Clin Microbiol Rev 12* (1999) 405-428.

[21] C.J. Thorns, M.J. Woodward, Fimbriae of Salmonella, p. 35. In C. Wray and A. Wray (ed.), Salmonella in domestic animals, CABI Publishing., (2000).

[22] I. Rychlik, D. Gregorova, H. Hradecka, Distribution and function of plasmids in Salmonella enterica, *Vet Microbiol* 112 (2006) 1-10.

[23] C. Winstanley, C.A. Hart, Type III secretion systems and pathogenicity islands, *J Med Microbiol* 50 (2001) 116-126.

[24] J.E. Galan, Salmonella interactions with host cells: type III secretion at work, Annu. *Rev. Cell Dev. Biol.* 17 (2001) 53-86.

[25] I. Hansen-Wester, M. Hensel, Salmonella pathogenicity islands encoding type III secretion systems, *Microbes Infect.* 3 (2001) 549-559.

[26] S.L. Marcus, J.H. Brumell, C.G. Pfeifer, B.B. Finlay, Salmonella pathogenicity islands: big virulence in small packages, *Microbes Infect.* 2 (2000) 145-156.

[27] M. Hensel, Evolution of pathogenicity islands of Salmonella enterica, *Int J Med Microbiol* 294 (2004) 95-102.

[28] E.J. McGhie, L.C. Brawn, P.J. Hume, D. Humphreys, V. Koronakis, Salmonella takes control: effector-driven manipulation of the host, *Curr Opin Microbi*ol 12 (2009) 117-124.

[29] S.Y. He, K. Nomura, T.S. Whittam, Type III protein secretion mechanism in mammalian and plant pathogens, *Biochim Biophys Acta.* 1694 (2004) 181-206.

[30] J. Garmendia, G. Frankel, V.F. Crepin, Enteropathogenic and enterohemorrhagic Escherichia coli infections: translocation, translocation, translocation, Infect. *Immun.* 73 (2005) 2573-2585.

[31] T.C. Marlovits, T. Kubori, A. Sukhan, D.R. Thomas, J.E. Galan, V.M. Unger, Structural insights into the assembly of the type III secretion needle complex, *Science* 306 (2004) 1040-1042.

[32] J.E. Galan, A. Collmer, Type III secretion machines: bacterial devices for protein delivery into host cells, *Science* 284 (1999) 1322-1328.

[33] B. Blaylock, O. Schneewind, Microbiology: loading the type III cannon, *Nature* 437 (2005) 821.

[34] J.R. Ellermeier, J.M. Slauch, Adaptation to the host environment: regulation of the SPI1 type III secretion system in Salmonella enterica serovar Typhimurium, Curr. *Opin. Microbiol.* 10 (2007) 24-29.

[35] A. Sukhan, T. Kubori, J. Wilson, J.E. Galan, Genetic analysis of assembly of the Salmonella enterica serovar Typhimurium type III secretion-associated needle complex, *J Bacteriol* 183 (2001) 1159-1167.

[36] T. Kubori, A. Sukhan, S.I. Aizawa, J.E. Galan, Molecular characterization and assembly of the needle complex of the Salmonella typhimurium type III protein secretion system, Proc. *Natl. Acad. Sci.* U S A 97 (2000) 10225-10230.

[37] M. Lara-Tejero, J.E. Galan, Salmonella enterica serovar typhimurium pathogenicity island 1-encoded type III secretion system translocases mediate intimate attachment to nonphagocytic cells, *Infect Immun* 77 (2009) 2635-2642.

[38] J. Pettersson, R. Nordfelth, E. Dubinina, T. Bergman, M. Gustafsson, K.E. Magnusson, H. Wolf-Watz, Modulation of virulence factor expression by pathogen target cell contact, *Science* 273 (1996) 1231-1233.

[39] F.G. van der Goot, G. Tran van Nhieu, A. Allaoui, P. Sansonetti, F. Lafont, Rafts can trigger contact-mediated secretion of bacterial effectors via a lipid-based mechanism, *J Biol Chem* 279 (2004) 47792-47798.

[40] R. Kenjale, J. Wilson, S.F. Zenk, S. Saurya, W.L. Picking, W.D. Picking, A. Blocker, The needle component of the type III secreton of Shigella regulates the activity of the secretion apparatus, *J Biol Chem* 280 (2005) 42929-42937.

[41] T.D. Pollard, G.G. Borisy, Cellular motility driven by assembly and disassembly of actin filaments, *Cell* 112 (2003) 453-465.

[42] Z. Ye, E.O. Petrof, D. Boone, E.C. Claud, J. Sun, Salmonella effector AvrA regulation of colonic epithelial cell inflammation by deubiquitination, *Am J Pathol* 171 (2007) 882-892.

[43] R.M. Jones, H. Wu, C. Wentworth, L. Luo, L. Collier-Hyams, A.S. Neish, Salmonella AvrA Coordinates Suppression of Host Immune and Apoptotic Defenses via JNK Pathway Blockade, *Cell Host Microbe* 3 (2008) 233-244.

[44] A.P. Liao, E.O. Petrof, S. Kuppireddi, Y. Zhao, Y. Xia, E.C. Claud, J. Sun, Salmonella type III effector AvrA stabilizes cell tight junctions to inhibit inflammation in intestinal epithelial cells, PLoS One 3 (2008) e2369.

[45] D. Zhou, M.S. Mooseker, J.E. Galan, An invasion-associated Salmonella protein modulates the actin-bundling activity of plastin, *Proc Natl Acad Sci* U S A 96 (1999) 10176-10181.

[46] E.J. McGhie, R.D. Hayward, V. Koronakis, Control of actin turnover by a salmonella invasion protein, *Mol Cell* 13 (2004) 497-510.

[47] A.N. Layton, E.E. Galyov, Salmonella-induced enteritis: molecular pathogenesis and therapeutic implications, *Expert Rev. Mol. Med.* 9 (2007) 1-17.

[48] D.M. Wall, W.J. Nadeau, M.A. Pazos, H.N. Shi, E.E. Galyov, B.A. McCormick, Identification of the Salmonella enterica serotype typhimurium SipA domain responsible for inducing neutrophil recruitment across the intestinal epithelium, *Cell Microbiol* 9 (2007) 2299-2313.

[49] L.C. Brawn, R.D. Hayward, V. Koronakis, Salmonella SPI1 effector SipA persists after entry and cooperates with a SPI2 effector to regulate phagosome maturation and intracellular replication, *Cell Host Microbe* 1 (2007) 63-75.

[50] D. Hersh, Monack, D.M., Smith, M.R., Ghori, N., Falkow, S., and Zychlinsky, A., The Salmonella invasin SipB induces macrophage apoptosis by binding to caspase-1, *PNAS* 96 (1999) 2396-2401.

[51] L.D. Hernandez, M. Pypaert, R.A. Flavell, J.E. Galan, A Salmonella protein causes macrophage cell death by inducing autophagy, *J Cell Biol* 163 (2003) 1123-1131.

[52] S.L. Fink, B.T. Cookson, Pyroptosis and host cell death responses during Salmonella infection, *Cell Microbiol* 9 (2007) 2562-2570.

[53] R.D. Hayward, R.J. Cain, E.J. McGhie, N. Phillips, M.J. Garner, V. Koronakis, Cholesterol binding by the bacterial type III translocon is essential for virulence effector delivery into mammalian cells, *Mol Microbiol* 56 (2005) 590-603.

[54] R.D. Hayward, V. Koronakis, Direct nucleation and bundling of actin by the SipC protein of invasive Salmonella, *EMBO J* 18 (1999) 4926-4934.

[55] Y. Zhang, W. Higashide, S. Dai, D.M. Sherman, D. Zhou, Recognition and ubiquitination of Salmonella type III effector SopA by a ubiquitin E3 ligase, HsRMA1, *J Biol Chem* 280 (2005) 38682-38688.

[56] Y. Zhang, W.M. Higashide, B.A. McCormick, J. Chen, D. Zhou, The inflammation-associated Salmonella SopA is a HECT-like E3 ubiquitin ligase, *Mol Microbiol* 62 (2006) 786-793.

[57] F.A. Norris, Wilson, M.P., Wallis, T.S., Galyov, E.E., and Majerus, P.W., Sop B, a protein required for virulence of Salmonella dublin, is an inositol phosphate phosphatase, *PNAS* 95 (1998) 14057-14059.

[58] D. Zhou, L.M. Chen, L. Hernandez, S.B. Shears, J.E. Galan, A Salmonella inositol polyphosphatase acts in conjunction with other bacterial effectors to promote host cell

actin cytoskeleton rearrangements and bacterial internalization, *Mol Microbiol* 39 (2001) 248-259.

[59] M.A. Bakowski, J.T. Cirulis, N.F. Brown, B.B. Finlay, J.H. Brumell, SopD acts cooperatively with SopB during Salmonella enterica serovar Typhimurium invasion, *Cell Microbiol* 9 (2007) 2839-2855.

[60] S. Hobbie, L.M. Chen, R.J. Davis, J.E. Galan, Involvement of mitogen-activated protein kinase pathways in the nuclear responses and cytokine production induced by Salmonella typhimurium in cultured intestinal epithelial cells, *J Immunol* 159 (1997) 5550-5559.

[61] A. Haraga, M.B. Ohlson, S.I. Miller, Salmonellae interplay with host cells, *Nat. Rev. Microbiol.* 6 (2007) 53-66.

[62] G.V. Mallo, M. Espina, A.C. Smith, M.R. Terebiznik, A. Aleman, B.B. Finlay, L.E. Rameh, S. Grinstein, J.H. Brumell, SopB promotes phosphatidylinositol 3-phosphate formation on Salmonella vacuoles by recruiting Rab5 and Vps34, *J Cell Biol* 182 (2008) 741-752.

[63] A. Friebel, H. Ilchmann, M. Aepfelbacher, K. Ehrbar, W. Machleidt, W.D. Hardt, SopE and SopE2 from Salmonella typhimurium activate different sets of RhoGTPases of the host cell, *J Biol Chem* 276 (2001) 34035-34040.

[64] Y. Fu, J.E. Galan, A salmonella protein antagonizes Rac-1 and Cdc42 to mediate host-cell recovery after bacterial invasion, *Nature* 401 (1999) 293-297.

[65] J.C. Patel, J.E. Galan, Manipulation of the host cytoskeleton by Salmonella - all in the name of entry, *Curr. Opin. Microbiol.* 8 (2005) 10-15.

[66] S. Murli, R.O. Watson, J.E. Galan, Role of tyrosine kinases and the tyrosine phosphatase SptP in the interaction of Salmonella with host cells, *Cell Microbiol* 3 (2001) 795-810.

[67] S.L. Lin, T.X. Le, D.S. Cowen, SptP, a Salmonella typhimurium type III-secreted protein, inhibits the mitogen-activated protein kinase pathway by inhibiting Raf activation, *Cell Microbiol* 5 (2003) 267-275.

[68] J. Bernal-Bayard, F. Ramos-Morales, Salmonella type III secretion effector SlrP is an E3 ubiquitin ligase for mammalian thioredoxin, *J Biol Chem* 284 (2009) 27587-27595.

[69] A. Haraga, S.I. Miller, A Salmonella type III secretion effector interacts with the mammalian serine/threonine protein kinase PKN1, *Cell Microbiol* 8 (2006) 837-846.

[70] J.R. Rohde, A. Breitkreutz, A. Chenal, P.J. Sansonetti, C. Parsot, Type III secretion effectors of the IpaH family are E3 ubiquitin ligases, *Cell Host Microbe* 1 (2007) 77-83.

[71] K. Geddes, M. Worley, G. Niemann, F. Heffron, Identification of new secreted effectors in Salmonella enterica serovar Typhimurium, *Infect Immun* 73 (2005) 6260-6271.

[72] D. Zhou, Mooseker, M.S., and Galan, J.E., Role of the S. typhimurium actin-binding protein SipA in bacterial internalization, *Science* 283 (1999) 2092-2095.

[73] S. Etienne-Manneville, A. Hall, Rho GTPases in cell biology, *Nature* 420 (2002) 629-635.

[74] M.C. Schlumberger, W.D. Hardt, Salmonella type III secretion effectors: pulling the host cell's strings., *Curr. Opin. Microbiol.* 9 (2005) 1-9.

[75] J. Diao, Y. Zhang, J.M. Huibregtse, D. Zhou, J. Chen, Crystal structure of SopA, a Salmonella effector protein mimicking a eukaryotic ubiquitin ligase, *Nat Struct Mol Biol* 15 (2008) 65-70.

[76] C. Kuijl, N.D. Savage, M. Marsman, A.W. Tuin, L. Janssen, D.A. Egan, M. Ketema, R. van den Nieuwendijk, S.J. van den Eeden, A. Geluk, A. Poot, G. van der Marel, R.L. Beijersbergen, H. Overkleeft, T.H. Ottenhoff, J. Neefjes, Intracellular bacterial growth is controlled by a kinase network around PKB/AKT1, *Nature* 450 (2007) 725-730.

[77] C.D. Ellermeier, J.M. Slauch, RtsA and RtsB coordinately regulate expression of the invasion and flagellar genes in Salmonella enterica serovar Typhimurium, *J Bacteriol* 185 (2003) 5096-5108.

[78] L.A. Pratt, W. Hsing, K.E. Gibson, T.J. Silhavy, From acids to osmZ: multiple factors influence synthesis of the OmpF and OmpC porins in Escherichia coli, *Mol Microbiol* 20 (1996) 911-917.

[79] C.D. Ellermeier, J.R. Ellermeier, J.M. Slauch, HilD, HilC and RtsA constitute a feed forward loop that controls expression of the SPI1 type three secretion system regulator hilA in Salmonella enterica serovar Typhimurium, *Mol Microbiol* 57 (2005) 691-705.

[80] B.M. Ahmer, J. van Reeuwijk, P.R. Watson, T.S. Wallis, F. Heffron, Salmonella SirA is a global regulator of genes mediating enteropathogenesis, *Mol Microbiol* 31 (1999) 971-982.

[81] J.R. Ellermeier, J.M. Slauch, Fur regulates expression of the Salmonella pathogenicity island 1 type III secretion system through HilD, *J Bacteriol* 190 (2008) 476-486.

[82] D.A. Pegues, M.J. Hantman, I. Behlau, S.I. Miller, PhoP/PhoQ transcriptional repression of Salmonella typhimurium invasion genes: evidence for a role in protein secretion, *Mol Microbiol* 17 (1995) 169-181.

[83] C. Altier, Genetic and environmental control of salmonella invasion, *J Microbiol* 43 Spec No (2005) 85-92.

[84] V. Bajaj, R.L. Lucas, C. Hwang, C.A. Lee, Co-ordinate regulation of Salmonella typhimurium invasion genes by environmental and regulatory factors is mediated by control of hilA expression, *Mol Microbiol* 22 (1996) 703-714.

[85] M.N. Giacomodonato, S. Uzzau, D. Bacciu, R. Caccuri, S.H. Sarnacki, S. Rubino, M.C. Cerquetti, SipA, SopA, SopB, SopD and SopE2 effector proteins of Salmonella enterica serovar Typhimurium are synthesized at late stages of infection in mice, *Microbiology* 153 (2007) 1221-1228.

[86] S.B. Porter, R. Curtiss III, Effect of inv mutations on Salmonella virulence and colonization in 1-day-old White Leghorn chicks, *Avian Dis*. 41 (1997) 45-57.

[87] L. Bohez, R. Ducatelle, F. Pasmans, N. Botteldoorn, F. Haesebrouck, F. Van Immerseel, Salmonella enterica serovar Enteritidis colonization of the chicken caecum requires the HilA regulatory protein, *Vet. Microbiol*. 116 (2006) 202-210.

[88] M.A. Jones, S.D. Hulme, P.A. Barrow, P. Wigley, The Salmonella pathogenicity island 1 and Salmonella pathogenicity island 2 type III secretion systems play a major role in pathogenesis of systemic disease and gastrointestinal tract colonization of *Salmonella enterica* serovar Typhimurium in the chicken, *Avian Pathol*. 36 (2007) 199-203.

[89] C.T. Parker, J. Guard-Petter, Contribution of flagella and invasion proteins to pathogenesis of Salmonella enterica serovar enteritidis in chicks, FEMS Microbiol. *Lett*. 204 (2001) 287-291.

[90] T.S. Desin, P.K. Lam, B. Koch, C. Mickael, E. Berberov, A.L. Wisner, H.G. Townsend, A.A. Potter, W. Köster, Salmonella enterica serovar enteritidis pathogenicity island 1 is not essential for but facilitates rapid systemic spread in chickens, *Infect Immun* 77 (2009) 2866-2875.

[91] V. Kuhle, M. Hensel, Cellular microbiology of intracellular Salmonella enterica: functions of the type III secretion system encoded by Salmonella pathogenicity island 2, *Cell Mol Life Sci* 61 (2004) 2812-2826.

[92] M. Hensel, Salmonella pathogenicity island 2, *Mol. Microbiol.* 36 (2000) 1015-1023.

[93] M. Hensel, E. Kuhle, Cellular microbiology of intracellular Salmonella enterica: functions of the type III secretion system encoded by Salmonella pathogenicity island 2, *Cell. Mol. Life Sci.* 61 (2004) 2812-2826.

[94] N.F. Brown, B.A. Vallance, B.K. Coombes, Y. Valdez, B.A. Coburn, B.B. Finlay, Salmonella pathogenicity island 2 is expressed prior to penetrating the intestine, *PLoS Pathog.* 1 (2005) 1-7.

[95] K. Uchiya, M.A. Barbieri, K. Funato, A.H. Shah, P.D. Stahl, E.A. Groisman, A Salmonella virulence protein that inhibits cellular trafficking, *Embo J* 18 (1999) 3924-3933.

[96] O. Steele-Mortimer, The Salmonella-containing vacuole: moving with the times, *Curr Opin Microbiol* 11 (2008) 38-45.

[97] J. Ruiz-Albert, X.J. Yu, C.R. Beuzon, A.N. Blakey, E.E. Galyov, D.W. Holden, Complementary activities of SseJ and SifA regulate dynamics of the Salmonella typhimurium vacuolar membrane, *Mol Microbiol* 44 (2002) 645-661.

[98] E.A. Miao, M. Brittnacher, A. Haraga, R.L. Jeng, M.D. Welch, S.I. Miller, Salmonella effectors translocated across the vacuolar membrane interact with the actin cytoskeleton, *Mol Microbiol* 48 (2003) 401-415.

[99] J. Poh, C. Odendall, A. Spanos, C. Boyle, M. Liu, P. Freemont, D.W. Holden, SteC is a Salmonella kinase required for SPI-2-dependent F-actin remodelling, *Cell Microbiol* 10 (2008) 20-30.

[100] V. Kuhle, G.L. Abrahams, M. Hensel, Intracellular Salmonella enterica redirect exocytic transport processes in a Salmonella pathogenicity island 2-dependent manner, *Traffic* 7 (2006) 716-730.

[101] L.A. Knodler, O. Steele-Mortimer, The Salmonella effector PipB2 affects late endosome/lysosome distribution to mediate Sif extension, *Mol Biol Cell* 16 (2005) 4108-4123.

[102] B.K. Coombes, M.E. Wickham, N.F. Brown, S. Lemire, L. Bossi, W.W. Hsiao, F.S. Brinkman, B.B. Finlay, Genetic and molecular analysis of GogB, a phage-encoded type III-secreted substrate in Salmonella enterica serovar typhimurium with autonomous expression from its associated phage, *J Mol Biol* 348 (2005) 817-830.

[103] L.A. Knodler, J. Celli, W.D. Hardt, B.A. Vallance, C. Yip, B.B. Finlay, Salmonella effectors within a single pathogenicity island are differentially expressed and translocated by separate type III secretion systems, *Mol Microbiol* 43 (2002) 1089-1103.

[104] J.A. Freeman, M.E. Ohl, S.I. Miller, The Salmonella enterica serovar typhimurium translocated effectors SseJ and SifB are targeted to the Salmonella-containing vacuole, *Infect Immun* 71 (2003) 418-427.

[105] X. Jiang, O.W. Rossanese, N.F. Brown, S. Kujat-Choy, J.E. Galan, B.B. Finlay, J.H. Brumell, The related effector proteins SopD and SopD2 from Salmonella enterica serovar Typhimurium contribute to virulence during systemic infection of mice, *Mol Microbiol* 54 (2004) 1186-1198.

[106] J.H. Brumell, S. Kujat-Choy, N.F. Brown, B.A. Vallance, L.A. Knodler, B.B. Finlay, SopD2 is a novel type III secreted effector of Salmonella typhimurium that targets late endocytic compartments upon delivery into host cells, *Traffic* 4 (2003) 36-48.

[107] X.J. Yu, M. Liu, D.W. Holden, SsaM and SpiC interact and regulate secretion of Salmonella pathogenicity island 2 type III secretion system effectors and translocators, *Mol Microbiol* 54 (2004) 604-619.

[108] J. Deiwick, S.P. Salcedo, E. Boucrot, S.M. Gilliland, T. Henry, N. Petermann, S.R. Waterman, J.P. Gorvel, D.W. Holden, S. Meresse, The translocated Salmonella effector proteins SseF and SseG interact and are required to establish an intracellular replication niche, *Infect Immun* 74 (2006) 6965-6972.

[109] S.L. Kujat Choy, E.C. Boyle, O. Gal-Mor, D.L. Goode, Y. Valdez, B.A. Vallance, B.B. Finlay, SseK1 and SseK2 are novel translocated proteins of Salmonella enterica serovar typhimurium, *Infect Immun* 72 (2004) 5115-5125.

[110] G. Le Negrate, B. Faustin, K. Welsh, M. Loeffler, M. Krajewska, P. Hasegawa, S. Mukherjee, K. Orth, S. Krajewski, A. Godzik, D.G. Guiney, J.C. Reed, Salmonella secreted factor L deubiquitinase of Salmonella typhimurium inhibits NF-kappaB, suppresses IkappaBalpha ubiquitination and modulates innate immune responses, *J Immunol* 180 (2008) 5045-5056.

[111] A. Rytkonen, J. Poh, J. Garmendia, C. Boyle, A. Thompson, M. Liu, P. Freemont, J.C. Hinton, D.W. Holden, SseL, a Salmonella deubiquitinase required for macrophage killing and virulence, *Proc Natl Acad Sci* U S A 104 (2007) 3502-3507.

[112] P. Mazurkiewicz, J. Thomas, J.A. Thompson, M. Liu, L. Arbibe, P. Sansonetti, D.W. Holden, SpvC is a Salmonella effector with phosphothreonine lyase activity on host mitogen-activated protein kinases, *Mol Microbiol* 67 (2008) 1371-1383.

[113] H. Li, H. Xu, Y. Zhou, J. Zhang, C. Long, S. Li, S. Chen, J.M. Zhou, F. Shao, The phosphothreonine lyase activity of a bacterial type III effector family, *Science* 315 (2007) 1000-1003.

[114] J. Deiwick, T. Nikolaus, S. Erdogan, M. Hensel, Environmental regulation of Salmonella pathogenicity island 2 gene expression, *Mol Microbiol* 31 (1999) 1759-1773.

[115] D. Walthers, R.K. Carroll, W.W. Navarre, S.J. Libby, F.C. Fang, L.J. Kenney, The response regulator SsrB activates expression of diverse Salmonella pathogenicity island 2 promoters and counters silencing by the nucleoid-associated protein H-NS, *Mol Microbiol* 65 (2007) 477-493.

[116] E. Fass, E.A. Groisman, Control of Salmonella pathogenicity island-2 gene expression, *Curr Opin Microbiol* 12 (2009) 199-204.

[117] X. Feng, D. Walthers, R. Oropeza, L.J. Kenney, The response regulator SsrB activates transcription and binds to a region overlapping OmpR binding sites at Salmonella pathogenicity island 2, *Mol Microbiol* 54 (2004) 823-835.

[118] A.K. Lee, C.S. Detweiler, S. Falkow, OmpR regulates the two-component system SsrA-ssrB in Salmonella pathogenicity island 2, *J Bacteriol* 182 (2000) 771-781.

[119] E.A. Groisman, The pleiotropic two-component regulatory system PhoP-PhoQ, *J Bacteriol* 183 (2001) 1835-1842.

[120] J.J. Bijlsma, E.A. Groisman, The PhoP/PhoQ system controls the intramacrophage type three secretion system of Salmonella enterica, *Mol Microbiol* 57 (2005) 85-96.

[121] R.T. Dame, The role of nucleoid-associated proteins in the organization and compaction of bacterial chromatin, *Mol Microbiol* 56 (2005) 858-870.

[122] M.W. Mangan, S. Lucchini, V. Danino, T.O. Croinin, J.C. Hinton, C.J. Dorman, The integration host factor (IHF) integrates stationary-phase and virulence gene expression in Salmonella enterica serovar Typhimurium, *Mol Microbiol* 59 (2006) 1831-1847.

[123] A. Kelly, M.D. Goldberg, R.K. Carroll, V. Danino, J.C. Hinton, C.J. Dorman, A global role for Fis in the transcriptional control of metabolism and type III secretion in Salmonella enterica serovar Typhimurium, *Microbiology* 150 (2004) 2037-2053.

[124] S. Lim, B. Kim, H.S. Choi, Y. Lee, S. Ryu, Fis is required for proper regulation of ssaG expression in Salmonella enterica serovar Typhimurium, *Microb Pathog* 41 (2006) 33-42.

[125] J.E. Shea, M. Hensel, C. Gleeson, D.W. Holden, Identification of a virulence locus encoding a second type III secretion system in Salmonella typhimurium, *Proc Natl Acad Sci* U S A 93 (1996) 2593-2597.

[126] J.E. Shea, C.R. Beuzon, C. Gleeson, R. Mundy, D.W. Holden, Influence of the Salmonella typhimurium pathogenicity island 2 type III secretion system on bacterial growth in the mouse, *Infect Immun* 67 (1999) 213-219.

[127] B.K. Coombes, B.A. Coburn, A.A. Potter, S. Gomis, K. Mirakhur, Y. Li, B.B. Finlay, Analysis of the contribution of Salmonella pathogenicity islands 1 and 2 to enteric disease progression using a novel bovine ileal loop model and a murine model of infectious enterocolitis, *Infect. Immun.* 73 (2005) 7161-7169.

[128] B. Coburn, Y. Li, D. Owen, B.A. Vallance, B.B. Finlay, Salmonella enterica serovar Typhimurium pathogenicity island 2 is necessary for complete virulence in a mouse model of infectious enterocolitis, *Infect. Immun.* 73 (2005) 3219-3227.

[129] L. Bohez, I. Gantois, R. Ducatelle, F. Pasmans, J. Dewulf, F. Haesebrouck, F. Van Immerseel, The Salmonella Pathogenicity Island 2 regulator ssrA promotes reproductive tract but not intestinal colonization in chickens, *Vet Microbiol* 126 (2008) 216-224.

[130] Y. Dieye, K. Ameiss, M. Mellata, R. Curtiss III, The Salmonella Pathogenicity Island (SPI) 1 contributes more than SPI2 to the colonization of the chicken by *Salmonella enterica* serovar Typhimurium, *BMC Microbiol.* 9 (2009).

[131] C. Poppe, Salmonella in domestic animals, in: C. Wray, A. Wray (Eds.), Salmonella infections in the domestic fowl, *Oxford University Press*, New York, 2000, pp. 107-132.

[132] J.C. McAllister, C.D. Steelman, J.K. Skeeles, Reservoir competence of the lesser mealworm (Coleoptera: Tenebrionidae) for Salmonella typhimurium (Eubacteriales: Enterobacteriaceae), *J Med Entomol* 31 (1994) 369-372.

[133] A.R. Olsen, T.S. Hammack, Isolation of Salmonella spp. from the housefly, Musca domestica L., and the dump fly, Hydrotaea aenescens (Wiedemann) (Diptera: Muscidae), at caged-layer houses, *J Food Prot* 63 (2000) 958-960.

[134] W.C. Hazeleger, N.M. Bolder, R.R. Beumer, W.F. Jacobs-Reitsma, Darkling beetles (Alphitobius diaperinus) and their larvae as potential vectors for the transfer of Campylobacter jejuni and Salmonella enterica serovar paratyphi B variant Java between successive broiler flocks, *Appl Environ Microbiol* 74 (2008) 6887-6891.

[135] Y.M. Tatfeng, M.U. Usuanlele, A. Orukpe, A.K. Digban, M. Okodua, F. Oviasogie, A.A. Turay, Mechanical transmission of pathogenic organisms: the role of cockroaches, *J Vector Borne Dis* 42 (2005) 129-134.
[136] G.A. Grassl, B.B. Finlay, Pathogenesis of enteric Salmonella infections, *Curr. Opin. Gastroenterol.* 24 (2007) 22-26.
[137] H.R. Juul-Madsen, B. Viertlboeck, A.L. Smith, T.W.F. Gobel, Avian innate immune response, p. 129-158. In F. Davison, B. Kaspers and K. A. Schat (ed.), Avian Immunology, Academic Press, UK., (2008).
[138] F. Van Immerseel, J. De Buck, I. De Smet, J. Mast, F. Haesebrouck, R. Ducatelle, The effect of vaccination with a Salmonella Enteritidis aroA mutant on early cellular responses in caecal lamina propria of newly hatched chickens, *Vaccine* 20 (2002) 3034-3041.
[139] F. Van Immerseel, J. De Buck, I. De Smet, J. Mast, F. Haesebrouck, R. Ducatelle, Dynamics of immune cell infiltration in the caecal lamina propria of chickens after neonatal infection with a Salmonella Enteritidis strain, *Dev. Comp. Immunol.* 26 (2002) 355-364.
[140] M.H. Kogut, G. Tellez, E.D. McGruder, B.M. Hargis, J.D. Williams, D.E. Corrier, J.R. DeLoach, Heterophils are decisive components in the early responses of chickens to Salmonella enteritidis infections, *Microb. Pathog.* 16 (1994) 141-151.
[141] M.H. Kogut, G. Tellez, B.M. Hargis, D.E. Corrier, J.R. DeLoach, The effect of 5-flourouracil treatment of chicks: a cell depletion model for the study of avian polymorphonuclear leukocytes and natural host defenses, *Poult. Sci.* 72 (1993) 1873-1880.
[142] A. van Dijk, M.H. Tersteeg-Zijderveld, J.L. Tjeerdsma-van Bokhoven, A.J. Jansman, E.J. Veldhuizen, H.P. Haagsman, Chicken heterophils are recruited to the site of Salmonella infection and release antibacterial mature Cathelicidin-2 upon stimulation with LPS, *Mol Immunol* 46 (2009) 1517-1526.
[143] M. Iqbal, V.J. Philbin, G.S. Withanage, P. Wigley, R.K. Beal, M.J. Goodchild, P. Barrow, I. McConnell, D.J. Maskell, J. Young, N. Bumstead, Y. Boyd, A.L. Smith, Identification and functional characterization of chicken toll-like receptor 5 reveals a fundamental role in the biology of infection with Salmonella enterica serovar typhimurium, *Infect Immun* 73 (2005) 2344-2350.
[144] M.H. Kogut, H. He, P. Kaiser, Lipopolysaccharide binding protein/CD14/ TLR4-dependent recognition of salmonella LPS induces the functional activation of chicken heterophils and up-regulation of pro-inflammatory cytokine and chemokine gene expression in these cells, *Anim Biotechnol* 16 (2005) 165-181.
[145] M.H. Kogut, M. Iqbal, H. He, V. Philbin, P. Kaiser, A. Smith, Expression and function of Toll-like receptors in chicken heterophils, *Dev Comp Immunol* 29 (2005) 791-807.
[146] K.J. Genovese, H. He, V.K. Lowry, D.J. Nisbet, M.H. Kogut, Dynamics of the avian inflammatory response to Salmonella following administration of the Toll-like receptor 5 agonist flagellin, *FEMS Immunol Med Microbiol* 51 (2007) 112-117.
[147] R.K. Beal, C. Powers, P. Wigley, P.A. Barrow, A.L. Smith, Temporal dynamics of the cellular, humoral and cytokine responses in chickens during primary and secondary infection with Salmonella enterica serovar Typhimurium, *Avian Pathol.* 33 (2004) 25-33.

[148] L. Chappell, P. Kaiser, P. Barrow, M.A. Jones, C. Johnston, P. Wigley, The immunobiology of avian systemic salmonellosis, *Vet Immunol Immunopathol* 128 (2009) 53-59.

[149] G.S. Withanage, P. Wigley, P. Kaiser, P. Mastroeni, H. Brooks, C. Powers, R. Beal, P. Barrow, D. Maskell, I. McConnell, Cytokine and chemokine responses associated with clearance of a primary Salmonella enterica serovar Typhimurium infection in the chicken and in protective immunity to rechallenge, *Infect Immun* 73 (2005) 5173-5182.

[150] R.K. Beal, C. Powers, P. Wigley, P.A. Barrow, P. Kaiser, A.L. Smith, A strong antigen specific T cell response is associated with age and genetically dependent resistance to avian enteric salmonellosis, *Infect. Immun*. 73 (2005) 7509-7516.

[151] B.G. Carvajal, U. Methner, J. Pieper, A. Berndt, Effects of Salmonella enterica serovar Enteritidis on cellular recruitment and cytokine gene expression in caecum of vaccinated chickens, *Vaccine* 26 (2008) 5423-5433.

[152] A. Berndt, A. Wilhelm, C. Jugert, J. Pieper, K. Sachse, U. Methner, Chicken cecum immune response to Salmonella enterica serovars of different levels of invasiveness, *Infect Immun* 75 (2007) 5993-6007.

[153] P. Kaiser, P. Staheli, *Avian cytokines and chemokines*, p. 203. In F. Davison, B. Kaspers, and K. A. Schat (ed.), Avian Immunology, 1st ed., Academic Press, Elsevier Ltd., U.K., (2008).

[154] M.B. Farnell, M. El Halawani, S. You, A.P. McElroy, B.M. Hargis, D.J. Caldwell, In vivo biologic effects of recombinant turkey interferon gamma in neonatal chicks: protection against Salmonella enteritidis organ invasion, *Avian Dis*. 45 (2001) 473-478.

[155] A. Berndt, U. Methner, Gamma/delta T cell response of chickens after oral administration of attenuated and non-attenuated Salmonella typhimurium strains, *Vet. Immunol. Immunopathol*. 78 (2001) 143-161.

[156] R.K. Beal, A.L. Smith, Antibody response to Salmonella: its induction and role in protection against avian enteric salmonellosis, *Expert Rev. Anti Infect. Ther.* 5 (2007) 873-881.

[157] M. Desmidt, R. Ducatelle, J. Mast, B.M. Goddeeris, B. Kaspers, F. Haesebrouck, Role of the humoral immune system in Salmonella enteritidis phage type four infection in chickens, *Vet. Immunol. Immunopathol*. 63 (1998) 355-367.

[158] R.K. Beal, C. Powers, T.F. Davison, P.A. Barrow, A.L. Smith, Clearance of Salmonella enterica serovar Typhimurium in chickens is indpendent of B-cell function, *Infect. Immun*. 74 (2006) 1442-1444.

[159] A. Wales, M. Breslin, R. Davies, Assessment of cleaning and disinfection in Salmonella-contaminated poultry layer houses using qualitative and semi-quantitative culture techniques, *Vet Microbiol* 116 (2006) 283-293.

[160] R.K. Gast, Serotype-specific and serotype-independent strategies for preharvest control of food-borne Salmonella in poultry, *Avian Dis*. 51 (2007) 817-828.

[161] P.E. Whistler, B.W. Sheldon, Comparison of ozone and formaldehyde as poultry hatchery disinfectants, *Poult Sci* 68 (1989) 1345-1350.

[162] D.J. Henzler, H.M. Opitz, The role of mice in the epizootiology of Salmonella enteritidis infection on chicken layer farms, *Avian Dis* 36 (1992) 625-631.

[163] L. Garber, M. Smeltzer, P. Fedorka-Cray, S. Ladely, K. Ferris, Salmonella enterica serotype enteritidis in table egg layer house environments and in mice in U.S. layer houses and associated risk factors, *Avian Dis* 47 (2003) 134-142.

[164] M.P. Doyle, M.C. Erickson, Reducing the carriage of foodborne pathogens in livestock and poultry, *Poult Sci* 85 (2006) 960-973.

[165] H. Kinde, D.H. Read, A. Ardans, R.E. Breitmeyer, D. Willoughby, H.E. Little, D. Kerr, R. Gireesh, K.V. Nagaraja, Sewage effluent: likely source of Salmonella enteritidis, phage type 4 infection in a commercial chicken layer flock in southern California, *Avian Dis* 40 (1996) 672-676.

[166] R.P. Johnson, C.L. Gyles, W.E. Huff, S. Ojha, G.R. Huff, N.C. Rath, A.M. Donoghue, Bacteriophages for prophylaxis and therapy in cattle, poultry and pigs, *Anim Health Res Rev* 9 (2008) 201-215.

[167] R.J. Atterbury, M.A. Van Bergen, F. Ortiz, M.A. Lovell, J.A. Harris, A. De Boer, J.A. Wagenaar, V.M. Allen, P.A. Barrow, Bacteriophage therapy to reduce salmonella colonization of broiler chickens, *Appl Environ Microbiol* 73 (2007) 4543-4549.

[168] R.D. Wagner, Efficacy and food safety considerations of poultry competitive exclusion products, *Mol Nutr Food Res* 50 (2006) 1061-1071.

[169] J.S. Bailey, N.J. Stern, N.A. Cox, Commercial field trial evaluation of mucosal starter culture to reduce Salmonella incidence in processed broiler carcasses, *J Food Prot* 63 (2000) 867-870.

[170] P.A. Barrow, Salmonella infections: immune and non-immune protection with vaccines, *Avian Pathol.* 36 (2007) 1-13.

[171] J. De Buck, F. Van Immerseel, F. Haesebrouck, R. Ducatelle, Colonization of the chicken reproductive tract and egg contamination by Salmonella, *J Appl Microbiol* 97 (2004) 233-245.

[172] J.M. Collard, S. Bertrand, K. Dierick, C. Godard, C. Wildemauwe, K. Vermeersch, J. Duculot, F. Van Immerseel, F. Pasmans, H. Imberechts, C. Quinet, Drastic decrease of Salmonella Enteritidis isolated from humans in Belgium in 2005, shift in phage types and influence on foodborne outbreaks, *Epidemiol Infect* 136 (2008) 771-781.

[173] G.L. Cooper, L.M. Venables, M.J. Woodward, C.E. Hormaeche, Vaccination of chickens with strain CVL30, a genetically defined Salmonella enteritidis aroA live oral vaccine candidate, *Infect Immun* 62 (1994) 4747-4754.

[174] J.O. Hassan, R. Curtiss, 3rd, Development and evaluation of an experimental vaccination program using a live avirulent Salmonella typhimurium strain to protect immunized chickens against challenge with homologous and heterologous Salmonella serotypes, *Infect Immun* 62 (1994) 5519-5527.

[175] M.C. Cerquetti, M.M. Gherardi, Vaccination of chickens with a temperature-sensitive mutant of Salmonella enteritidis, *Vaccine* 18 (2000) 1140-1145.

[176] A. Feberwee, E.G. Hartman, J.J. de Wit, T.S. de Vries, The spread of Salmonella gallinarum 9R vaccine strain under field conditions, *Avian Dis* 45 (2001) 1024-1029.

[177] I. Gantois, R. Ducatelle, L. Timbermont, F. Boyen, L. Bohez, F. Haesebrouck, F. Pasmans, F. van Immerseel, Oral immunisation of laying hens with the live vaccine strains of TAD Salmonella vac E and TAD Salmonella vac T reduces internal egg contamination with Salmonella Enteritidis, *Vaccine* 24 (2006) 6250-6255.

[178] M.J. Woodward, G. Gettinby, M.F. Breslin, J.D. Corkish, S. Houghton, The efficacy of Salenvac, a Salmonella enterica subsp. Enterica serotype Enteritidis iron-restricted bacterin vaccine, in laying chickens, *Avian Pathol* 31 (2002) 383-392.

[179] R.A. Penha Filho, J.B. de Paiva, Y.M. Arguello, M.D. da Silva, Y. Gardin, F. Resende, A.B. Berchieri Junior, L. Sesti, Efficacy of several vaccination programmes in

commercial layer and broiler breeder hens against experimental challenge with Salmonella enterica serovar Enteritidis, *Avian Pathol* 38 (2009) 367-375.

[180] A.Y. Inoue, A. Berchieri, Jr., A. Bernardino, J.B. Paiva, E.V. Sterzo, Passive immunity of progeny from broiler breeders vaccinated with oil-emulsion bacterin against Salmonella enteritidis, *Avian Dis* 52 (2008) 567-571.

[181] W. Liu, Y. Yang, N. Chung, J. Kwang, Induction of humoral immune response and protective immunity in chickens against Salmonella enteritidis after a single dose of killed bacterium-loaded microspheres, *Avian Dis* 45 (2001) 797-806.

[182] M. Meenakshi, C.S. Bakshi, G. Butchaiah, M.P. Bansal, M.Z. Siddiqui, V.P. Singh, Adjuvanted outer membrane protein vaccine protects poultry against infection with Salmonella enteritidis, *Vet Res Commun* 23 (1999) 81-90.

[183] M.I. Khan, A.A. Fadl, K.S. Venkitanarayanan, Reducing colonization of Salmonella Enteritidis in chicken by targeting outer membrane proteins, *J Appl Microbiol* 95 (2003) 142-145.

[184] J. De Buck, F. Van Immerseel, F. Haesebrouck, R. Ducatelle, Protection of laying hens against Salmonella Enteritidis by immunization with type 1 fimbriae, *Vet Microbiol* 105 (2005) 93-101.

[185] Y. Toyota-Hanatani, Y. Kyoumoto, E. Baba, T. Ekawa, H. Ohta, H. Tani, K. Sasai, Importance of subunit vaccine antigen of major Fli C antigenic site of Salmonella enteritidis II: a challenge trial, *Vaccine* 27 (2009) 1680-1684.

[186] T.S. Desin, C. Mickael, P.K. Lam, A.A. Potter, W. Köster, Protection of epithelial cells from Salmonella enterica serovar Enteritidis by antibodies against the SPI-1 Type 3 Secretion System, Can. *J. Microbiol.* 56 (2010) 522-526.

[187] T.S. Desin, A.L. Wisner, P.K. Lam, E. Berberov, C.S. Mickael, A.A. Potter, W. Köster, Evaluation of Salmonella enterica serovar Enteritidis pathogenicity island-1 proteins as vaccine candidates against S. Enteritidis challenge in chickens, *Vet Microbiol* 148 (2011) 298-307.

[188] R.J. Atterbury, J.J. Carrique-Mas, R.H. Davies, V.M. Allen, Salmonella colonisation of laying hens following vaccination with killed and live attenuated commercial Salmonella vaccines, *Vet Rec* 165 (2009) 493-496.

[189] P. Luber, Cross-contamination versus undercooking of poultry meat or eggs - which risks need to be managed first?, *Int J Food Microbiol* 134 (2009) 21-28.

In: Salmonella: Classification, Genetics and Disease Outbreaks ISBN: 978-1-61942-928-4
Editors: Adelaide S. Monte, Paulo Eduardo De Santos

Chapter 3

HAZARD OF *SALMONELLA* IN THE INTACT SHELL EGG AND ITS POSSIBLE REMOVAL FROM IT

Juan A. Ordóñez, M. Isabel Cambero, M. Luisa Garcí and M. Concepción Cabeza
Departamento de Nutrición, Bromatología y Tecnología de los Alimentos. Madrid, Spain

ABSTRACT

It is well known that the main microbiological hazard derived from egg consumption is the presence of *Salmonellae*, being the serovars *S.* Enteritidis and *S.* Typhimurium the most frequently implicated in the outbreaks. Although bacteria can reach the inside of the eggs by transovarian or through the shell pores, the main way of contamination probably occurs from organisms located in the shell, which can attain the inner part of the egg when it is broken for cooking other foods, e.g. custard, salads, desserts. In developed countries, the outbreaks of salmonellosis increased until 2004, observing a clear decline afterward, which is attributed to the success of implementing programs to control *Salmonella* in poultry populations. In spite of this, salmonellosis is still the main cause of foodborne illness. Therefore, the decontamination of shell eggs remains of public health concern yet.

Many chemical (e.g. washing, hydrogen peroxide, ozone and electrolyzed water) and physical (e.g. water boiling, pasteurization, ionizing and ultraviolet radiation, pulsed light, high pressure,) methods for shell eggs sanitation have been envisaged, being the pasteurization that of the most concern. Many heat treatment conditions have been proposed to remove *Salmonellae* from eggshells, but none have been completely satisfactory due to the adverse effects of the heat on the functional properties of the white and yolk.

An attempt to develop a procedure to reach this goal has been recently performed by our group. The ability of thermoultrasonication (ultrasounds and heat simultaneously applied) to eliminate *Salmonella* from eggshell was studied, using *S.* Enteritidis and *S.* Senftenberg as models. The thermoultrasonication dramatically reduced the heat resistant of *Salmonella*. E.g., the D-value of *S.* Enteritidis at 55 ºC (2.89 minutes for the heat treatment alone) was reduced a 77.16 %, i.e. it passed to 0.66 minutes when the thermoultrasonication was applied. In the case of *S.* Senftenberg the reduction was lower. The same figures at 57 °C were 10.54 and 3.92 minutes, respectively.

No effects of the thermoultrasonication on several attributes (shelf-life, loss of freshness, eggshell breaking strength, emulsifying and foaming abilities, etc.) were observed.

The fundamentals of the new process for shell egg sanitation have been established at a laboratory scale. As an ultrasonic treatment added to an existing heat process would increase its bactericidal efficiency, the process might have important practical implications for the egg industry. It is now necessary to validate the process at a higher scale to confirm the results.

Eggs: General Considerations

The eggs most commonly consumed worldwide by humans are hen (*Gallus gallus*) eggs and are a high quality food. Their albumin is used as a reference to assess the quality of other proteins. In addition to the albumin, the egg also contains other proteins and a balanced proportion of carbohydrates, fats, mineral elements (selenium, potassium, phosphorus, iodine, magnesium, calcium, sodium, zinc, copper, etc.) and vitamins (folic acid, cobalamins, biotin, pantotenic acid, riboflavin, niacin, thiamine, retinol, tocopherols and calciferols) (Stadelman, 1995; Watkins, 1995; Volmer *et al.*, 1999). The fat from eggs contains a high proportion of essential fatty acids belonging mainly to the n-6 and, to a lesser extent, to the n-3 family, both essential for several biological functions (Lesckanich and Noble, 1997). The mean weight of an egg is 57 g, of which 11% corresponds to the eggshell, 58% the white and 31% the yolk (Li-Chan *et al.*, 1995). These percentages are similar for all eggs, regardless of their weight. Fresh egg compounds are widely used in the food industry, owing to their high nutritional value and excellent functional properties including their water holding capacity, gel formation, the fact that they can be whisked and form foam, and their emulsifying properties (Robinson, 1987; Kato *et al.*, 1993; Montjoie, 1993; Yang and Baldwin, 1995). They, also, control the growth of sugar crystals, slowing down crystallization in jams and confectionary and can be used to enhance the flavor and color of some products (Anonymous, 2000). Therefore, the egg may be considered as a multifunctional ingredient since it plays several roles simultaneously, proving superior to other food products or ingredients that only present some of these qualities.

Eggs are unfertilized hen ovules that have their own natural container, the eggshell. After being laid, the inside of the egg is usually sterile for two main reasons: the eggshell and its membranes provide resistance to microbial penetration and, secondly, the presence of antimicrobial substances in the white makes it a hostile environment for bacterial growth. The egg has three structures that, to some degree, prevent it from becoming contaminated: the cuticle, the shell and the membranes (Garibaldi and Stokes, 1958; Kraft *et al.*, 1958; Mayes and Takeballi, 1983). The cuticle is a fine invisible layer that covers the entire shell. It is a protein structure with a sponge-like appearance, which facilitates the passage of air but prevents the entry of microorganisms. However, it is a very sensitive layer that is easily removed by extreme desiccation, washing, moisture, dirt, friction and ageing, among other factors. Hence, any manipulation of the shell that could constitute an aggression may lead to loss of the cuticle (Hartung and Stadelman, 1962), leaving the shell pores uncovered, permitting the entry through them of microorganisms present on the shell to the egg interior, thus contaminating the egg (Board *et al.*, 1964).

Egg white contains a number of antimicrobial agents: lisozyme, avidine, conalbumin and ovoflavoprotein. In addition, it also has a high viscosity and an alkaline pH (Mayes y Takeballi, 1983; Board *et al.*, 1994; Wesierska, 2006). Lisozyme is especially effective against Gram-positive bacteria but its bactericidal action disappears when the white and yolk are mixed (Ibrahim *et al.,* 1991). Avidine and ovoflavoprotein fix the biotin and riboflavin, respectively, which become no longer available for microorganisms that require them (Baron *et al.*, 2000). The same occurs with conalbumin, which forms complexes with different metal ions such as iron, copper, zinc (Bezkorovainy, 1981). The pH of the white is slightly alkaline but, due to the loss of carbon dioxide from the egg during storage, this rises with time (even to 9.3) becoming a dysgenic factor for microbial growth. By contrast, the pH of the yolk and its nutrient compounds make it an ideal medium for the growth of most microorganisms. *Salmonella*, for example, grow rapidly at room temperature in the yolk and reach the stationary phase after two days, which is maintained during the period of egg storage (Humphrey *et al.*, 1989b). In spite of the natural barriers which an egg has to prevent the entry of microorganisms through the eggshell, the presence of *Salmonella* has been detected in the egg interior, owing to the weakening of these barriers from numerous causes, such as humidification of the shell, storage at room temperature, cracks in the shell, and the loss of integrity of the cuticle.

The most likely mechanisms described for contamination of the egg interior are: a) through pores and fissures in the shell (horizontal contamination), which reach the shell from ether the oviduct or contact with fecal matter often present at the site of egg laying, or b) by transovarian route (vertical contamination), during egg formation (in infected animals). Once inside the egg, they can multiply rapidly, since *Salmonella* has a generation time of approximately half an hour at 37 °C and of 3.5 hours at 15-5 °C (Ruzickova, 1994; Braun y Fehlhaber, 1995; ICMSF, 1998). Hence, starting with just one cell, populations of around one million cells are reached in 10 and 70 hours, respectively. Eggs with these rates of contamination are a major risk for the consumer's health if they are eaten after insufficient heat treatment, or if they are used to make sauces, deserts or confectionary. This risk persists when the contamination only affects the eggshell, since the *Salmonella* will inevitably pass to the egg interior when the shell is broken, and the microorganism will multiply if the egg products are not manipulated and chilled appropriately. Furthermore, there is evidence indicating that cross-contamination of egg shells can occur at the processing level (egg grading, packing, etc.). The probability of this cross-contamination depends on the proportion of *Salmonella* contaminated eggs, and is further influenced by the type of technology used and the hygienic practices applied (EFSA, 2009).

SALMONELLOSIS AND PUBLIC HEALTH

Salmonellosis is a foodborne illness caused by some species of the *Salmonella* genus, especially by *Salmonella enterica*. It has been considered an important public health problem from the last forty years. It has been estimated to affect around 3 million people each year, causing 200,000 deaths (Anjum, 2007). *Salmonella enterica* is the main causal agent of foodborne infections and accounts for 99% of the *Salmonella* isolated in man. Although more than 2,000 serovars of *S. enterica* are known, most infections in humans are caused by only a few serovars, the most common of which, in developed countries, corresponds to *S.* Enteritidis and *S.* Typhimurium. A recent report (Hendriksen *et al.*, 2011) deals with the distribution of the 15 most frequently identified serovars of *Salmonella* isolated during the period 2001 to 2007. In all geographic areas throughout the study period, with the exception of Oceanic and North American regions, *Salmonella* serovars Enteritidis and Typhimurium ranked the first and second most common serovars, respectively. In the North American and Oceanic (Australia and New Zealand) regions, the same serovars were the most frequent, but in the opposite order. The percentage of *S.* Enteritidis isolates from humans was 43.5% (range: 40.6% [2007] to 44.9% [2003]) and that of *S.* Typhimurium was 17.1% (range: 15% [2007] to 18.9% [2001]). Other serovars (Newport, Infantis, Virchow, Hadar and Agona) were also isolated with an overall proportion of 3.5%, 1.8%, 1.5%, 1.5%, and 0.8%, respectively.

In developed countries, outbreaks of salmonellosis increased until 2004, after which there was a clear decline in the notification of outbreaks. For example, in Europe there were 108,614 reported outbreaks of salmonellosis (23.7 cases per 100,000 inhabitants), representing a decrease of 17.4% compared to 2008, corresponding to the fifth consecutive year in which the number of cases of this disease had dropped, with an average decrease of 12% over the five-year period (EFSA, 2011). This reduction was mainly attributed to the success of implementing national programs to control *Salmonella* in poultry populations, which reduced the presence of *Salmonella* in eggs (EFSA, 2011), but was also due to the application of other control measures in the food chain (EFSA, 2011). In spite of this, salmonellosis is still the main cause of foodborness illness in man.

Eggs and food produce containing raw eggs are still the main source of contagion of this accounting for almost 50% of salmonella cases illness with *S.* Enteritidis being the serovar most frequently involved, accounting for a 76% of cases (EFSA, 2011). Hence, egg consumption is considered to be the primary cause of human salmonellosis worldwide. Its ubiquitous condition and the existence of asymptomatic carriers in the human and animal populations, make it especially difficult to control, and, together with its high level of prevalence in industrialized countries, this microorganism is a priority target in public health.

STRATEGIES TO CONTROL *SALMONELLA*

In the light of this situation, it is necessary to control *Salmonella* to prevent, or at least to reduce outbreaks of salmonellosis caused by contaminated eggs or foods prepared with them. Different chemical and physical methods have been tried, including ones in which the water used to clean them contains a variety of cleaning agents (Worley *et al.*, 1992; Knape *et al.*, 2001) such as hydrogen peroxide (Padron, 1995), chlorine and iodine (Knape *et al.*, 1999), ozone (Koidis *et al.*, 2000) and electrolyzed water (Russell, 2003), or boiled water (Himathongkham *et al.*, 1999), ultraviolet rays (Kuo *et al.*, 1997), light pulses (Dunn, 1996), gamma radiation (Téllez *et al.*, 1995), X-rays (Serrano *et al.*, 1997) and gaseous plasma (Davies and Breslin, 2003). Hale and Kirk (1997) applied a combined treatment of heat and ionizing radiation and achieved three decimal reductions in the number of salmonella present.

However, initially the most appropriate and convenient processes appear to be refrigeration, cleaning the shell and pasteurization.

Refrigeration is effective for inhibiting the growth of *Salmonella*, since the minimum growth temperature is about 7 ºC (Mackey *et al.*, 1980; ICMSF, 1996) and they cannot penetrate the shell at temperatures of around 10 ºC (Simmons *et al.* 1970; Ruzickova, 1994; ICMSF, 1996). However, it is probably only applied in practice in the home. They are usually sold in the shops at room temperature, since the condensation produced by this storage can, on the one hand, result in partial loss of the cuticle, favoring the entry of microorganisms and, on the other hand, because the cold does not eliminate the risk of *Salmonellae* on the eggshell since, although these do not multiply they do not die either. Therefore, the risk of infection remains since the bacteria are in a viable state (Saeed and Koons, 1993).

Although cleaning the eggshell by washing improves the appearance of the eggs and reduces the microbial load present on the eggshell, an incorrect operation can result in *S.* Enteritidis penetrating the egg through the pores (Kim and Slavik, 1996). While in the European Union (EFSA, 2005) it is not permitted to wash eggs to be used for direct human consumption, in the United States this practice has been employed since the start of the Seventies. It is also a common practice in Canada, Australia and Japan. The arguments maintained by those who advice against washing eggs are based on the following premises (Stadelman, 1994; ICMSF, 1996): a) washing with a liquid that is at a lower temperature than the eggs can result in aspiration (liquid + bacteria) through the pores, b) any operation that moistens the shell increases the alteration, presumably based on the argument of water penetrating the pores by capillarity, c) it increases disorganization of the cuticle with increased microbial penetration and d) washing water that contains iron (> 2 ppm of Fe III) increases the level of this metal in albumen, neutralizing the antimicrobial effect of conalbumin.

The pasteurization would appear to be the most logical option to sanitize intact eggs, since all species of the *Salmonella* genus except for *S.* Senftenberg, are thermolabile bacteria. However, the pasteurization has not been consistently used at an industrial level because the temperature required to achieve safe levels of decontamination changes the functional properties of the egg white and yolk, invalidating them for many culinary and technological uses.

Nonetheless, there have been endless attempts to do this, since it was first attempted around a century and a half ago, in 1867 (ICMSF, 1980). Many studies have been carried out to try to find a method to apply heat treatment to intact eggs of a sufficient thermal intensity to guarantee microbiological safety, but without altering the physical and functional properties (Kato *et al.*, 1995; Handa and Kuroda, 1999). Some of these studies are described below:

One of the most attractive was that conducted by Funk (1947) who patented a process consisting in immersing intact eggs in water or oil at a temperature of 59 ºC for 5 to 10 minutes. This method was reasonably effective, but eggs consumed today are fresher and they have a lower pH, which increases the heat-resistance of the salmonellae, so nowadays these treatment conditions would be insufficient to reduce the load of this microorganism to an acceptably safe level. A longer heating time, or a higher temperature, would be required, which would have negative effects on the egg compounds.

The application of temperatures of around 71 ºC for a few minutes would destroy *S.* Enteritidis; although the white begins to coagulate at 60 to 65.5 ºC, so prolonged heating would result in denaturation of the proteins, with adverse effects on the functionality of the egg's components (Hou *et al.*, 1996; Gosal and Ross-Murphy, 2000). For example, pasteurization at 64 °C for 2 minutes can cause some proteins to denaturize and precipitate during the acidification phase, e.g., when making mayonnaise, reducing its stability (Campbell *et al.*, 2003).

Humphrey *et al.* (1990) inoculated eggs with the *S.* Enteritidis PT4 strain using 10^8 cells per egg and treated them thermally at 57 and 58 °C, obtaining decimal reduction times (D-values) of 6 and 3.7 minutes, respectively. These values are very high, since to achieve at least the 5 decimal reductions required to guarantee microbiological safety, longer times are required that adversely affect the functional properties of the egg. Similarly, Schuman *et al.* (1997) applied pasteurization treatments at 57 and 58 °C to shell eggs by immersing them in hot water and obtained D-values for the *Salmonella* strain they used of 6.0 and 4.5 minutes, respectively. Taking into consideration the normal *Salmonella* load present in egg, 5 decimal reductions gives the consumer a broad safety margin. To achieve this, according to the D-values estimated by these authors, it would be necessary to apply heat treatments for 30 and 23 minutes at 57 and 58 °C, respectively, which are very long times if the eggs' thermolabile compounds are to remain unaltered.

Van Lith *et al.* (1995) heated shell eggs with an initial contamination in the yolk of 10^1 - 10^3 cells of *S.* Enteritidis PT4, with water at 57 °C for 20 - 30 minutes, but concluded that the treatment was not sufficient to reduce the microbial load to safe levels. Moreover, heating to temperatures above 57 °C for longer than 20 minutes caused the albumen to coagulate (Stadelman *et al.*, 1996; Mermelstein, 2001).

Hou *et al.* (1996) studied the survival of *S.* Enteritidis ATCC 13076 in shell eggs when heated in a water bath at 57 °C for 25 minutes and achieved only 3 decimal reductions, without denaturation of the proteins. Afterwards, they used a combined system of heating the eggs in a water bath at 57 °C for 25 minutes, followed by treating with hot air at 55 °C for 1 hour, and obtained 7 decimal reductions, but the viscosity of the white decreased, its turbidity increased compared with untreated eggs and the lisozyme activity was also reduced by half.

In short, none of the methods mentioned have proved completely satisfactory to reduce the presence of *S.* Enteritidis to safe levels (Catalano and Knabel, 1994) since the conditions required to do this would have a negative effect on the egg quality. Finally, it is worth noting that the ICMSF (1980) has reported a list of conditions (time-temperature binomial and heating medium) proposed by around fifteen authors for the pasteurization of shell eggs. Taking into account all data recorded in this ICMSF book, a "limit equation" (I) can be approximated

$$\text{(I)} \qquad \log t = 5.77 - 0.085\,T$$

where t is the treatment time and T the temperature of the treatment.

This can be used to approximately estimate the maximum heating conditions that can be applied to the egg to reduce the load of *Salmonella*, without producing changes in the sensorial and functional properties of the egg compounds. Hence, at 52, 55 and 58 °C, the treatment times would be lower than 22.4, 12.4 and 6.9 minutes, respectively. The most common D-values offered in egg (or that can be estimated from original works) refer to *S.* Enteritidis, at 55 °C are in the 4 to 11 minutes interval (Schaffner *et al.*, 1989; Humphrey *et al.*, 1990; Shah *et al.*, 1991; Palumbo *et al.*, 1995; Michalski *et al.*, 1999). Considering that 5D reductions are sufficient to decrease the salmonella load to achieve the food safety objective (FSO), not even the lowest D-value (4 minutes) would fulfill this target. Similar considerations can also be made for temperatures of 52 and 58 °C assuming a z-value of 4 – 5 °C for this serovar (Humphrey *et al.*, 1990; Palumbo *et al.*, 1995; Michalski *et al.*, 1999).

As far as the authors are aware, there is only one case where pasteurized shell eggs were marketed. In 1998, a patent was filed (U.S. patent 5.843.505) to hygienize shell eggs that were sold by the Pasteurized Eggs Corp. of New Hampshire under the commercial name of "Davidson´s Pasteurized Eggs" (Mermelstein, 2001). The treatment consisted in a heating by immersing in water or air at 56 – 62 °C, conditions that produced 5 decimal reductions in the initial load of *Salmonella* and maintained the functionality of the albumen (Schuman, 2000; Zeidler, 2001; Brackett *et al.*, 2001). Next, after the eggs had been cooled, inspected and rinsed they were coated and packaged to prevent possible recontaminations (Schuman, 2000). Eggs treated in this way could be kept for 6 months at 5 °C. This is the only hygienizing method that has been used commercially, but requires eggs to be stored under refrigeration after treatment.

Later, however, Baron *et al.* (2003) once again concluded that it was impossible to achieve a level of microbiological safety that permitted an adequate level of protection (ALOP) to the consumer, while maintaining optimal functional properties of the egg compounds.

However, the attempts have not ceased and a new process to pasteurize shell eggs have been recently developed (Perry *et al.*, 2011). It is based on combining heating at 56 °C for 10 minutes and ozone. The physical quality and functionality of shell eggs, pasteurized with heat or a combination of heat and ozone, were assessed during eight weeks of heating and ozone stored at 4 or 25 °C. Eggs were treated as follows: (1) immersion heating that mimics commercial pasteurization processes (egg internal temperature of 56 ± 0.1 °C for 32 minutes), or (2) a newly-developed combination process comprised of heating (56 ± 0.1 °C, internal, for 10 minutes) followed by gaseous ozone treatment. These time-temperature conditions are at the limit of producing modifications in the functional properties of egg compounds. Indeed, the values were rudely consistent with the former "limit equation" (I). In fact, after pasteurization, regardless of the method, the first negative effects of heating corresponded to increased albumen opacity and decreased albumen overrun. Authors notified detrimental effects on quality markers, which were more severe in heat-pasteurized eggs than those treated with the ozone-based process. The authors concluded that heat-ozone pasteurization, by virtue of its less severe heat treatment, yields a safe final product that more closely resembles untreated shell eggs. However, it seems that the food safety objective cannot be achieved with this combined process because on several occasions (Schaffner *et al.*, 1989; Shah *et al.*, 1991; Michalski *et al.*, 1999) D-values at 56 °C close to 10 minutes have been reported for *S.* Enteritidis, so, only one decimal reduction may be achieved at this temperature. It would be necessary to attain a reduction in the level of at least 4D – 5D to guarantee an acceptably low level of *Salmonella*.

It can, therefore, be said that, to date, no acceptable method has been developed to remove *Salmonella* from shell eggs due to the adverse effects of the temperatures required on the functional properties of the white and yolk, and the difficulty of achieving a homogeneous heating of the egg. This is because shell eggs, unlike liquid egg, cannot be stirred during the pasteurization process to distribute the heat and prevent the proteins from coagulating. This can, therefore, result in problems associated with overheating and coagulation of the white near the shell.

THE THERMOULTRASONICATION AS AN ALTERNATIVE METHOD FOR SANITIZING INTACT SHELL EGGS

It was previously concluded that, in spite of the different types of heat treatment devised to eliminate *Salmonella* from shell eggs, none have been used on an industrial scale. Given, on the one hand, the number of outbreaks of salmonellosis still occurring worldwide and, on the other, the difficulty of sanitizing shell eggs, the need to develop an effective method to remove salmonella from eggshells is still an unresolved technological problem. Any reduced intensity of the heat treatment, combined with a more lethal effect will always be beneficial for the safety and quality of the treated egg. One recent attempt to achieve this objective has been the combination of ultrasound and heat, a process called thermoultrasonication (Ordóñez *et al.*, 1987). The simultaneous application of both agents lead to a synergic effect in which the ultrasound sensitizes the microorganisms to the lethal action of heat, significantly reducing the thermoresistance of sporulated and vegetative bacteria. This synergic effect of ultrasound and heat has been demonstrated in several microorganisms, including sporeforming organisms, such as *Bacillus subtilis* (García *et al.*, 1989) and vegetative forms, such as enterococci (Ordóñez *et al.*, 1984) and *Staphylococcus aureus* (Ordóñez *et al.*, 1987). In this latter work, for example, the D-value at 53.5 ºC dropped from 6.3 minutes to 2.5 minutes applying ultrasound during the heat treatment, in other words, the D-value decreased by 60%, meaning that if, for example, the initial population is around 10^6 cell/ml, this will be reduced to 2.5×10^4 with the heat treatment and to 1×10^2 with the thermoultrasonic treatment. In other words, around 4 decimal reductions will be produced by thermoultrasonication, compared to only 1.6 reductions with the heat treatment. On the basis of these data, it was postulated that if *Salmonella* are affected by thermoultrasonication in a similar way, then this could be of great value to reduce the bacterial load on the eggshell to statistically negligible levels.

RESPONSE OF *SALMONELLA SPP.* TO HEAT AND ULTRASONIC TREATMENTS

Heat Resistance of *Salmonella*

Several studies have focused on the heat resistance of *Salmonella*, both in foods and in laboratory media, and on the effect of several factors such as environmental ones (Hills *et al.*, 1997; Jung and Beuchat, 1999; Kwon and Ricke, 1998; Weissinger *et al.*, 2000), water activity (Baird-Parker *et al.*, 1970; Goepfert *et al.*, 1970), pH (Anellis *et al.*, 1954) and the nature of the solutes in the heating medium (Hansen and Rieman, 1963; Cotterill and Glauert, 1968; Tuncan and Scott, 1989; Fletcher and Csonka, 1998). Table 1 shows the heat resistance at 55 and 60 ºC in egg or egg compounds (values taken from original articles or estimated from their data) for some strains of *S.* Enteritidis and *S.* Seftenberg.

S. Enteritidis presents a similar heat resistance to the other *Salmonella* commonly associated with eggs and significantly lower (around 10-fold) than that of *S.* Senftenberg (Osborne *et al.*, 1954; Humphrey *et al.*, 1989b, 1990; Chantarapanont *et al.*, 2000; Doyle and Mazzotta, 2000; Breeuwer *et al.*, 2003; Mañas *et al.*, 2003a, 2003b, Cabeza *et al.*, 2004; Cabeza *et al.*, 2005a).

Table 1. Thermal parameters of *S.* Enteritidis and *S.* Senftenberg in different egg compounds. The values for comparative purposes have been extrapolated from the original data

Microorganism	Medium	z (ºC)	D_{55} (min)	D_{60} (min)	Ref.
S. Enteritidis	Líquid whole egg	9.56	10.14	3.06	1
S. Enteritidis	"	3.87-6.04	3.91-5.93	0.22-0.75	2
S. Enteritidis	"	3.38	11.84	0.39	3
S. Enteritidis	"	5.38	1.85	0.22	4
S. Enteritidis	"	3.59	11.05	0.45	5
S. Enteritidis 13076	"	3.95	2.19	0.12	6
S. Enteritidis PT4	Yolk, pH 6.3	3.90	21.00	1.10	2
S. Enteritidis	"	4.61-6.55	3.29-8.46	0.51-0.70	7
S. Enteritidis	"	4.33	8.59	0.60	5
S. Enteritidis	Yolk + 10% salt	5.47	10.03	1.22	5
S. Enteritidis	Yolk + 5% salt + 5% sucrosa	4.31	182.39	12.65	5
S. Enteritidis PT4	Albumen	5.71	1.50	0.20	2
S. Enteritidis	"	5.01	1.18	0.12	5
S. Enteritidis 13076	"	4.44	0.83	0.06	6
S. Enteritidis	Albumen, pH 9.2	W.D.	0.72	W.D.	8
S. Enteritidis 13076	Distilled water	4.57	2.89	0.23	9
S. Senftenberg 775W	Líquid whole egg	8.17	30.30	7.40	2
S. Senftenberg	"	W.D.	2.80	W.D.	10
S. Senftenberg 775W	Líquid whole egg, pH 7.7	5.60	36.22	4.56	11
S. Senftenberg 775W	Yolk, pH 6.3	9.07	42.00	11.80	2
S. Senftenberg	Yolk	4.07	11.02	0.65	7
S. Senftenberg 775W	Liquid albumen	8.71	3.00	0.80	2
S. Senftenberg 775W	Liquid albumen, pH 9	4.67	7.17	0.61	12
S. Senftenberg 775W	Liquid albumen, pH 9.5	2.69	2.33	0.03	12
S. Senftenberg 775W	Liquid albumen + polyphosphate, pH 9	4.66	0.78	0.07	12
S. Senftenberg 775W	Liquid albumen + polyphosphate, pH 9.5	4.58	0.36	0.03	12
S. Senftenberg 43845	Distilled water	6.26	21.99	3.50	13

W.D.: Without enough data.

1. Schaffner *et al.*, 1989; 2. Humphrey *et al.*, 1990; 3. Shah *et al.*, 1991; 4. Muriana *et al.*, 1996; 5. Michalski *et al.*, 1999; 6. Jin *et al.*, 2008; 7. Palumbo *et al.*, 1995; 8. Boziaris *et al.*, 1998; 9. Cabeza *et al.*, 2004; 10. Mañas *et al.*, 2003b; 11. Mañas *et al.*, 2003a; 12. Kohl, 1971; 13. Cabeza *et al.*, 2005a.

For example, at 55 °C, the D-value of the latter serovar is around 34.3 minutes versus 6.4 minutes for S. Enteritidis PT4 (Humphrey *et al.*, 1990). In distilled water, D-values of 21.9 minutes have been reported for *S.* Senftenberg (Cabeza *et al.*, 2005a) and 2.89 minutes for *S.* Enteritidis (Cabeza *et al.*, 2004) at the same temperature.

It has been repeatedly shown that the lower the water activity, the higher the heat resistance (Goepfert *et al.*, 1970; Gibson, 1973; Corry, 1974; Summer *et al.*, 1991; Mattick *et al.*, 2001; Álvarez *et al.*, 2003; Aljarallah and Adams, 2007; Chiewchan *et al.*, 2007). Also, the structure and composition of the food matrix affect the heat resistance of *Salmonella* (Mattick *et al.*, 2001; Smith *et al.*, 2001), which is higher in complex media. For example, it has been reported for *S.* Senftenberg 775W, D values at 60 °C of 3.6 - 7.5 minutes and 5 - 10 minutes in a 0.5% NaCl water solution and peas soup, respectively (Thomas *et al.*, 1966). In addition, when bacteria are attached to tissues, they have a higher heat resistance than those are free bacteria or dispersed in a food or broth (Murphy *et al.*, 2002). Similarly, a greater heat resistance has also been observed for this organism in high fat content foods (Shachar and Yaron, 2007). The *S. enterica* serovars Agona, Enteritidis and Typhimurium inoculated in peanut butter showed a high heat resistance, resulting in a D-value of only 3.2 minutes at 90 °C. The heat resistance of *Salmonella* in different egg compounds also depends on the pH and the nature of the compounds, and is generally higher in the egg yolk than the white (Osborne *et al.*, 1954; Anellis *et al.*, 1954; Ng, 1966, Garibaldi *et al.*, 1969; USDA, 1969; Cotterill *et al.*, 1973; Humphrey *et al.*, 1990; Shah *et al.*, 1991; Palumbo *et al.*, 1995; Michalski *et al.*,1999) with a particularly marked destruction in the albumen (Jung and Beuchat, 2000; Doyle and Mazzota, 2000; Jin *et al.*, 2008). In contrast, the results of Schuman *et al.* (1997) and Schuman and Sheldon (1997) found that different strains of *Salmonella* presented a greater heat resistance in the albumen. However, the D-values calculated in egg yolk from 60 to 62.2 °C by Palumbo *et al.* (1995) were 1.8 to 2.6 times higher than those obtained by previous authors. Muriana *et al.* (1996) suggested that *S.* Enteritidis could use proteins and lipids from the yolk to maintain the integrity of its membrane against the thermal inactivation. Table 1 shows the thermal parameters (D-value at 55 and 60 °C and z value) of *S.* Enteritidis and *S.* Senftenberg in several egg compounds and other media under different conditions.

Response of *Salmonella* to Ultrasonic Treatment

The influence of the treatment medium on the inactivation of microorganisms by ultrasonic treatment has been studied by several authors. Lee *et al.* (1989) applied ultrasounds to chocolate inoculated with *S.* Eastbourne for 10 and 30 minutes and only achieved reductions of 26 and 74%, respectively, probably mainly due to the high fat and sugar contents. However, these same authors obtained 4 decimal reductions in the *Salmonella* counts when they applied the treatment for 10 minutes in peptone water, which clearly demonstrates the influence of the medium on the inactivation of microorganisms by ultrasounds. Most microorganisms are highly resistant to ultrasounds in standard treatment conditions so (Raso *et al.*, 1998; Pagán *et al.*, 1999), as also occurs with heat treatment, the intensity required to obtain microbiologically-safe products (Sanz *et al.*, 1985; Mason, 1998) produces important changes in the composition and physical and sensorial properties of the foods (Williams, 1994; Sala *et al.*, 1995), without producing a significant reduction in the microbial load (Mason *et al.*, 1996; Seymour *et al.*, 2002; Huang *et al.*, 2006).

It has also been found that the combination of ultrasounds and other agents (e.g. chemical and pressure) can increase its bactericidal power. Hence, ultrasound increased the efficacy of chlorine at decontaminating chicken breasts (Lillard, 1993; 1994). When this author applied ultrasounds and chlorine simultaneously he found a reduction from 2.5 to 4 logarithmic units of the bacterial load, while ultrasounds and immersion in chlorine applied separately only achieved reductions of 1 – 1.5 and less than 1 log units, respectively. Seymour *et al.* (2002) studied the behavior of *S.* Typhimurium in iceberg lettuce against different treatments: rinsing with water, rinsing with chlorinated water, ultrasounds combined with water and ultrasounds combined with chlorinated water, and obtained reductions of 0.7, 1.7, 1.5 and 2.7 log units, respectively. The greater effect of the combination of ultrasounds and chlorinated water can be explained by the fact that the gaseous cavitation produced releases the microorganisms adhered to the food, making them more vulnerable to the chemical agents. Wrigley and Llorca (1992) studied the effect of ultrasounds on *S.* Typhimurium in brain-heart infusion broth and skimmed milk and obtained between 2 and 3 decimal reductions depending on the treatment time. When ultrasounds were applied at 50 °C an even greater reduction was achieved. However, in whole liquid egg the microorganisms were more resistant, and the decimal reduction achieved by applying s at 50 °C for 30 minutes was lower than 1D. The protective effect of liquid egg is probably caused by the reduced intensity of the cavitation resulting from the higher viscosity of this product (Hülsen, 1999). However, Huang *et al.* (2006) obtained the same reduction in the *S.* Enteritidis load in the same product with only 5 minutes of treatment, possibly because in this case the ultrasounds were applied directly to the egg.

Mañas *et al.* (2000) studied the resistance of *S.* Enteritidis, *S.* Typhimurium and *S.* Senftenberg to the action of ultrasounds under pressure (0.2 MPa) at sublethal (40°C, manosonication) and lethal temperatures (60°C, manothermosonication), in citrate-phosphate buffer and in liquid egg. They also determined the effect of the amplitude, relative pressure and temperature of the treatment on the inactivation rate by manosonication. The D-values obtained for *S.* Enteritidis, *S.* Typhimurium and *S.* Senftenberg at 60 °C in buffer solution were 0.068, 0.12 and 1.0 minutes, respectively; and in liquid egg were 0.12, 0.20 and 1.4 minutes. At sublethal temperatures (40 °C), the D-values obtained in buffer were 0.73, 0.78 and 0.84 minutes, whereas for the same treatment in liquid egg the D-values were 0.76, 0.84 and 5.5 minutes. A linear increase in the amplitude of the ultrasounds waves was associated with an exponential increase in the rate of inactivation by manosonication. The data obtained at 60 °C are interesting. When the D-values obtained at this temperature for *S.* Enteritidis and *S.* Senftenberg are compared with those shown in Table 1, these tend to be lower, which can be explained by the combined action of ultrasounds and heat (Ordóñez *et al.*, 1987), although in this work an additional agent, pressure, must also be taken into account. In any case, this result supports a generalization of the sensitizing effect of ultrasounds to the lethal action of heat on bacterial spores.

Recently, the destruction of *S.* Enteritidis in whole liquid egg has been studied by electric pulses, high pressure and ultrasounds, applying these agents individually and in combination (Huang *et al.*, 2006). The electric pulses seemed to have no effect, even when the number of pulses and the treatment temperature were increased, due to the high viscosity of the egg. The high pressures applied in multiple cycles had a greater effect than when these were applied in a single cycle for an equivalent time, the effect increased with the number of cycles and also with temperatures higher than 20°C.

RESPONSE OF *SALMONELLA* SPP. TO THERMOULTRASONIC TREATMENT

S. Enteritidis ATCC 13076

Both ultrasounds and heat resistance of vegetative bacteria is easily determined in jacketed vessels, in which the suspending medium is heated to reach a constant temperature, which is controlled by a water bath connected to the vessel. The same system might be used to assay the heat resistance of bacteria attached to the eggshell, but it must be ensured that the egg is completely submerged, since the heating medium acts as heating agent and ultrasounds transmission. However, when the ultrasonic treatment was applied, the cell disruptor tip was found to erode, and even crack, the egg shell. It was necessary, therefore, to design a special vessel (Figure 1) to physically separate the egg from the tip (Cabeza *et al.*, 2004). Essentially, the system consists of a jacketed vessel for continuous circulation of the heating medium and two compartments separated by a thermostable plastic net with holes of 2 mm diameter to prevent contact between the egg and the tip, while the water flows freely. Additionally, the cavitation bubbles provoke a great turbulence, which result in a rapid homogenization of the temperature of the heating medium. Since higher sonication volumes have been associated with reduced lethal power (Huang *et al.*, 2006), an experiment was conducted to study the relationship between the sonication power and the volume. This phenomenon was reflected in the heat destruction graph obtained with *S.* Enteritidis suspended in various water volumes (Figure 2), for which the corresponding equations are shown in Table 2.

Table 2. Thermoultrasonic destruction equations and z-values for *S.* Enteritidis ATCC 13076 suspended in different volumes of distilled water

V (ml)	Destruction equation	R^2	z (°C)
100	log D = 6.5897 - 0.1217 T	0.99	8.22
200	log D = 7.0901 - 0.128 T	0.98	7.81
500	log D = 9.3066 - 0.1629 T	0.99	6.14
750	log D = 10.224 - 0.1787 T	0.99	5.60
1200	log D = 11.855 - 0.2067 T	0.99	4.84

Plotting the inverse logarithm of the slopes of the above equations (Table 2) as a function of temperature produced the straight line in Figure 3, for which the equation is:

$$\text{(II)} \qquad \frac{\Delta V}{\Delta D} = 0.252\,T - 11.113$$

where $\frac{\Delta V}{\Delta D}$ is $\frac{1}{tg\alpha}$; V the volume (ml); D the decimal reduction time (minutes) and T the temperature (°C).

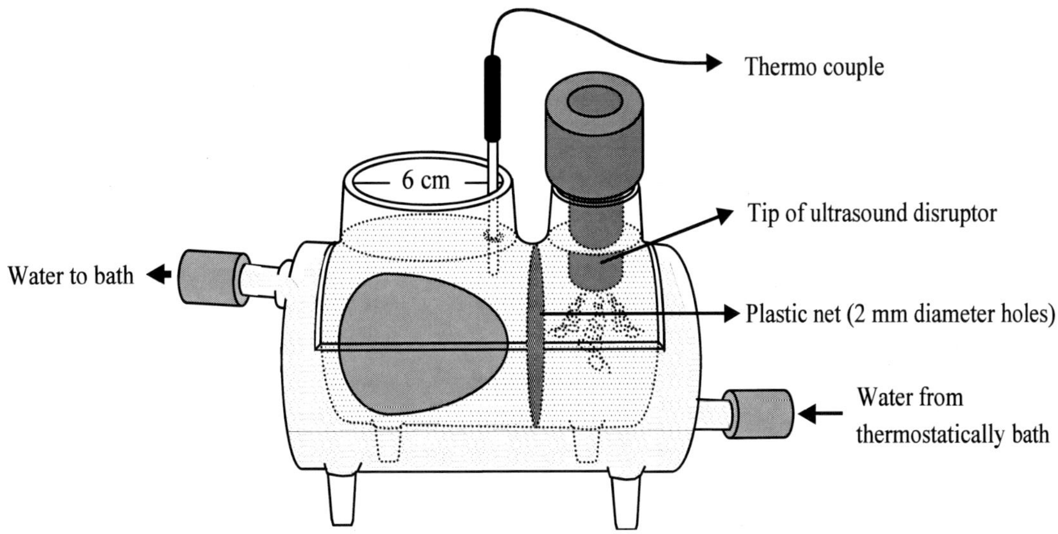

Figure 1. Jacketed vessel designed for thermoultrasonicating intact egg (Cabeza *et al.*, 2004).

In our conditions, 200 ml was the most convenient volume to use. The vessel was constructed, therefore, to contain one egg submerged in 200 ml of water so that the volume of the heating/sonication medium were the same as that used in the experiments performed to determine the heat resistance of bacterial suspensions (Cabeza *et al.*, 2004).

The efficacy of thermoultrasonication on the viability of the salmonellae was studied in both the bacterial suspensions and also in the egg, using *S.* Enteritidis as model, since this is the commonest serovar involved in human outbreaks of salmonella, and *S.* Senftenberg, because of its unusually high heat resistance.

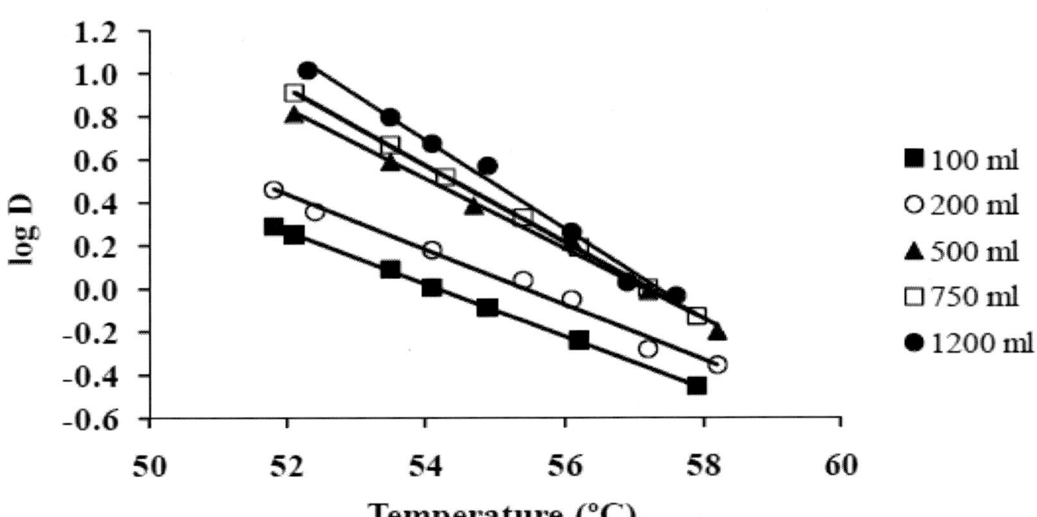

Figure 2. Thermoultrasonic destruction curves of *Salmonella enterica* serovar Enteritidis ATCC 13076 suspended in different volumes of distilled water.

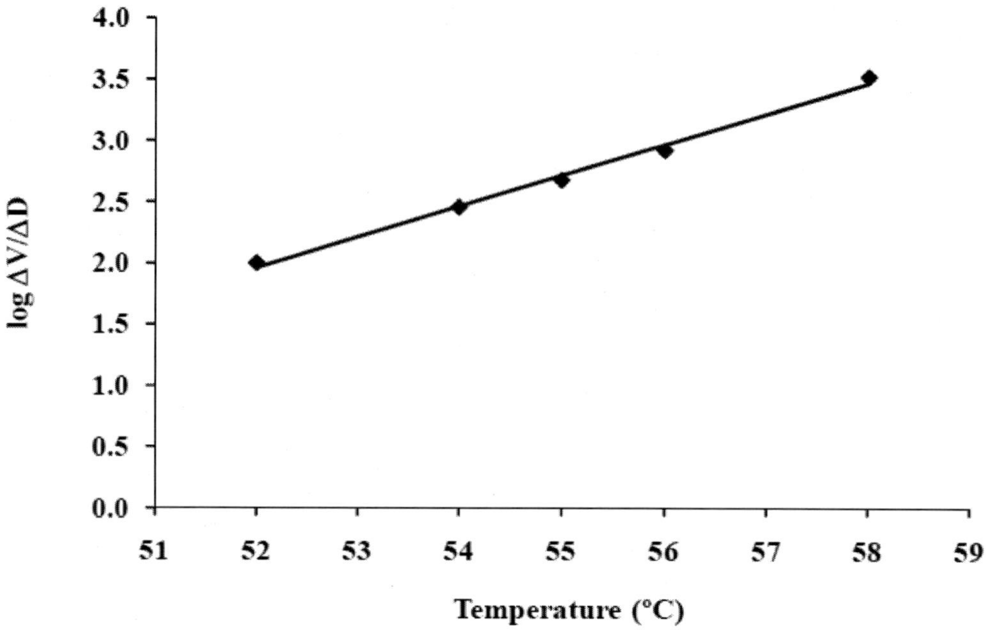

Figure 3. Relationship between sonication volume, treatment temperature and D-values.

Figure 4 shows the ultrasonic, heat and thermoultrasonic treatment resistances of *S.* Enteritidis at different temperatures and Table 3 the destruction curves and the z- values for the former treatments (Cabeza *et al.*, 2004).

It is unnecessary to examine in depth the heat resistance of *S.* enteritidis as the thermal parameters for this species are well-documented in the literature (see Table 1). The z-values reported vary in the range of 3.54 – 4.33 °C (Schuman and Sheldon, 1997; Jin *et al.*, 2008). The equations shown in Table 2 are in total agreement with those reported in the afore-mentioned references.

Table 3. Destruction equations and z-values for *Salmonella enterica* serovar Enteritidis ATCC 13076

Destruction equation [a]		z-value (°C) [b]	95% CL [c]
$\log D_s = 1.4457 - 0.0231\,T$	($R^2 = 0.99$)	43.29	41.39-45.79
$\log D_h = 12.500 - 0.2189\,T$	($R^2 = 0.99$)	4.57	4.19-5.03
$\log D_t = 8.3632 - 0.1534\,T$	($R^2 = 0.95$)	6.52	5.16-8.92
$\log D_{te} = 7.4527 - 0.1388\,T$	($R^2 = 0.98$)	7.20	6.54-8.03

[a] D_s, D-value for ultrasonic treatment; D_h, D-value for heat treatment; D_t, D-value for thermoultrasonic treatment; D_{te}, D-value for thermoultrasonic treatment of eggs immersed in water; T, temperature (°C).

[b] Increase in temperature for the D-value to decrease by 1 log cycle.

[c] 95% confidence limits.

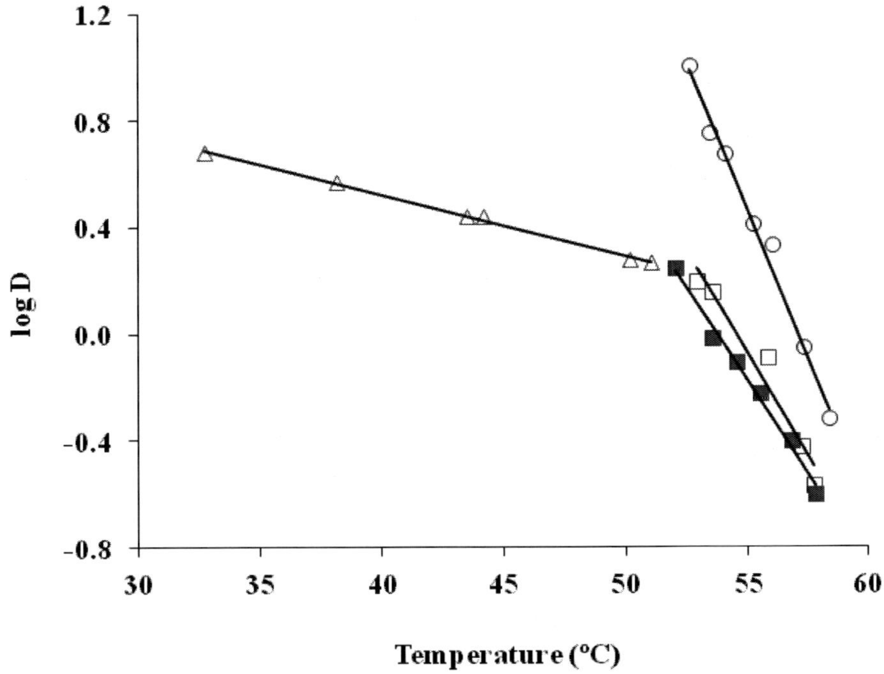

Figure 4. Destruction curves of *Salmonella enterica* serovar Enteritidis ATCC 13076 suspended in distilled water and attached on shell eggs. Ultrasonic treatment (Δ), heat treatment (O), and, thermoultrasonic treatment in distilled water (□). Thermoultrasonic treatment on intact eggs inmersed in distilled water (■).

From the equations shown in Table 3, it is evident that the thermoultrasonic treatment caused a higher killing effect than the heat treatment; D-values at 52 °C of 2.44 minutes and 13.10 minutes were respectively estimated. Therefore, the D-value for the thermoultrasonic treatment was 5.37-fold lower than that of the heat treatment, which means that the original bacterial load of a suspension of *S.* Enteritidis is reduced by more than 99.999% (10^5-fold) by applying thermoultrasonic treatment compared to the decrease of 1D (10-fold or 90%) with the heat treatment. However, this was not the same intensity throughout the temperature range studied (52.55 – 57.75 °C). For example, at 56 °C, the D-values were 0.61 and 2.17 minutes, respectively, i.e. the thermoultrasonic treatment was only 3.56-fold lower i.e. around a 99.96% reduction. Figure 4 shows that when the temperature rose above 52 °C, the thermoultrasonic destruction curve will intersect the heat destruction curve at the theoretical temperature of 63.2 °C. At this point, the thermoultrasonic treatment becomes a heat treatment alone, lacking the sensitizing effect of ultrasound. This phenomenon has been previously reported for both *Staphylococcus aureus* in the range 50 – 57 °C (Ordoñez *et al.*, 1987) and *Bacillus subtilis* spores in the interval 70 – 95 °C (García *et al.*, 1989). An explanation for this is based on the effect of different factors affecting the gaseous cavitation (García *et al.*, 1989), the most important being the surface tension, viscosity and vapor pressure which, in turn, depend of the temperature (Alliger, 1975; Sala *et al.*, 1995; Piyasena *et al.*, 2003). As the sonication temperature rises, the cavitation bubbles form and grow more quickly due to the reduced surface tension and viscosity; therefore, more bubbles are produced, although the violence of bubble collapse is lower since the higher vapor pressure of the gas in the bubble acts a cushion (Berliner, 1984). As the temperature increases, all these phenomena are accelerated, minimizing the efficacy of the ultrasonic treatment (Alliger, 1975; Berliner, 1984).

The thermoultrasonication destruction curve obtained for *S.* Enteritidis attached to the eggshell (Table 3) predicts that the D-values at 52 and 58 °C are 1.77 and 0.25 minutes, respectively. However, when the treatment was applied to a bacterial suspension the same figures calculated from the corresponding equation (Table 3) are 2.44 and 0.29 minutes. The values are very similar and the small differences are due to the different z-values found, 6.52 °C for bacterial suspension and 7.79 °C for the treatment of intact eggs. This minor deviation might be explained by the difficulty of applying the treatment to eggs in homogeneous conditions. Despite this deviation, the effect follows the same pattern.

S. Senftenberg ATCC 43845

The behavior of *S.* Senftenberg in response to thermoultrasonication was investigated in the range of 57.8 to 67 °C. Figure 5 and Table 4 show the destruction curves and the corresponding equations, respectively. As expected, *S.* Senftenberg presented a greater heat resistance than *S.* Enteritidis and the lethal parameters are in accordance with those reported in the literature (Gibson, 1973; Goepfert and Biggie, 1968; Thomas *et al.,* 1966).

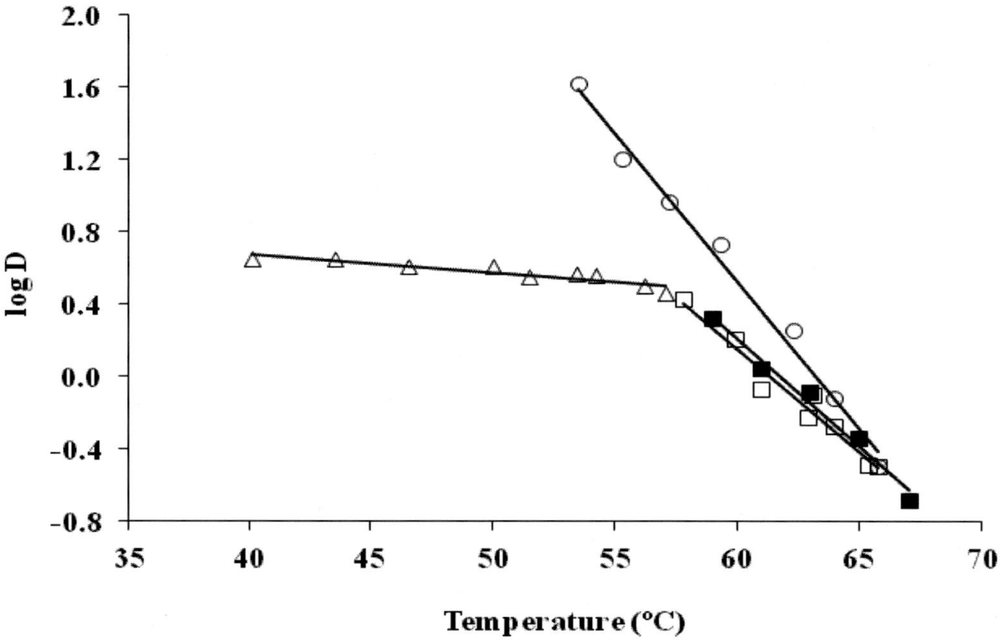

Figure 5. Destruction curves of *Salmonella* Senftenberg ATCC 43845 suspended in distilled water and attached to shell eggs. Ultrasonic (Δ), heat (O), and thermoultrasonic treatments of bacteria suspended in distilled water (□). Thermoultrasonic treatment (■) of bacteria attached to the shell of intact eggs immersed in distilled water.

Table 4. Destruction equations and z-values for *Salmonella enterica* serovar Senftenberg ATCC 43845

Destruction equation [a]	R^2	z-value (°C) [b]	95% CL [c]
$\log D_s = 1.0714 - 0.0099\,T$	0.84	101.2	76.78-148.42
$\log D_h = 10.1257 - 0.1597\,T$	0.99	6.26	5.85-6.74
$\log D_t = 6.7409 - 0.1098\,T$	0.97	9.11	8.06-10.47
$\log D_{te} = 8.0033 - 0.13\,T$	0.98	7.69	6.82-8.81

[a] D_s, D-value for ultrasonic treatment; D_h, D-value for heat treatment; D_t, D-value for thermoultrasonic treatment; D_{te}, D-value for thermoultrasonic treatment of eggs immersed in water; T, temperature (°C).

[b] Increase in temperature for the D-value to decrease by 1 log cycle.

[c] 95% confidence limits.

As with *S.* Enteritidis, it was observed that the thermoultrasonic treatment applied to *S.* Senftenberg had a more lethal effect than heat treatment alone, and its intensity varied over the temperature range studied. However, the degree of reduction was much higher in the case of *S.* Enteritidis since the percentage reductions in D-values between 81.4 and 47.9% were determined in the 6 degree centigrade (52 – 58.4 °C) interval assayed (Cabeza *et al.*, 2004) while reductions observed for the killing of *S.* Senftenberg were between 65.2 and 11.1% in the 57.8 – 67 °C temperature interval (Cabeza *et al.*, 2005a). Therefore, the D-value at 57.8 °C for the heat treatment was 7.77 minutes (90% reduction) *vs* 2.7 minutes obtained for the thermoultrasonic treatment, i.e. 2.87-fold lower or a reduction in load of nearly 99.9%. Without considering the differences in heat resistance between both salmonella serovars, the thermoultrasonication of eggs with attached cells shows a similar behavior, as it can be deduced by comparing Figures 4 and 5. As the kinetics follow the same pattern, all considerations made for *S.* Enteritidis may also be extended to *S.* Senftenberg.

EFFECT OF THE THERMOULTRASONICATION ON THE FUNCTIONAL PROPERTIES OF EGG COMPOUNDS

The overall conclusion for thermoultrasonication treatment is that this technology can increase the lethal effectiveness of heat treatments without increasing the temperature or treatment time. This can reduce the levels of salmonella present on the eggshell to statistically negligible levels. However, the effect of this technology on the functional properties of egg compounds has not been established. The effect of heat on these properties is well-known and it is explained, more or less descriptively, in many publications, although very few describe the precise conditions in which these effects are produced. The kinetics of these events have not been described either, but rather they are explained in a overall kind according to the phenomenon under consideration. Hence, it has been reported that the yolk is more thermostable than the white, since the latter begins to denature at 62 °C and the yolk at 65 °C (Belitz and Grosch, 1988); the pasteurization of shell eggs increases the whipping time required to form the foam (Kline *et al.*, 1965); the ovoalbumin readily denaturizes but the conalbumin coagulates at an even lower temperature (Belitz and Grosch, 1988); the ovomucoid is very stable to heat coagulation because it contains nine disulphide bonds (Belitz and Grosch, 1988); the ovoalbumin becomes more stable with increasing storage time owing to a change from sulphydric groups to disulphide bonds (Takahashi *et al.*, 1991; Mamathambika and Bardwell, 2008), etc. Among the few publications reporting precisely the beginning of events derived from heat application to shell eggs, it is worth citing the one that describes how whipping time increases after a heat treatment of 53 °C for 2 - 3 minutes (Kline *et al.*, 1965), another describes an increased opacity of the white at 57 °C (Stadelman *et al.*, 1996) and, perhaps, the most relevant is that related to the conalbumin (the most termolabile compound), specifying that it begins to denaturize at 57.3 °C (Belitz and Grosch, 1988). If this were established as the critical temperature, the "limit equation" (I) predicts that no more than 8 minutes a 57.3 °C must be applied to retain the functional properties of the egg.

Since heat-denaturation of proteins is a strictly temperature-dependent phenomenon, it can be said in general that the Q10 of the event is of the order of 2 (z-value = 33 °C). This parameter predicts that at 54 °C, the conalbumin starts to denature at 10 minutes. Similar considerations can be made about the loss of transparency of the ovoalbumin, since the values published are similar to those relating to denaturation of the conalbumin (see above). By applying the former equation, the heat-treatment time necessary to eliminate the salmonella would be 15 minutes, which is 1.5-fold the time it takes for the conalbumin to begin to denaturize.

All these calculations suggest that the possibility of reducing the treatment temperature (or time) when using thermoultrasonication, would help to maintain the functional properties of egg. Cabeza *et al.* (2005b) carried out a study for this purpose and applied thermoultrasonic treatment at 54 °C for 5 minutes, at which 5.5 D reductions of the population are achieved. This is one more decimal reduction than that required to obtain the FSO, thus guaranteeing a microbiologically safe product. The most important parameters of fresh (untreated) eggs were compared with values obtained for eggs thermoultrasonicated in the aforementioned conditions. These corresponded to: shelf-life during storage in different conditions of temperature and relative humidity, emulsifying and foaming abilities, rheological properties (hardness, springiness, adhesiveness, cohesiveness, gumminess and chewiness) of a gel formed with egg white by thermal coagulation, resistance of the shell to breakages and sensorial properties of cooked egg. Statistically significant differences were not found in any case (number of samples between 10 and 50, depending of the feature analyzed). It was even observed (although without significant differences) in studies on shelf-life that, as the severity of the storage conditions was increased, (temperature and relative humidity), the loss of moisture from the egg was slower in the treated than in the fresh egg, which it has been attributed to sealing of the pores in the shell during thermoultrasonic treatment by the protein layer (cuticle) located on the outside surface of the shell.

Consequently, the thermoultrasonic treatment applied (54 °C, 5 minutes) did not produce any changes in the properties of the egg compounds, and reduced the salmonella population to values which easily the FSO is achieved.

The effect of thermoultrasonication on the ultrastructure and physical properties of the eggshell, and the possible salmonella penetration was also studied (Cabeza *et al.*, 2011). No effect was found on the physical properties of shells stored in different conditions nor was the structure of the eggshell affected, except for the cuticle. Most of the outer surface, including pores, of the thermoultrasonicated eggshell lacked the cuticle outer layer, but cuticle residues remained within the mouth of the pore. This probably resulted in the eggshell pores remaining blocked, since both yolk and white remained sterile after three weeks of storage under several temperature and relative humidity conditions.

PRACTICAL CONSIDERATIONS

The temperature interval selected for studies with *S.* Enteritidis was between 52 °C and 58 °C and the most concern result at the moment is that thermoultrasonic treatment of *S.* Enteritidis in eggs immersed in water had a much stronger bactericidal effect than heat treatment alone (D values at 52 °C and at 57.8 °C of the heat treatment were 13.10 and 0.70 minutes, respectively, versus 1.77 and 0.25 minutes of the thermoultrasonic treatment). In other words, at these temperatures, the D values decreased by 86.5% and 64.3%, respectively, which means that at 52 °C, a reduction of one logarithmic unit is achieved with the heat treatment (reduction in the original number of bacteria by 90%), while with the thermoultrasonic treatment 7.4 D reductions are achieved, i.e., 99.999999%. The z-values were different for the heat (4.57°C) and the thermoultrasonic (7.2 °C) treatments. Then, at 58 °C these differences are significantly less, but still important, approaching a reduction of 3 logarithmic units. This corresponds to a reduction of 1 D (90% of original number) with the heat treatment versus 2.8 D with thermoultrasonic treatment, i.e. a reduction greater than 99.5% with the latter treatment.

The increased bactericidal efficiency of the thermoultrasonic treatments has very important practical implications. The data reported in the literature referring to the percentage of eggs in the market contaminated with *S.* Enteritidis are not consistent. The same can also be said about the number of bacteria present on a contaminated egg (ICMSF, 1980), but some publications (Humphrey *et al.*, 1989a; 1991) indicate that a common contamination would be in the order of 100 cells/egg. Let us consider, for reasons of safety for the consumer, a level of contamination of 10-fold this figure, i.e., 10^3 C.F.U./egg. If an intermediate temperature from the aforementioned interval (for example, 54°C) for 15 minutes is applied [the most frequently recommended maximum conditions to prevent the adverse effects of heating on the egg's functional properties (ICMSF, 1980)], the heat treatment would only achieve a bactericidal effect equivalent to a reduction of 3.14 D (D at 54 °C = 4.78 minutes) of the original population. This would result in a rate of surviving bacteria of around 1 cell per egg, which would be totally unsatisfactory from a hygienic perspective. However, the thermoultrasonic treatment would cause the bacterial load to decrease by 16.6 D (D at 54 °C = 0.9 minutes), in other words, to around 10^{-13} cells/egg, a completely safe level, since it would correspond to a statistically negligible level of contamination. Moreover, this level is so insignificant that it would the temperature or the treatment time could be significantly reduced, which would help maintain the functional properties of the egg compounds.

D-values at 54 °C for *S.* Enteritidis higher than those recorded for the strain used here as a model (*S.* Enteritidis ATCC13076) have been reported (Schaffner *et al.*, 1989; Shah *et al.*, 1991; Michalski *et al.*, 1999) of around 10 minutes. In this case, the microbial load reductions for the heat and the thermoultrasonic treatments would be 1.5 D and about 8.3 D, since a D-value a 54 °C of 1.8 minutes may be estimated (assuming that the strains of the D-value at 54

°C = 10 minutes have the same response against the thermoultrasonic treatment as *S.* Enteritidis ATCC13076). The reduction is much lower but very important, because the final load would be about 10^{-6} cells/egg.

The Food Safety Objective (FSO) and its Achievement with Thermoultrasonic Treatment

The health authorities in western societies have developed strict regulations in an attempt to obtain maximum microbiological safety of food products to protect the consumer's health. To collaborate with this worthy goal, two concepts have been recently introduced. One is the Food Safety Objective (FSO), and the other is that this objective must result in an ALOP (Appropriate Level of Protection), in other words, an adequate level of protection for the consumer. The FSO is defined as the maximum frequency or concentration that a microbiological hazard can have in a food at the time of its consumption, which offers an adequate level of protection to the consumer (ICMSF, 2002; Gorris, 2005). Hence, the FSO converts the ALOP into parameters that can be controlled by the industries and monitored by government agencies. The setting of a specific FSO for a given food, and the fulfillment of this objective by a treatment depends on several factors, including the infective dose of the microorganism or microorganisms most important for health in the product, the generation time in the case that environmental conditions allow microbial growth, the usual initial level per unit of product, the microbiological criterion, and the normal conditions in which the products are to be stored or distributed for sale.

FSO for *S.* Enteritidis

Let us consider the conditions to establish the minimum thermoultrasonic treatment should be applied to shell eggs in order to reach a product *S.* Enteritidis free to an adequate level of consumer protection (FSO), it could be used the same arguments and criteria that some organisms and authors have employed to estimate the FSO in hamburgers (FDA, 1999), Frankfurt sausages (ICMSF, 2002) and ready-to-eat foods (RTE) (Cabeza *et al.*, 2009; Hoz *et al.*, 2008) to determine the heat treatment (in the case of hamburgers and Frankfurt sausages) or E-beam treatment (in the case of RTE products) that must be applied to achieve the corresponding FSO. In the present case, these would be related to the thermoultrasonic treatment of shell eggs.

When shell eggs are considered, the situation is different to that of the aforementioned food. In the previous cases, the FSO is expressed in terms of CFU/g which cannot be done in the case of shell eggs and it must be established per unit. In spite of this, the concepts and reasoning followed by these organizations to estimate the FSO are suitable for shell eggs.

Salmonella are Gram-negative rods that can multiply at aw higher than 0.95, at a pH higher than 4.9 and at temperatures between 8 and 45 °C (ICMSF, 1998). The infective doses of salmonella vary in relation to the species and serovar. In experiments with human volunteers, very high infective doses have been found, of more than 10,000 salmonellae (McCullough and Eisele, 1951; Hornick *et al.*, 1970). However, outbreaks of food illness have always been associated with less than 100 cells/g in the food (D'Aoust *et al.*, 1975;

Gangarosa, 1978; Blaser and Newman, 1982; Silliker and Gabis, 1986; Hockin *et al.*, 1989), for example, in the case of *S. enterica*, values as low as 28 cells/g has been recorded (Vought and Tatini, 1998). The differences in infective doses estimated by the different authors appear to be caused by the variable number of bacteria that survive during transit through the digestive tract, especially through the stomach. For example, water ingested without food passes through the stomach more quickly than when the bacteria are trapped in a food substance. Similarly, very fatty foods protect the *Salmonella* from being destroyed by the gastric juices (ICMSF, 1996).

S. Enteritidis has a generation time (g-value) of approximately 30 minutes at 37 ºC and 3.5 h at 15.5 ºC (Ruzickova, 1994; Braun and Fehlhaber, 1995) so, after starting with only one cell, the infective dose (30 – 100 cells) would be reached in between 3 and 20 hours, respectively, and populations of around 1 million would be reached in around 10 hours at 37 ºC or 66 hours at 15.5ºC. However, g values of 26 minutes have also been obtained at temperatures above 20ºC (Instituto de Estudios del Huevo, 2006).

The available data relating to the percentage of eggs on the market contaminated with salmonella are not consistent. Values about has been offered (ICMSF, 1980) although in the last few years lower levels (1 – 3%) has been reported (EFSA, 2011). There is also some variability in the number of bacteria present on contaminated eggs (ICMSF, 1980) but some publications (Humphrey *et al.*, 1989a; 1991) have suggested that a common rate of contamination is around 100 cells/egg.

Let us consider a hypothetical extreme case so that an FSO can be established to cover the most unfavorable conditions referred to in the previous paragraph, and the achievement of this FSO by any treatment will guarantee the supply of eggs free of *S.* Enteritidis.

Consider that a mayonnaise salad is being prepared for 200 people 8 hours before it is to be eaten, and that during this time it is exposed to temperatures of around 25ºC. Imagine that one egg provides 6 individual portions (therefore, 34 eggs would be used). According to the most unfavorable scenario, 5% of the eggs will be contaminated by 100 cells of *S.* Enteritidis, with a g-value of around 26 minutes and an infective dose of 28 bacteria. Then, the total number of bacteria in the whole product is estimated to be around 170 cells of *S.* Enteritidis, i.e., around 0.85 per portion, and 18.5 generations will be generated after 8 hours of exposure, which would produce a population of around 3.15×10^5 CFU per portion. Taking into account the infective dose, there will certainly be an outbreak of salmonella. Since the infective dose is 28 cells, by applying a simple operation it can be deduced that there should be fewer than 7.55×10^{-5} CFU per portion, i.e., 4.5×10^{-4} (log = 4.223) cells/egg to be at the moment of consumption lower than the infective dose. As it is starting with 5 cells/egg (log = 0.699), the treatment would have to produce 4.1 decimal reductions.

Compare the sanitation of shell eggs submitted to heat and thermoultrasonic treatments at 54 ºC. Equations (III) and (IV) can be applied to establish the conditions of each treatment, respectively.

$$\text{(III)} \quad \log D = 12.500 - 0.219\ T \qquad D = 4.78 \text{ min.}$$

$$\text{(IV)} \quad \log D = 7.453 - 0.139\ T \qquad D = 0.91 \text{ min.}$$

where D is the decimal reduction time and T is the temperature applied.

Since, according to the "limit equation" (I), the maximum time for pasteurization of shell eggs is 15 minutes at 54 °C if the egg functional properties are to be maintained, a total of 3.14 decimal reductions would be produced in the heat treatment, which is less than the 4.1 decimal reductions required. This would produce a post-treatment load of 3.62×10^{-3} CFU/egg that would result in contamination of the product at the time of consumption of 222 cells per portion. This is more than 8-fold the infective dose which is completely unsatisfactory from a hygienic perspective. However, with the thermoultrasonic treatment, a reduction of 16.48D would be produced, i.e., a contamination of 1.66 cell per 10^{16} eggs, which is statistically negligible. This level of safety is even greater than that achieved with the 12D reductions in *Clostridium botulinum* obtained for the industrial production of canned foods with a pH over 4.5. Even, it could be reduced either the temperature or the treatment time or both. In relation to the treatment time, the FSO could be achieved at 54 °C with a thermoultrasonication time of around 3.73 minutes. In other words, almost a quarter of the time would be sufficient to obtain the FSO, which would have a negligible negative effect on the sensorial and functional properties of the egg compounds. Alternatively, the treatment temperature could be reduced. This was proposed in the article by Cabeza *et al.* (2004), who applied a thermoultrasonication treatment for 12 minutes at 52 °C. At this temperature the D-value deduced from equation (IV) is around 1.72 minutes, which would provoke around 7 decimal reductions. This treatment would be less aggressive for the egg compounds but the FSO would be equally achieved.

FSO for *S.* Senftenberg

There are very few data about the incidence, percentage of contaminated eggs and level of contamination by this serovar since the 95% of salmonella outbreaks produced by eating eggs or egg products are caused by *S.* Enteritidis, followed by *S.* Tiphymurium (EFSA, 2011; Hendriksen *et al.*, 2011). However, from the report of EFSA (2007) it may be deduced that about 1.67% of laying hen flocks contaminated belong to the serovar *S.* Senftenberg. Assuming, a contamination of eggs of 5%, the incidence of *S.* Senftenberg would be about 0.1%, i.e., at level of contamination of around 500 times lower than that of *S.* Enteritidis. Nonetheless, to increase the level of safety in the practical example proposed for *S.* Senftenberg we have assumed a contamination per egg approximately 250 times lower, i.e, of approximately 2.0×10^{-2} cells/egg, although the FSO would remain the same, given that all the other parameters (such as multiplication rate, mesophilia etc.) are similar for both serovars. The most important difference is the atypical heat resistance of *S.* Senftenberg, around ten times higher than that of *S.* Enteritidis as can be deduced from the correspondent aforementioned kinetics since a D-value at 58 °C of 7.29 minutes may be determined for *S.* Senftenberg and 0.66 minutes for *S.* Enteritidis.

By making similar calculations to those carried out for *S.* Enteritidis it can be estimated that, after exposure of the product at room temperature, its contamination by *S.* Senftenberg at the time of consumption (18.5 generations) would be 1.24×10^3 cells per portion. The infective dose is unknown but for safety reasons it could be considered the same as for *S.* Enteritidis and the population would have to be reduced to the previously mentioned levels, i.e., 4.5×10^{-4} cells/egg to ensure that the infective dose is not reached when the eggs are consumed.

The maxima load to be present in the eggs to reach the infective dose is the same than that of S. Enteritidis approximately 4 cells of *S.* Senftenberg for every 10^4 eggs (log = -3.397). Since the initial contamination is 2.0 x 10^{-2} cells/egg (log = -1.699), the treatment would have to produce 1.7 decimal reductions.

Equations (V) and (VI) define the behavior of *S.* Senftenberg in response to heat and thermoultrasonic treatments, respectively. Since this *Salmonella* is highly heat-resistant, a heat treatment of 54 ºC is non-lethal because the D-value, as can be calculated from equation (V) is 32 minutes, which would exceed the recommended treatment time, at this temperature, of 15 minutes. It would, therefore, be necessary to apply the treatment at a higher temperature at which *S.* Senftenberg would be more sensitive. For example, at 58 ºC for which the maximum treatment time, limited by the adverse effects to the egg compounds, would be 7 minutes. The D-values can be calculated from equations (V) and (VI) and are shown at the side of the equations

(V) $\log D = 10.126 - 0.159\ T$ D = 7.29 min.

(VI) $\log D = 8.003 - 0.130\ T$ D = 2.90 min.

where D is the decimal reduction time and T is the temperature applied.

With the heat treatment alone, not even a decimal reduction would be achieved and the FSO would not be reached. After treatment, there would still be a surviving population of 2.22 x 10^{-3} CFU/egg, corresponding to 137.2 viable cells per portion at the time of consumption, which is higher than the infective dose considered. It is unsatisfactory from a health perspective. However, with the thermoultrasonic treatment a reduction of 2.4D would be obtained. This would meet the FSO, although with only a small safety margin, i.e., the residual contamination would be 8 x 10^{-5} cells/egg (in practice 80 cells per 10^4 eggs). In other words, 1.3 x 10^{-5} cells/portion which, after 8 hours of growth, would correspond to 4.82 cells per portion, which is lower than the infective dose, so the FSO would also be fulfilled for *S.* Senftenberg.

For the elimination of *S.* Enteritidis, a thermoultrasonic treatment at 52ºC has been proposed for 12 minutes (Cabeza *et al.*, 2004). This temperature is barely lethal for *S.* Senftenberg, since, according to equation (IV) the D value is 66 minutes. However, focusing on the response of this latter *Salmonella* serovar to ultrasonic treatment alone, defined by equation (VII), a D-value of 3.6 minutes is obtained at 52 ºC.

(VII) $\log D = 1.071 - 0.010\ T$ D = 3.6 min.

where D is the decimal reduction time and T the temperature applied.

This means that the treatment proposed to eliminate *S.* Enteritidis (52 ºC, 12 minutes), would correspond to only ultrasonic treatment for *S.* Senftenberg. This would cause reductions in the population of this serovar of 3.3 D, which is higher than the 1.7 D required to achieve the FSO. In this case, the FSO would be fulfilled with a much greater safety margin than that obtained with the thermoultrasonic treatment at 58 ºC. Clearly, since this treatment is less aggressive the functional properties of the egg components would be conserved better. Other combinations could also be assayed that would achieve similar results.

In conclusion, thermoultrasonic treatment of eggs immersed in water for 12 minutes at 52 ºC would produce eggs free from *S.* Enteritidis and *S.* Senftenberg. If it can be assumed that *S. enterica*, Thiphymurium [the next most frequent serovar in egg after *S.* Enteritidis (ICMSF, 1998)], presents a similar heat-resistance to *S.* Enteritidis, it can be generalized that thermoultrasonic treatment would eliminate salmonella on eggs to levels that can guarantee a microbiologically safe product.

FINAL CONSIDERATIONS

The results reported here have demonstrated the great lethal efficiency of thermoultrasonic treatment at temperatures that the functional properties of the egg white and yolk are maintained. This treatment eliminates the salmonella present on the eggshell to levels that the food safety objective is reached, producing eggs with an adequate safety level to protect the consumer.

Now, it is necessary to design a system for the continuous processing of eggs and also to optimize the parameters that determine the effectiveness of the thermoultrasonic treatment. One of these parameters corresponds to the volume of water used to immerse the eggs during the treatment, since this greatly affects the effectiveness of the process. For this purpose, equation (II) has been developed that relates the thermoultrasonication volume and decimal reduction times. In this case, the volume of the thermosonication medium was adjusted to 200 ml, because this was sufficient to demonstrate the formulated hypothesis. This volume is evidently not appropriate for a process, even on a pilot scale, although an equation has been devised that can be used to model for calculating the precise volume of treatment. It is necessary to carefully define the operational conditions and to develop an equipment to demonstrate the efficiency of the thermoultrasonication at a pilot scale, to subsequently apply the results on an industrial scale.

REFERENCES

Aljarallah, K. M. and Adams, M. R. (2007). Mechanisms of heat inactivation in *Salmonella* serotype Typhimurium as affected by low water activity at different temperatures. *Journal of Applied Microbiology*, 102, 153-160.

Alliger, H. (1975). Ultrasonic disruption. American Laboratory, 10, 75-85.

Álvarez, I.; Mañas, P.; Sala, F. J. and Condón, S. (2003). Inactivation of *Salmonella* enterica serovar Enteritidis by ultrasonic waves under pressure at different water activities. *Applied and Environmental Microbiology*, 69, 668-672.

Anellis, A.; Lubas, J. and Rayman, M. M. (1954). Heat resistance in liquid egg of some strains of the genus *Salmonella*. *Food Research*, 19, 377-395.

Anjum, M. F. (2007). Revealing the mosaic nature of *Salmonella* genomes using microarrays. In M. Rhen, D. Maskell, P. Mastroeni, and J. Threlfall (Eds.), Salmonella: *molecular biology and pathogenesis* (pp. 169-190). Norfolk, United Kingdom: Horizon Bioscience, Wymondham.

Anonymous. (2000). Egg Outlook is. *Prepared Foods,* 169, 71-74.

Baird-Parker, A. C.; Boothroyd, M. and Jones, E. (1970). The effect of water activity on the heat resistance of heat sensitive and heat resistant strains of salmonellae. *Journal of Applied Bacteriology*, 33, 515-522.

Baron, F.; Fauvel S., and Gautier, M. (2000). Behaviour of *Salmonella* Enteritidis in industrial egg white: egg naturally contains factors inhibitory to *Salmonella* growth. In J. S. Sim, N. Nakai, and W. Guenter (Eds), *Egg Nutrition and Biotechnology* (pp. 417-430). Oxon, U.K.: CAB International.

Baron, F.; Nau, F.; Guerín-Dubiard, C.; Gonnet, F.; Dubois, J. J. and Gautier, M. (2003). Effect of dry heating on the microbiological quality, functional properties, and natural bacteriostatic ability of egg white after reconstitution. *Journal of Food Protection*, 66, 825-832.

Belitz, H. D., and Grosch, W. (1988). *Química de los Alimentos* (pp. 433-446). Zaragoza, Spain: Acribia.

Berliner, S. (1984). Application of ultrasonic processors. *International Biotechnology Laboratory*, 2, 42-49.

Bezkorovainy, A. (1981). Antimicrobial properties of iron-binding proteins. *Advances in Bladder Research*, 135, 139-154.

Blaser, M. J. and Newman, L. S. (1982). A review of human salmonellosis. I. Infective dose. *Reviews of Infectious Diseases*, 4, 1096-1106.

Board, R. G., Clay, C., Lock, J., and Dolman, J. (1994). The eggs: a compartmentalized aseptically packaged food. In R. G. Board, and R. Fuller (Eds.), *Microbiology of the Avian Egg* (pp. 43-61). London: Chapman and Hall.

Boziaris, I. S.; Humpheson, L. and Adams, M. R. (1998). Effect of nisin on heat injury and inactivation of *Salmonella enteritidis* PT4. *International Journal of Food Microbiology*, 43, 7-13.

Brackett, R. E.; Schuman, J. D.; Ball, H. R. and Scouten, A. J. (2001). Thermal inactivation kinetics of *Salmonella* spp. within intact eggs heated using humidity-controlled air. *Journal of Food Protection*, 64, 934-938.

Braun, P. and Fehlhaber, K. (1995). Migration of *Salmonella enteritidis* from the albumen into the egg yolk. *International Journal of Food Microbiology*, 25, 95-99.

Breeuwer, P.; Lardeau, A.; Peterz, M. and Joosten, H. M. (2003). Desiccation and heat tolerance of *Enterobacter sakazakii*. *Journal of Applied Microbiology*, 95, 967-973.

Cabeza, M. C.; Ordóñez, J. A.; Cambero, I.; de la Hoz, L. and García, M. L. (2004). Effect of thermoultrasonication on *Salmonella enterica* serovar Enteritidis in distilled water and intact shell eggs. *Journal of Food Protection*, 67, 1886-1891.

Cabeza, C.; García, M. L.; Hoz, L.; Cambero, M. I. and Ordóñez, J. A. (2005a). Destruction of *Salmonella* Senftenberg on the shells of intact eggs by thermoultrasonication. *Journal of Food Protection*, 68, 841-844.

Cabeza, M. C.; García, M. L.; de la Hoz, L.; Cambero, M. I. and Ordóñez, J. A. (2005b). Thermoultrasonication eliminates *Salmonellae* from the intact eggshell without changing the functional properties of their components. *Journal of Food Science*, 70, 292-295.

Cabeza, M. C.; de la Hoz, L.; Velasco, R.; Cambero, M. I. and Ordóñez, J. A. (2009). Safety and quality of ready-to-eat dry fermented sausages subjected to E-beam radiation. *Meat Science*, 83, 320-327.

Cabeza, M. C.; Cambero, M. I.; de la Hoz, L.; García, M. L. and Ordóñez, J. A. (2011). Effect of the thermoultrasonic treatment on the eggshell integrity and their impact on the microbial quality. *Innovative Food Science and Emerging Technologies*, 12, 111-117.

Campbell, L.; Raikos, V. and Euston, S. R. (2003). Modification of functional properties of egg-white proteins. *Nahrung Food*, 47, 369-376.

Catalano, C. R. and Knabel, S. J. (1994). Destruction of *Salmonella enteritidis* in high pH and rapid chilling during simulated commercial egg processing. *Journal of Food Protection*, 57, 592-595.

Chantarapanont, W.; Slutsker, L; Tauxe, R. V. and Beuchat, L. R. (2000). Factors influencing inactivation of *Salmonella* Enteritidis in hard-cooked-eggs. *Journal of Food Protection*, 63, 36-43.

Chiewchan, N.; Pakdee, W. and Devahastin, S. (2007). Effect of water activity on thermal resistance of *Salmonella* Krefeld in liquid medium and on rawhide surface. *International Journal of Food Microbiology*, 114, 43-49.

Corry, J. E. L. (1974). The effects of sugars and polyols on the heat resistance of salmonellae. *Journal of Applied Bacteriology*, 37, 31-43.

Cotterill, O. J. and Glauert, J. (1968). Thermal resistance of salmonellae in egg yolk products containing sugar and salt. *Poultry Science*, 48, 1156-1166.

Cotterill, O. J.; Glauert, J. and Krause, G. F. (1973). Thermal destruction curves for *Salmonella oranienburg* in egg products. *Poultry Science*, 52, 568-577.

D´Aoust, J. Y.; Aris, B. J.; Thisdele, P.; Durante, A.; Brisson, N.; Dragon, D.; Lachapelle, G.; Johnston, M. and Laidley, R. (1975). *Salmonella eastborne* outbreak associated with chocolate. *Canadian Institute of Food Science and Technology Journal*, 8, 181-184.

Davies, R. H. and Breslin, M. (2003). Investigations into possible alternative decontamination methods for *Salmonella* Enteritidis on the surface of table eggs. *Journal of Veterinary Medicine*, 50, 38-41.

De la Hoz, L.; Cambero, M. I.; Cabeza, M. C.; Herrero, A. M. and Ordóñez, J. A. (2008). Elimination of *Listeria monocytogenes* from vacuum-packed dry-cured ham by E-beam radiation. *Journal of Food Protection*, 7, 2001-2006.

Doyle, M. E. and Mazzotta, A. S. (2000). Review of studies on the thermal resistance of *Salmonella*. *Journal of Food Protection*, 63, 779-795.

Dunn, J. (1996). Pulsed light and pulsed electric field for foods and eggs. *Poultry Science*, 75, 1133-1136.

EFSA (European Food Safety Authority). (2005). Opinion of the Scientific Panel on Biological Hazards on the request from the Commission related to the Microbiological Risks on Washing of Table Eggs. *The EFSA Journal,* 269, 1-39.

EFSA (European Food Safety Authority). (2007). Report of the task force on zoonoses data collection on the analysis of the baseline survey on the prevalence of *Salmonella* in holdings of broiler flocks of *Gallus gallus*, Part B. *The EFSA Journal*, 101, 1-86.

EFSA (European Food Safety Authority). (2009). Special measures to reduce the risk for consumers through *Salmonella* in table eggs – e.g. cooling of table eggs. Scientific Opinion of the Panel on Biological Hazards. (Question No EFSA-Q-2007-198). Adopted on 22 January 2009. *The EFSA Journal*, 957, 1-29.

EFSA (European Food Safety Authority). (2011). Authority, European Centre for Disease Prevention and Control; The European Union Summary Report on Trends and Sources of

Zoonoses, Zoonotic Agents and Food-borne Outbreaks in 2009. *EFSA Journal*, 9(3), 2090.

FDA. (1999). Food Code. U.S. Department of Health and Human Services. Washington, DC 20204: Public Health Service Food and Drug Administration.

Fletcher, S. A. and Csonka, L. N. (1998). Characterization of the induction of increased thermotolerance by high osmolarity in *Salmonella*. *Food Microbiology*, 15, 307-317.

Funk, E. M. (1947). Process for preserving eggs for edible consumption. U.S. Patent 2,423,233.

Gangarosa, E. J. (1978). What have we learned from 15 years of *Salmonella* surveillance?. *Proceedings of National Salmonellosis Seminar* (January 10-11, pp. 1-28). Washington, D.C., U.S.: Department of Agriculture.

García, M. L.; Burgos, J.; Sanz, B. and Ordóñez, J. A. (1989). Effect of heat and ultrasonic waves on the survival of two strains of *Bacillus subtilis*. *Journal of Applied Bacteriology*, 67, 619-628.

Garibaldi, J. A. and Stokes, J. L. (1958). Protective role of shell membranes in bacterial spoilage of eggs. *Food Research*, 23, 283-290.

Garibaldi, J. A.; Straka, R. P. and Ijichi, K. (1969). Heat resistance of *Salmonella* in various egg products. *Applied Microbiology*, 17, 491-496.

Gibson, B. (1973). The effect of high sugar concentrations on the heat resistance of vegetative micro-organisms. *Journal of Applied Bacteriology*, 36, 365-376.

Goepfert, J. M. and Biggie, R. A. (1968). Heat resistance of *Salmonella typhimurium* and *Salmonella senftenberg* 775W in milk chocolate. *Applied Microbiology*, 16, 1939-1940.

Goepfert, J. M.; Iskander, I. K. and Amundson, C. H. (1970). Relation of the heat resistance of *Salmonellae* to the water activity of the environment. *Applied Microbiology*. 19, 429-433.

Gorris, L. G. M. (2005). Food safety objective: An integral part of food chain management. *Food Control*, 16, 801–809.

Gosal, W. S. and Ross-Murphy, S. B. (2000). Globular protein gelation. *Current Opinion in Colloid and Interface Science*, 5, 188-194.

Hale, Jr. and Kirk, K. (1997). Method for maintaining interior quality of irradiated shell eggs. Patent No 5700504. USA.

Handa, A. and Kuroda, N. (1999). Functional improvements in dried egg white through the Maillard reaction. *Journal of Agriculture and Food Chemistry,* 47, 1845-1850.

Hansen, N. H. and Riemann, H. (1963). Factors affecting the heat resistance of nonsporing organisms. *Journal of Applied Bacteriology*, 26, 314-333.

Hartung, T. E. and Stadelman, W. J. (1962). The influence of metallic cations on the penetration of the egg shell membranes by *Pseudomonas fluorescens*. *Poultry Science*, 41, 1590-1596.

Hendriksen, R. S.; Vieira, A. R.; Karlsmose, S.; Lo Fo Wong, D. M. A.; Jensen, A. B.; Wegener, H. C.; and Aarestrup, F. M. (2011). Global monitoring of *Salmonella* serovar distribution from the World Health Organization global foodborne infections network country data bank: results of quality assured laboratories from 2001 to 2007. *Foodborne Pathogens and Disease,* 8, 887-900.

Hills, B. P.; Manning, C. E.; Ridge, Y. and Brocklehurst, B. (1997). Water availability and the survival of *Salmonella typhimurium* in porous systems. *International Journal of Food Microbiology*, 36, 187-198.

Himathongkham, S.; Riemann, H. and Ernst, R. (1999). Efficacy of disinfection of shell eggs externally contaminated with *Salmonella* Enteritidis. Implications for egg testing. *International Journal of Food Microbiology,* 49, 161-167.

Hockin, J. C.; D´Aoust, J. Y.; Bowering, D.; Jessop, J. H.; Khanna, B.; Lior, H. and Milling, M. E. (1989). An international outbreak of *Salmonella nima* from imported chocolate. *Journal of Food Protection*, 52, 51-54.

Hornick, R. B.; Greisman, S. E.; Woodward, T. E.; DuPont, H. L.; Dawkins, A. T. and Snyder, M. J. (1970). Typhoid fever: pathogenesis and immunologic control. *New England Journal of Medicine*, 283, 686-691.

Hou, H.; Singh, R. K.; Muriana, P. M. and Stadelman, W. J. (1996). Pasteurization of intact shell eggs. *Food Microbiology*, 13, 93-101.

Huang, E.; Mittal, G. S. and Griffiths, M. W. (2006). Inactivation of *Salmonella enteritidis* in liquid whole egg using combination treatments of pulsed electric field, high pressure and ultrasound. *Biosystems Engineering,* 94, 403-413.

Hülsen, U. (1999). Alternative heat treatment processes. *European Dairy Magazine*, 3, 20-24.

Humphrey, T. J.; Baskerville, A.; Mawer, S.; Rowe, B. and Hopper, S. (1989a). *Salmonella enteritidis* phage type 4 from the contents of intact eggs: a study involving naturally infected hens. *Epidemiology and Infection.* 103: 415-423.

Humphrey, T. J.; Greenwood, M.; Gilbert, R. J.; Rowe, B. and Chapman, P. A. (1989b). The survival of salmonellas in shell eggs cooked under simulated domestic conditions. *Epidemiology and Infection*, 103, 35-45.

Humphrey, T. J.; Chapman, P. A.; Rowe, B. and Gilbert, R. J. (1990). A comparative study of the heat resistance of salmonellas in homogenized whole egg, egg yolk or albumen. *Epidemiology and Infection*, 104, 237-241.

Humphrey, T. J.; Whitehead, A.; Gawler, A. H. L.; Henley, A. and Rowe, B. (1991). Numbers of *Salmonella enteritidis* in the contents of naturally contaminated hens´ eggs. *Epidemiology and Infection*, 106, 489-496.

Ibrahim H. R.; Kato A. and Kobayashi K. (1991). Antimacrobial effects of lysozyme against Gram-negative bacteria due to covalent binding of palmitic acid. *Journal of Agricultural and Food Chemistry*, 39, 2077-2082.

ICMSF (International Commission on Microbiological Specifications for Foods). (1980). *Microbial ecology of foods*, 2: Food Commodities (pp. 521-566). New York: Academic Press.

ICMSF (International Commission on Microbiological Specifications for Foods). (1996). Microorganisms in Food, 5: Microbiological specifications of food pathogens. New York: Blackie Academic and Professional.

ICMSF (International Commission on Microbiological Specifications for Foods). (1998). *Microorganisms in Food*, 6. Microbial ecology of food commodities: Egg and egg products (pp. 475-520). London: Blackie Academic and Professional.

ICMSF (International Commission on Microbiological Specification for Foods). (2002). *Microorganisms in foods*, 7: Microbiological testing in food safety management: *Listeria monocytogenes* in cooked sausage (frankfurters) (pp. 285-312). New York: Kluivert Academic/Plenum publishers.

Instituto de Estudios del Huevo. (2006). Seguridad Alimentaria en Huevos y Ovoproductos (pp. 45-52). Madrid, Spain: Instituto de Estudios del Huevo.

Jin, T.; Zhang, H.; Boyd, G. and Tang, J. (2008). Thermal resistance of *Salmonella enteritidis* and *Escherichia coli* K12 in liquid egg determined by thermal-death-time disks. *Journal of Food Engineering*, 84, 608-614.

Jung, Y. S. and Beuchat, L. R. (1999). Survival of multidrug-resistant *Salmonella* Typhimurium DT104 in egg powders as affected by water activity and temperature. *International Journal of Food Microbiology*, 49, 1-8.

Jung, Y. S. and Beuchat, L. R. (2000). Sensivity of multidrug-resistant *Salmonella typhimurium* DT104 to organic acids and thermal inactivation in liquid egg products. *Food Microbiology*, 17, 63-71.

Kato, A.; Minaki, K. and Kobayashi, K. (1993). Improvement of emulsifying properties of egg white proteins by the attachment of polysaccharide through Maillard reaction in a dry state. *Journal of Agricultural and Food Chemistry*, 41, 540-543.

Kato, A.; Aoki, T., Kato, N.; Nakamura, R. and Matsuda, T. (1995). Modification of ovoalbumin with glucose 6-phosphate by aminocarbonyl reaction. Improvement of protein heat stability and emulsifying activity. *Journal of Agricultural and Food Chemistry*, 43, 301-305.

Kim, J. W. and Slavik, M. F. (1996). Changes in eggshell surface microstructure after washing with cetylpyridinium chloride or trisodium phosphate. *Journal of Food Protection*, 59, 859-863.

Kline, L.; Sugihara, T. F.; Bean, M. L. and Ijichi, K. (1965). Heat pasteurization of raw liquid egg white. *Food Technology*, 19, 1709-1718.

Knape, K. D.; Carey, J. B.; Burgess, R. P.; Kwon, Y. M. and Ricke, S. C. (1999). Comparison of chlorine with an iodine-based compound on eggshell surface microbial populations in a commercial egg washer. *Journal of Food Safety,* 19, 185-194.

Knape, K. D.; Carey, J. B. and Ricke, S. C. (2001). Response of foodborne *Salmonella* spp. marker strains inoculated on egg shell surfaces to disinfectants in a commercial egg washer. *Journal of Environmental Science and Health,* 36, 219-227.

Kohl, W. F. (1971). Pasteurizing egg whites permits effective destruction of salmonellae at pasteurization temperatures of 126-131°F. *Food Technology*, 25, 102-110.

Koidis, P.; Bori, M. and Vareltzis, K. (2000). Efficacy of ozone treatment to eliminate *Salmonella* Enteritidis from eggshell surface. *Archiv für Lebensmittelhygiene*, 51, 4-6.

Kraft, A. A.; Elliot, L. E. and Brant, A. W. (1958). The shell membranes as a barrier to bacterial penetration of eggs. *Poultry Science*, 37, 238-240.

Kuo, F. L.; Carey, J. B. and Ricke, S. C. (1997). UV irradiation of shell eggs: effect on populations of anaerobes, moulds, and inoculated *Salmonella* Typhimurium. *Journal of Food Protection*, 60, 639-643.

Kwon, Y. M. and Ricke S. C. (1998). Induction of acid resistance of *Salmonella* Typhimurium by exposure to short-chain fatty acids. *Applied and Environmental Microbiology*, 64, 3458-3463.

Lee, B. H.; Kermasha, S. and Baker, B. E. (1989). Thermal, ultrasonic and ultraviolet inactivation of *Salmonella* in thin films of aqueous media and chocolate. *Food Microbiology*, 6, 143-152.

Lesckanich, C. D. and Noble, R. C. (1997). Manipulation of n-3 polyunsaturated fatty acid composition of avian eggs and meat. *World's Poultry Science Journal*, 53, 156-183.

Li-Chan, E. C. Y., Powrie, W. D., and Nakai, S. (1995). The chemistry of eggs and egg products. In W. J. Stadelman, and O. J. Cotterill (Eds.), *Egg Science and Technology* (pp. 105-175). New York: The Haworth Press.

Lillard, H. S. (1993). Bactericidal effect of chlorine on attached *Salmonellae* with and without sonication. *Journal of Food Protection*, 56, 716-717.

Lillard, H. S. (1994). Decontamination of poultry skin by sonication. *Food Technology,* 48, 72-73.

Mackey, B. M.; Roberts, T. A.; Mansfield, J. and Farkas, G. (1980). Growth of *Salmonella* on chilled meat. *Journal of Hygiene*, 85, 115-124.

Mamathambika, B. S. and Bardwell, J. C. (2008). Disulfide-linked protein folding pathways. *Annual Review of Cell and Developmental Biologyl*, 24, 211-235.

Mañas, P.; Pagán, R.; Raso, J.; Sala, F. J. and Condón, S. (2000). Inactivation of *Salmonella enteritidis, Salmonella typhimurium* and *Salmonella senftenberg* by ultrasonic waves under pressure. *Journal of Food Protection*, 63, 451-456.

Mañas, P.; Pagán, R.; Álvarez I. and Condón, S. (2003a). Survival of *Salmonella senftenberg* 775 W to current liquid whole egg pasteurization treatments Food Microbiology. *Food Microbiology*, 20, 593-600.

Mañas, P.; Pagán, R.; Raso, J. and Condón, S. (2003b). Predicting thermal inactivation in media of different pH of *Salmonella* grown at different temperatures. *International Journal of Food Microbiology*, 87, 45-53.

Mason, T. J. (1998). Power ultrasound in food processing – The way forward. In M. J. W. Povey, and T. J. Mason (Eds.), *Ultrasound in Food Processing* (pp. 104-126). London: Blackie Academic and Professional.

Mason, T. J.; Paniwnyk, L. and Lorimer, J. P. (1996). The uses of ultrasound in food technology. *Ultrasonics Sonochemistry,* 3, S253-S260.

Mattick, K. L.; Jorgensen, F.; Wang, P.; Pound, J.; Vandeven, M. H. and Ward, L. R. (2001). Effect of challenge temperature and solute type on heat tolerance of *Salmonella* serovars at low water activity. *Applied and Environmental Microbiology*, 67, 4128-4136.

Mayes, F. J. and Takeballi, M. A. (1983). Microbial contamination of the hen's egg: a review. *Journal of Food Protection*, 46, 1092-1098.

McCullough, N. B. and Eisele, C. W. (1951). Experimental human salmonellosis. Pathogenicity of strain of *Salmonella newport, Salmonella derby* and *Salmonella bareilli* obtained from spray-dried whole egg. *Journal of Infectious Diseases*, 89, 209-213.

Mermelstein, N. H. (2001). Pasteurization of shell eggs. *Food Technology*, 55, 72-73, 79.

Michalski, C. B.; Brackett, R. E.; Hung, Y. C. and Ezeike, G. O. I. (1999). Use of capillary tubes and plate heat exchanger to validate U.S. Department of Agriculture pasteurization protocols for elimination of *Salmonella* Enteritidis from liquid egg products. *Journal of Food Protection*, 62, 112-117.

Montjoie, Y. (1993). Ovoproduits: sur un marché en croissance, la qualité est la première des exigeances. *Aviculteur*, 540, 56-59.

Muriana, P. M.; Hou, H. and Singh, R. K. (1996). A flow-injection system for studying heat inactivation of *Listeria monocytogenes* and *Salmonella enteritidis* in liquid whole egg. *Journal of Food Protection*, 59, 121-126.

Murphy, R. Y.; Duncan, L. K.; Johnson, E. R.; Davis, M. D. and Marcy, J. A. (2002). Thermal inactivation of *Salmonella* Senftenberg and *Listeria innocua* in beef/turkey blended patties cooked via fryer and/or air convection oven. *Journal of Food Science*, 67, 1879-1885.

Ng, H. (1966). Heat sensitivity of 300 *Salmonella* isolates. In: U.S. Department of Agriculture, Agricultural Research Service ARS 74-37, The Destruction of *Salmonellae*: *A Report of the Western Experiment Station Collaborators Conference* (pp. 39-41). Washington, DC: U.S. Department of Agriculture.

Ordóñez, J. A.; Sanz, B.; Hernández, P. E. and López-Lorenzo, P. (1984). A Note on the effect of combined ultrasonic and heat treatments on the survival of thermoduric *Streptococci*. *Journal of Applied Bacteriology*, 56, 175-177.

Ordóñez, J. A.; Aguilera, M. A.; García, M. L. and Sanz, B. (1987). Effect of combined ultrasonic and heat treatment (thermoultrasonication) on the survival of a strain of *Staphylococcus aureus*. *Journal of Dairy Research*, 54, 61-67.

Osborne, W. W.; Straka, R. P. and Lineweaver, H. (1954). Heat resistance of strains of *Salmonella* in liquid whole egg, egg yolk and egg white. *Food Research*, 19, 451-463.

Padron, M. (1995). Egg dipping in hydrogen peroxide solution to eliminate *Salmonella typhimurium* from eggshell membranes. *Avian Diseases*, 39, 627-630.

Pagán, R.; Mañas, P.; Álvarez, I. and Condón, S. (1999). Resistance of *Listeria monocytogenes* to ultrasonic waves under pressure at sublethal (manosonication) and lethal (manothermosonication) temperatures. *Food Microbiology*, 16, 139-148.

Palumbo, M. S.; Beers, S. M.; Bhaduri, S. and Palumbo, S. A. (1995). Thermal resistance of *Salmonella* spp. and *Listeria monocytogenes* in liquid egg yolk and egg yolk products. *Journal of Food Protection*, 58, 960-966.

Perry, J. J.; Rodriguez-Saona, L. E. and Yousef, A. E. (2011). Quality of shell eggs pasteurized with heat or heat-ozone combination during extended storage. *Journal of Food Science*, 76, S437-S444.

Piyasena, P.; Mohareb, E. and McKellar, R. C. (2003). Inactivation of microbes using ultrasound: a review. *International Journal of Food Microbiology*, 87, 207-216.

Raso, J.; Pagán, R.; Condón, S. and Sala, F. J. (1998). Influence of temperature and pressure on the lethality of ultrasound. *Applied and Environmental Microbiology*, 64, 465-471.

Robinson, D. S. (1987). The chemical basis of albumen quality. In R. G. Wells, and C. G. Belyavin (Eds.), Egg Quality - Current Problems and Recent Advances (pp. 171-191). London: Butterworths.

Russell, S. M. (2003). The effect of electrolyzed oxidative water applied using electrostatic spraying on pathogenic and indicator bacteria on the surface of eggs. *Poultry Science*, 82, 158-162.

Ruzickova, V. (1994). Growth and survival of *Salmonella enteritidis* in selected egg foods. *Veterinary Medicine*, 39, 187-195.

Saeed, M. A. and Koons, C. W. (1993). Growth and heat resistance of *Salmonella enteritidis* in refrigerated and abused eggs. *Journal of Food Protection*, 56, 927-931.

Sala, F. J, Burgos, J., Condón, S., López, P., and Raso, J. (1995). Effect of heat and ultrasound on microorganisms and enzymes. In G. W. Gould (Ed.), *New Methods of Food Preservation* (pp. 176-204). London: Blackie Academic and Professional.

Sanz, B., Palacios, P., López, P., and Ordóñez, J. A. (1985). Effect of ultrasonic waves on the heat resistance of *Bacillus stearothermophilus* spores. In G. J. Dring, D. J. Ellar, and G. W. Gould (Eds.), *Fundamental and Applied Aspects of Bacterial Spores* (pp. 251-259). London: Academic Press.

Schaffner, D. F.; Hamdy, M. K.; Toledo, R. T. and Tift, M. L. (1989). *Salmonella* inactivation in liquid whole egg by thermoradiation. *Journal of Food Science*, 54, 902-905.

Schuman, J. D. (2000). Methods for thermal processing of shell eggs. Presented in the 6th annual symposia series on Food Safety in the 21st century: Shell eggs and egg products – safety issues (May 18). Inst. Chicago, IL: Food technologists.

Schuman, J. D. and Sheldon, B. W. (1997). Thermal resistance *of Salmonella* spp. and *Listeria monocytogenes* in liquid egg yolk and egg white. *Journal of Food Protection*, 60, 634-638.

Schuman, J. D.; Sheldon, B. W.; Vandepopuliere, J. M. and Ball Jr., H. R. (1997). Immersion heat treatments for inactivation of *Salmonella enteritidis* with intact eggs. *Journal of Applied Microbiology*, 83, 438-444.

Serrano, L. E.; Murano, E. A.; Shenoy, K. and Olson, D. G. (1997). D values of *Salmonella* Enteritidis isolates and quality attributes of shell eggs and liquid whole eggs treated with irradiation. *Poultry Science*, 76, 202-205.

Seymour, I. J.; Burfoot, D.; Smith, R. L.; Cox, L. A. and Lockwook, A. (2002). Ultrasound decontamination of minimally processed fruits and vegetables. *International Journal of Food Science and Technology*, 37, 547-557.

Shachar, D. and Yaron, S. (2007). Heat tolerance of *Salmonella enterica* serovars Agona, Enteritidis, and Typhimurium in peanut butter. *Journal of Food Protection*, 69, 2687-2691.

Shah, B. D.; Bradshaw, J. G. and Peeler, J. T. (1991). Thermal resistance of egg-associated epidemic strains of *Salmonella enteritidis*. *Journal of Food Science*, 56, 391-393.

Silliker, J. H., and Gabis, D. A. (1986). *Salmonella*. In A. M., Pearson, and T. R. Duston (Eds.), *Advances in Meat Research*, vol 2: Meat and Poultry Microbiology (pp. 209-229). New York: Elsevier.

Simmons, E. R.; Ayres, J. C. and Kraft, A. A. (1970). Effect of moisture and temperature on ability of salmonellae to infect shell eggs. *Poultry Science*, 49, 761-768.

Smith, S. E.; Maurer, J. L.; Orta-Ramírez, A.; Ryser, E. T. and Smith, D. M. (2001). Thermal inactivation of *Salmonella* spp., *Salmonella* Typhimurium, and *Escherichia coli* O157:H7 in ground beef. *Journal of Food Science*, 66, 1164-1168.

Stadelman, W. J. (1994). Contaminants of liquid egg products. Contaminants of liquid egg products. In G. Board, and R. Fuller (Eds.), *Microbiology of the Avian Egg* (pp. 139-151). London: Chapman and Hall Ltd.

Stadelman, W. J. (1995). Quality identification of shell eggs. In W. J., and Stadelman O. J. Cotterill (Eds.), *Egg Science and technology* (pp. 39-66). New York: The Haworth Press.

Stadelman, W. J.; Singh, R. K.; Muriana, P. M. and Hou, H. (1996). Pasteurization of eggs in the shell. *Poultry Science*, 75, 1122-1125.

Summer, S. S.; Sandros, T. M.; Harmon, M. C.; Scott, V. N. and Bernard, D. T. (1991). Heat resistance of *Salmonella typhimurium* and *Listeria monocytogenes* in sucrose solutions of various water activities. *Journal of Food Science*, 56, 1741-1743.

Takahashi, N.; Koseki, T.; Doi, E. and Hirose, M. J. (1991). Role of an intrachain disulfide bond in the conformation and stability of ovalbumin. *Journal of Biochemistry*, 109, 846-851.

Téllez, I. G.; Trejo, R. M.; Sánchez, R. E.; Ceniceros, R. M.; Luna, Q. P.; Zazua, P. and Hargis, B. M. (1995). Effect of gamma irradiation on commercial eggs experimentally inoculated with *Salmonella* Enteritidis. *Radiation Physics and Chemistry*, 46, 789-792.

Thomas, C. T.; White, J. C. and Longreé, K. (1966). Thermal resistance of *Salmonellae* and *Staphylococci* in foods. *Applied Microbiology*, 14, 815-820.

Tuncan, E. U. and Scott, E. M. (1989). Combined effect of sucrose and heat treatment temperature in the thermal resistance of *Staphylococcus aureus* MF-31. *Journal of Food Science*, 54, 936-939.

USDA. 1969. Egg pasteurization manual. ARS 74-48. Poultry Laboratory, Department of Agriculture, Albany, California, Agriculture Research Service United States.

Van Lith, L. A. J. T.; Putirulan, F. F. and Mulder, R. W. A. W. (1995). Pasteurization of table eggs to eliminate salmonellae. *Archiv für Geflügelkunde*, 59, 157-160.

Volmer, G., Josst, G., Schenker, D., Sturm, N., and Vreden, N. (1999). Huevos, leche y quesos. *Elementos de Bromatología Descriptiva* (pp. 365-376). Zaragoza: Acribia, S.A.

Vought, K. J. and Tatini, S. R. (1998). *Salmonella enteritidis* contamination of ice cream associated with a 1994 multistate outbreak. *Journal of Food Protection*, 61, 5-10.

Watkins, B. A. (1995). The nutritive value of eggs. In W. J. Stadelman, and O. J. Cotterill (Eds.), *Egg Science and Technology* (pp. 177-194). New York: The Haworth Press.

Weissinger, W. R.; Chantarapanont, W. and Beuchat, L. R. (2000). Survival and growth of *Salmonella baildon* in shredded lettuce and diced tomatoes, and effectiveness of chlorinated water as a sanitizer. *International Journal of Food Microbiology*, 62, 123-131.

Wesierska E., (2006). Czynniki jakości mikrobiologicznej spożywczych jaj kurzych. *Medycyna Weterynaryjna*, 62, 1222–1228.

Williams, A. (1994). New technologies in food processing: Part II. *Nutrition and Food Science,* 1, 20-23.

Worley, B. S.; Wheatley, W. B.; Lauten, S. D.; Willians, D. E.; Mora, E. C. and Worley, S. D. (1992). Inactivation of *Salmonella* Enteritidis on shell eggs by novel N-halamine biocidal compounds. *Journal of Industrial Microbiology*, 11, 37-42.

Wrigley, D. M. and Llorca, N. G. (1992). Decrease of *Salmonella typhimurium* in skim milk and egg by heat and ultrasonic wave treatment. *Journal of Food Protection*, 55, 678-680.

Yang, S. C., and Baldwin, R. E. (1995). Functional properties of eggs in foods. In W. J. Stadelman, and O. J. Cotterill (Eds.), *Egg Science and Technology* (4 ed., pp. 405-463). Binghamton, NY: The Haworth Press, Inc.

Zeidler, G. (2001). Processing and packaging shell eggs. In D. D. Bell, and D. Weaver Jr. (Eds.), *Commercial chicken meat and egg production* (pp. 1129-1161). Norwell, MA: Kluwer Academic Publishers.

Zwietering, M. (2005). Practical considerations on food safety objectives. *Food Control*, 16, 817-823.

In: Salmonella: Classification, Genetics and Disease Outbreaks ISBN: 978-1-61942-928-4
Editors: Adelaide S. Monte, Paulo Eduardo De Santos

Chapter 4

SALMONELLA ENTERICA SURVIVAL TO BIOCIDES AND ANTIBIOTICS – AN OVERVIEW OF RESISTANCE MECHANISMS AND GENE EXPRESSION

Diana Rodrigues and Joana Azeredo
Institute for Biotechnology and Bioengineering,
Centre of Biological Engineering, University of Minho,
Campus de Gualtar, Braga, Portugal

ABSTRACT

Nowadays, *Salmonella* spp. is still considered one of the major foodborne pathogens, being responsible for thousands of deaths worldwide and widespread economic losses every year. *Salmonella enterica* strains have proven to be highly adaptable and able to survive in the external environment, and their ability to respond effectively to environmental changes is important in their survival in the food chain. Moreover, like many other microorganisms, *S. enterica* is able to adhere and form biofilms on several different surfaces, which increases its inherent resistance and, thus, significantly affects plant sanitation and product safety. Bacterial resistance to antimicrobial agents in general, as well as the underlying mechanisms, have been widely studied by several authors. Additionally, a number of scientists have recently expressed concern that the common and indiscriminate use of biocides may be a contributing factor to the development and selection of antibiotic-resistant strains, giving rise to a phenomenon known as "cross-resistance". In this context, the present chapter intends to review the scientific results concerning the mechanisms by which *S. enterica* planktonic and biofilm cells may become resistant to biocides action, as well as the relation between biocide and antibiotic resistance by this foodborne pathogen. Moreover, genomic aspects involved in such adaptive and resistant behaviours will also be considered.

List of Terms

Acquired resistance
Active compound
Active efflux
Adaptive resistance
Antibiotic
Antimicrobial agent
Antiseptics
Bacterial resistance
Bactericidal
Bacteriostatic
Biocide
Biofilm
Chemotherapeutic agent
Conjugative transfer
Cross-contamination
Cross-resistance
Disinfection
Efflux pump
Food safety
Genetic transformation
Horizontal gene transfer
Hydrophobicity
Integron
Intrinsic resistance
Mutation
Plasmid
Sub-inhibitory concentration
Sub-lethal concentration
Transmission vehicles
Transposon

Introduction

Bacterial food poisoning continues to be an important health problem worldwide, with numerous foodborne disease outbreaks and deaths recorded every year. The European Food Safety Authority [1] reported a total of 5,550 foodborne outbreaks in the European Union in 2008, causing 48,964 human infection cases, 4,356 hospitalizations, and 46 deaths. The same entity [1] also stated that most of the reported outbreaks were caused by *Salmonella enterica*, confirming that this organism is still one of the most important foodborne pathogens. Although primarily intestinal bacteria, *S. enterica* are widespread in the environment and commonly found in farm effluents, human sewage, and in any material subject to faecal contamination. Salmonellosis has been recognized in all countries but appears to be most prevalent in areas with intensive animal husbandry, especially poultry and swine production.

Inadequate cleaning and disinfection of food-processing facilities is the cause of major economic losses and represents a serious danger to public health. In fact, several studies have shown that the presence of microorganisms on food contact surfaces is one of the most common causes of food spoilage and transmission of foodborne diseases [2, 3, 4]. Moreover, bacteria ability to adhere and form biofilms makes disinfection even more difficult and challenging [5, 6, 7]. Accordingly, the efficacy of the most common commercial products used for surfaces cleaning and disinfection - which are mainly based on phenolic compounds, organic acids, alcohols, chlorine, quaternary ammonium compounds (QACs), and iodophors - has been reported to be higher against bacterial suspensions than against adhered cells and biofilms [8, 9, 10]. *S. enterica* fits this scenario perfectly, since there are numerous reports showing that this bacterium is able to adhere and form biofilms on many different surfaces found in food processing plants [2, 11, 12, 13], and is also capable to resist biocides action both as planktonic cells [14, 15, 16] and biofilms [17, 18, 19, 20].

Besides the serious problem of bacterial resistance to biocides, there are also studies that point out a possible relation between such resistance behaviour and a lower susceptibility to antibiotics, a phenomenon known as "cross-resistance". Indeed, it has been thought that some biocides and antibiotics may have similar behaviours and characteristics in the way they act and in the way bacteria develop resistance to them [21, 22, 23, 24]. Such occurrences have also been studied concerning *S. enterica* cells and, although only *in vitro* studies have been performed till know, there are evidence that these bacteria can indeed become more resistant to antibiotic when previously exposed to biocides [e.g. 15]. For *S. enterica*, as for bacteria in general, the resistance to biocides and/or antibiotics is based on various different mechanisms that have been discovered over the years. Such mechanisms can be intrinsic or acquired, include various different processes, and involve cellular modifications that can go as deep as the genetic level.

S. Enterica as a (Persistent) Food Safety Problem

Besides all efforts and improvements regarding food safety, foodborne illness outbreaks are still very often reported and have a really serious impact on public-health. As mentioned before, salmonellosis is one of most common foodborne illness, with numerous reports from worldwide confirming this fact every year. The chain of the events related with the occurrence of salmonellosis has been quite complex and dissimilar along the time. At the beginning of the 1970s, numerous reports of human salmonellosis caused by *S. enterica* Agona in Europe and in the United States of America were related with the ingestion of chicken from Peru which feed contained fish meal [25]. After that, in the 1980s, *S. enterica* Enteritidis found in eggs and contaminated chicken was the major responsible for worldwide outbreaks of human salmonellosis. In this case, it is believed that breeders and laying hens were infected by rodent faeces and urine, and the bacterium was vertically transmitted, infecting their progeny. Additionally, in the same epoch, outbreaks of human salmonellosis resultant from ingestion of pork and beef meat contaminated with *Salmonella* serovars have been reported in several nations [26, 27, 28], with *S. enterica* Typhimurium being the major serotype implicated. Both kinds of meat were possibly contaminated during the slaughter followed by insufficient cooking.

Although the infectious dose of *S. enterica* is believe to be about 1 to 10^9 cfu/g, single-food-source outbreaks indicate that just 1 to 10 cells can be enough to cause salmonellosis in people belonging to the YOPI (young, old, pregnant and immune-compromised) groups, which are more susceptibility to infection [29, 30]. Moreover, the infectious dose may also vary depending on the bacterial strain, serovar, growth condition and host susceptibility, this last including the condition of the intestinal tract, age and underlying diseases or immune insufficiencies. In general, humans get infected with *S. enterica* when eating food or drinking water contaminated with these bacteria through animal reservoirs. Concerning *S. enterica* Typhi and *S. enterica* Paratyphi A, although they do not have animal reservoir, contamination can occur by eating the inappropriately handled food by infected persons [31].

Main Transmission Vehicles

S. enterica are broadly disseminated in nature and they survive well in a diversity of foods. Dairy products, poultry, and eggs are the most ordinary vehicles of salmonellosis. Moreover, these bacteria are among the most commonly found in fresh fruit and vegetables [32], which is an important fact since, in recent years, the occurrence of foodborne outbreaks caused by the contamination of fresh fruits and vegetables has increased and become a huge concern in developed countries. Accordingly, outbreaks of salmonellosis have been related to an extensive diversity of vegetables and fresh fruits including parsley, alfalfa sprout, lettuce, tomato, apple, cantaloupe, melon, mango, and unpasteurized orange juice [33]. The human health risk is further enhanced by *Salmonella* favouritism to grow on fresh products during retail exhibition at ambient temperature. As an example, cantaloupe from Mexico was responsible for a *S.* Poona outbreak in USA, in 2000 [34, 35]. In this way, the role of vegetables as vehicle for pathogens diffusion has become clear and frequent, showing that significant health problems can occur from ingestion of contaminated vegetables if sanitation practices fail.

Disease surveillance reports frequently recognize poultry (ducks, chickens, geese, and turkeys) as the major vehicles in the salmonellosis outbreak. Moreover, *S. enterica* can penetrate eggs from the oviduct (particularly ducks), with infiltration into the egg being enhanced when the cuticle is damaged, the exterior of the egg is wet, temperature is reduced and/or specific gravity of the shell is low. Contamination of eggs, and principally egg contents by *S. enterica* Enteritidis, are assumed the main cause of the incidence of salmonellosis in Europe and North America since 1980s [30, 36]. The US Centres for Disease Control and Prevention had recently stated that there were about 1,469 diseases related with eggs infected by *S. enterica* Enteritidis accounted in Minnesota, California, and Colorado between May and August of 2010 [37].

Red-meat and red-meat products are also known as a significant source of human salmonellosis. In 2007 alone, for example, food items based on pork and beef meat that contained *Salmonella* were the cause of 37 outbreaks in Europe, with 800 cases of human salmonellosis reported [38]. Numerous other cases have been documented concerning human salmonellosis outbreaks related with ingestion of contaminated or improperly cooked red meat [39, 40, 41, 42, 43]. Due to their animal derivation, dairy products can as well be related with human foodborne salmonellosis. Since pasteurization of milk and dairy products kills *Salmonella* serovars, milk-borne salmonellosis is usuallly associated to the ingestion of unprocessed or improperly pasteurized milk. Nevertheless, *Salmonella* serovars can also contaminate dairy products following the pasteurization procedure [44]. As a recent example, an outbreak of human salmonellosis related with cheese was described in Switzerland, where a national outbreak of gastrointestinal illness caused by *S. enterica* Stanley (an uncommon serovar in Europe) took place between September 2006 and February 2007. The mentioned bacteria were found on a local soft cheese and in 94% of the infected persons, and the problem was solved by the removal of the cheese from the market [45].

On the other hand, the dissemination of this pathogen to the food processing plants and equipments for food preparation is also of great significance. As mentioned before, *S. enterica* cells can adhere to various different food contact surfaces, may then develop into a biofilm, and consequently cause cross-contamination. Therefore, these bacteria can enter the food chain at any point from animals feed, to food manufacturing, processing and transaction, as well food preparation in restaurants and in the home [46].

S. Enterica Resistance to Biocides and Cross-Resistance to Antibiotics

Antiseptics, disinfectants and preservatives (generally called "biocides") are freely obtainable without prescription, unlike antibiotics, and therefore are used on a daily basis in abattoirs, farms, homes, schools, restaurants, hospitals, other work places and in health care products [47, 48, 49, 50]. Moreover, increasing worries over the transmission of food-borne illnesses have led to a fast increase in the application of biocidal agents in industry and homes. This has raised the concern that the random and improper application of such products (including deficient cleaning prior to the application, inadequate concentrations, or the existence of sub-lethal remaining disinfectants following cleaning) might enhance not only the development of bacterial resistance to biocides but also the possible cross-resistance to certain therapeutic antibiotics. Several studies over this subject have been done and some of them proved the likelihood for this phenomenon to take place, inclusively as far as *S. enterica* is concerned [51, 52, 53].

Resistance to Biocides

Biocides are generally a mixture of active compounds and, as a result, usually have multiple, nonspecific modes of action to destroy bacteria. As a consequence, contrasting to what usually happens with antibiotic resistance, any resistance to biocides is improbable to occur by a single mutational step [48, 54]. So, for high-level biocide resistance to occur as a consequence of target site mutations it may be necessary that repeated selection events and modification of a number of target proteins take place. Nevertheless, low susceptibility of bacteria to biocides was first reported back in the 1950s and 1960s, and seems to be ever-increasing [49]. A general example concerns the use of cationic agents – such as triclosan (TLN), quaternary ammonium compounds (QACs), and chlorhexidine (CHX) - which are believed to be on the basis of the selection and persistence of bacterial cells that can resist antimicrobials and biocides action through mechanisms as active efflux, nonspecific alteration of the cell envelope, and degradation [47, 49, 51].

In the next sub-sections are presented in more detail three particular aspects involved in biocide resistance by *S. enterica*. The first one is related with biofilm associated tolerance, which is an ever-increasing worry among food producers and consumers, as well as a very interesting research subject due to the significant differences found between planktonic and biofilm cells' response to biocides. *S. enterica* cell surface alterations will also be addressed since the outer layer of bacterial cells is the first part of the organism to interacts with the foreign bodies, substances and compounds, playing a crucial role in cell interaction with the surrounding environment and being the first stage of cell defense. Finally, as one of the most common and relevant resistance mechanisms, active efflux could not be excluded from this chapter, and some more detailed information about *S. enterica* will be presented.

Biofilm Associated Tolerance

As mentioned above, *S. enterica* has the ability to form biofilms in several distinct food contact surfaces. This bacterial life form has been considered the best example of how physiological adjustment might be a factor in achieving intrinsic resistance [47, 55], and it is also accepted that diverse stresses (such as starvation, chemical stress, and desiccation) suffered by the surface associated microbes are favourable for the expansion of improved resistance to disinfection by *S. enterica* [56, 57]. Biofilms have been reported as possessing susceptibilities towards biocides that are 100–1000 times less than equivalent populations of free-floating counterparts [58], and there is mounting evidence that microorganisms in biofilms actively respond to chemical challenges [57]. Accordingly, there are reports that bacteria in biofilms can respond to biocide treatment by increasing the synthesis of extracellular polymeric substances (EPS) that contribute to the matrix of the biofilm [59, 60]. While biofilms are exposed to chemical agents, reaction-diffusion limited penetration might result in only low levels of the biocidal agent reaching the deeper regions of biofilms [57]. Thus, the sheltered cells are then able to enter an adapted-resistant state if the local time scale for adaptation is faster than that of disinfection, and this mechanism is not available to a planktonic population [57]. It has also been proposed that biofilm resistance can be achieved by the extracellular matrix capability to respond to the biocidal challenge and, consequently, neutralize the active agent involved [61]. Moreover, nutrient and oxygen reduction inside the biofilm lead some bacteria to go into a non-growing (i.e., stationary or even dormant) state [62, 63], in which they are less vulnerable to growth-dependent chemical killing [64]. Moreover, quorum-sensing (i.e., cell-to-cell signalling) molecules can make biofilm cells to alter their gene expression patterns, allowing a subpopulation of biofilm bacteria to differentiate into a phenotypically resistant state [65].

Mangalappalli-Illathu *et al.* [66] investigated the mechanisms underneath the adaptive resistance or tolerance in *Salmonella enterica* Enteritidis biofilms following exposure to sub-lethal concentration of benzalkonium chloride (BAC). BAC is a nitrogen-based surface-active QAC with a broad-spectrum antimicrobial activity, commonly used as a cationic surfactant and disinfectant for processing lines and surfaces in the food industry. Because of their positive charge, QACs establish electrostatic bonds with negatively charged sites on bacterial cell walls, destabilizing the cell wall and cytoplasmic membrane, promoting cell lysis, leakage and death [47, 67]. These compounds are known to be bacteriostatic at low concentrations and bactericidal at high concentrations [68], which means that low concentrations of this biocide can enhance the emergence of adaptive resistance. Diverse resistance mechanisms, such as slime production, modifications in membrane fatty acid composition, degradation of the biocides, efflux pumps, and the alteration of targets, are believed to be involved in the adaptive resistance against QACs [e.g. 67, 69, 70]. Mangalappalli-Illathu *et al.* [66] studied the capability of *S. enterica* Enteritidis biofilms to survive lethal exposure and to re-grow in the presence of BAC after adaptation to this biocide, as a way to get more information about the subjacent mechanisms of development of adaptive resistance. These authors also compared the protein expression patterns of adapted and wild-type *S. enterica* biofilm cells in order to clarify the major biochemical patterns involved in the acquisition of adaptive resistance to BAC. It was observed that BAC-adapted *S. enterica* Enteritidis biofilms gained the capacity to endure a usually lethal exposure to BAC and then re-grow [66]. Simultaneously to the adaptation process it was found a general increase in protein biosynthesis, including proteins from the energy metabolism (TpiA and Eno), amino acid and protein biosynthesis (WrbA, TrxA, RplL, Tsf, Tuf, DsbA, and RpoZ), nutrient binding (FruB), adaptation (CspA), and degradation of 1,2-propanediol (PduJ and PduA). Moreover, it was observed an up-regulation of key proteins related with detoxification (Tpx, SodB, and a possible peroxidise), cold shock response (DegQ), and stress response (YnaF). The up-regulation of such significant proteins by *S. enterica* Enteritidis biofilm cells clarifies the mechanisms involved in their adaptive resistance to BAC.

Cell Surface Alterations

The nature and composition of the surface differs between cell types (or entities), but might also change as a consequence of modifications in the environment [55, 71]. Although there can be major consequences on viability related with interaction at the cell surface [72, 73], the active agents of most biocides have intracellular targets [74, 75]. The outermost layers of microbial cells might, thus, have an important effect on their vulnerability (or resistance) to biocides and antibiotics. Chemical and physical agents interfere with the fatty acid profiles of bacterial cells, which modifications have been pointed out as a mechanism of adaptation and survival [76, 77, 78]. The first step of bactericidal action is connecting to the bacterial cell surface to then cross the outer membrane (gram negative) or cell wall (gram positive) in order to get to its site of action at the cytoplasm or cytoplasmic membrane. The gram negative cell envelope has adjusted itself in order to control the transport of compounds into and out of the cell to an extraordinary level of specificity. Apart from peptidoglycan (which is squishy and, thus, permeable), all the parts of the cell envelope have a function in the obstruction mechanisms. Moreover, cell surface charge has also been reported to be relevant for bacterial resistance mechanisms against positively charged antibacterial agents [79], and cell hydrophobicity has been considered a significant property for the bacterial cell, since changes of surface hydrophobicity influences the bacterial reaction to biocides [80].

Mangalappalli *et al.* [81] had examined the ability of BAC-adapted and non-adapted planktonic and biofilm *S. enterica* cell populations to adapt to and survive a range of BAC concentrations. These authors found that fatty acid composition was considerably influenced by phenotype (biofilm or planktonic cells) and BAC adaptation, and that cell surface roughness was also much higher on biofilm cells than on planktonic cells. It was also observed that adaptation to BAC lead to an up-regulation of key proteins, both in planktonic and biofilm *S. enterica* cells, which were related to cold adaptation, protein translation and modification, biosynthesis, and detoxification [81]. On another work, Braoudaki and Hilton [82] had studied the potential for adaptive resistance of *S. enterica* Enteritidis, Typhimurium and Virchow to increasing sub-lethal concentrations of TLN, erythromycin, and BAC, by assessing permeability modifications of the outer membrane, including hydrophobicity, lipopolysaccharides (LPS), and cell surface charge. Even though these authors had not found noteworthy alterations when examining the outer membrane and LPS, the majority of the pre-adapted strains were remarkably less hydrophobic than resistant strains. Moreover, it was observed an increased cell surface hydrophobicity related with erythromycin resistance in *S. enterica* Enteritidis and *S. enterica* Typhimurium, which was quite unpredicted as erythromycin is a hydrophobic compound [82]. Finally, concerning the cell surface charge, this parameter was observed to be extensively more negative in the erythromycin adapted *S. enterica* Virchow when contrasted to the parent strain. Likewise, even though without statistical meaning, all BAC- and TLN-resistant *S. enterica* strains had also noteworthy alteration in the charge of the cell [82].

Active Efflux

Bacterial cells can achieve a higher tolerance to biocides by triggering a system usually called efflux pump, which decreases the effectiveness of biocides by "pumping out" lethal compounds. Efflux pumps can perform on numerous chemically different compounds, [83], with efflux determinants of biocide resistance exhibiting broad substrate specificity, including a range of structurally dissimilar agents that might also comprise antibiotics [84, 85, 86, 87]. Efflux pumps are extremely conserved, are effective in a broad range of gram-negative organisms, and can also be carried on plasmids [85]. There are five main families of efflux pumps, each one of them including pumps that are specific for single agents as well as pumps that can perform multidrug efflux. Such families are: the multidrug and toxic compound extrusion (MATE) family [88], the small multidrug resistance (SMR) family [89] - now described as part of the larger drug/metabolite transporter (DMT) superfamily [90] -, the resistance-nodulation-division (RND) family [85, 91], the major facilitator superfamily (MFS) [92], and the ATP-binding cassette (ABC) family [93]. Multidrug efflux pumps have broader specificity and are able to eliminate from the cell a high variety of structurally unrelated antibiotics and disinfectants. It is likely that these exporters developed initially to eliminate endogenous metabolites, but that a coincident capability to extrude harmful compounds has shown to be an advantageous survival approach that has been selected for, and included, by nearly all identified genus and species of bacterium. It is also important to realize that efflux pumps as a resistance mechanism are not limited to gram-negative bacteria. The multidrug efflux pumps *qacA* to *qacG* are involved in biocide lower susceptibility in *Staphylococcus aureus* [94], as can be found in already published scientific reviews [95, 96].

Like other bacteria, *Salmonella* has a big set off of transporters with nine identified multidrug efflux systems [97]. AcrAB-TolC is the main multidrug efflux pump in numerous Gram-negative bacteria, and its over-expression in *Salmonella* cells has been reported to happen when these bacteria contacts with small dosages of biocide [98, 99]. While AcrAB is the most important system, expression of other RND pumps (AcrEF and AcrD) is co-ordinately regulated with AcrAB in *Salmonella*, and AcrEF is able to functionally complement AcrAB [100]. Randall *et al.* [98] had tried to determine if only one passage of *S. enterica* Typhimurium in the presence of farm biocides would selected for mutants with reduced vulnerability to biocides and/or antibiotics. The disinfectants tested were a tar oil phenol (which was a blend of high boiling point tar acids and organic acids), an oxidizing compound based disinfectant, an aldehyde based disinfectant, and a dairy sterilizing disinfectant (which comprised a quaternary ammonium biocide, non-ionic surfactant and excipients). Their results showed that efflux pumps are necessary for intrinsic resistance to some biocides, and that contact with such chemical agents might trigger expression of the AcrAB–TolC efflux system. In fact, after exposure to a tar oil phenol (one of the biocides tested) it was observed a significant over-expression of proteins related to efflux and its involvement in disinfectant tolerance, including the AcrAB/ TolC efflux pump, EmrA multidrug efflux pump, and others proteins involved in detoxification of hydroperoxides (AhpC and AhpE) and pyruvate dehydrogenase (AceE and AceF) [98]. Nevertheless, the authors also observed that a single contact between *S. enterica* cells and the biocides was not enough to select for multiply antibiotic-resistant (MAR) strains. In contrast, a very recent work performed by Whitehead *et al.* [101], aiming at analyzing *S. enterica* Typhimurium response to biocides with different modes of action, have shown that *S. enterica* cells can survive challenge with biocides at recommended-use concentration, and that a single contact with such biocide concentrations can be sufficient to select mutant cells with efflux mediated multidrug resistance. The authors confirmed these findings through gene expression examination which revealed AcrEF multidrug efflux pump to be de-repressed in the mutants that survived the biocides action [101].

Cross-Resistance to Antibiotics: Recent Studies and General Mechanisms Involved

Various organisms are resistant to some antimicrobial agents because of their natural metabolic characteristics (intrinsic resistance), while others can develop mechanisms to defend themselves [102]. Cell membrane function and the synthesis of cell wall, nucleic acid and protein are the four major targets for antibiotic action on bacteria. Although the overall mechanism of action of biocides is different from the antibiotics - as previously mentioned and reported by other authors [103, 104] -, adaptive resistance to QACs by long lasting sub-lethal exposure, as well as the cross-resistance of adapted strains to antimicrobial chemotherapeutic agents (such as trimethoprim, amoxicillin, tetracycline, and clavulanic acid, among others) and other biocides (CHX and TLN), have been reported concerning different bacteria as *Pseudomonas fluorescens* [67], *Serratia marcescens* [105], *Pseudomonas aeruginosa* [106, 107], *Escherichia coli* [51, 70, 108], and *Salmonella enterica* [51]. Accordingly, there have been increasing evidences that permanent and unrestrained use of antibacterial agents can considerably enhance bacterial resistance, and that there are numerous resemblances in the way bacteria are capable to defend themselves from antibiotics and biocides [52]. Such mechanisms can be of intrinsic or acquired nature and comprise, among others, modification of the antibiotic itself, reduced drug accumulation, alteration of the target, and reduced permeability (Table 1) [109]. Moreover, as also mentioned before, active efflux mechanisms are also gradually more implicated in bacterial drug resistance [83]. In fact, it has been thought that the cross-resistance between unrelated drugs can be caused by the expression of efflux mechanisms. A variety of structures concerning efflux pumps have been described, and a single protein can operate alone to perform efflux. Conventional efflux pumps expel just one drug or one class of drugs, while a multidrug efflux system is capable to propel out a broad variety of compounds [83, 110]. Taking into account this overall scenario, the rising concerns and the increasing interest of scientists regarding the relation between disinfectant exposures and selection of antibiotic resistant bacteria [49, 52] are perfectly justified. Some recent studies on this subject matter regarding *S. enterica* were selected and will now be presented here.

Table 1. Bacterial resistance mechanisms against biocides and antibiotics

Mechanism	Nature
Decrease of membrane permeability	Intrinsic
Active efflux	Intrinsic
Decreased accumulation (plasmid-mediated efflux)	Acquired
Enzymatic modification	Acquired
Enzymatic inactivation	Intrinsic / Acquired
Overproduction of target	Acquired
Alteration of the target site	Acquired
Bypass of sensitive step	Acquired
Absence of enzyme–metabolic pathway	Acquired

As mentioned above, the addition of biocides such as TLN, BAC, and CHX in home cleaning and sanitation products has turned into a worryingly common practice. Braoudaki and Hilton [111] studied the existence of a possible relation between adaptive resistance to biocides and cross-resistance to other antibacterial agents in *S. enterica*. In this study, when strains were recurrently exposed to sub-inhibitory amounts of biocides or antibiotics, it was found a significant level of cross-resistance to a variety of both kinds of antimicrobial agents in *S. enterica* Virchow, while an inferior level was found in *S. enterica* Typhimurium and *S. enterica* Enteritidis. The same authors have also observed that adaptive resistance was rapidly reached, and that cross-resistance in adaptively resistant *S. enterica* was different according with the serotype. In fact, *S. enterica* Typhimurium was cross-resistant to CHX, while *S. enterica* Enteritidis showed to be cross-resistant to chloramphenicol. Moreover, *S. enterica* Virchow resistant to BAC revealed a high resistance to CHX, but CHX-resistant *S. enterica* Virchow did not express cross-resistance to BAC, which indicates the existence of specific resistance mechanisms [111].

Multiply antibiotic-resistance (MAR) of *S. enterica* Typhimurium cells is related with lower susceptibility to disinfectants and antibiotics (as tetracyclines, β-lactams, fluoroquinolones, and chloramphenicol), and higher tolerance to organic solvents [112, 113, 114]. The selection of MAR corresponds to a serious problem since these kinds of strains can be the launching pad to high-level resistance in *S. enterica* [113, 114, 115]. Furthermore, it has been reported that chemicals that have phenolic rings can de-repress the multiple antibiotic resistance locus *marRAB* leading to a higher efflux [112] which, as mentioned before, is frequently pointed out as a resistance mechanism to both biocides and antibiotics [83]. Randall *et al* [115] have verified that growth of *S. enterica* with sub-inhibitory concentrations of farm disinfectants conduced to a low but statistically significant enhancement in isolation of MAR strains, which were latter distinguished when subjected to cyclohexane or antibiotics [115, 116]. Moreover, in several cases, the degree of resistance to antibiotics was even clinically significant, which was mainly clear for the MAR strains subjected to ciprofloxacin.

In a more recent study, Karatzas *et al.* [117] have also found that long-lasting exposure to disinfectants can lead to a lower susceptibility to numerous antibiotics and biocides, which can be related to reduced levels of outer membrane proteins and over-expression of acrAB-tolC. Since these are efflux pumps that have the ability to perform on a variety of chemically different compounds - biocides and antibiotics included [83] -, with this work the authors verified a earlier supposition that active efflux might be a linking relation between disinfectant resistance and antibiotic resistance [83, 113]. With the same work, Karatzas *et al.* [117] have also demonstrated that this outcome frequently takes place together with over-expression of numerous stress proteins, lower motility and invasiveness, and enhanced RNA and protein synthesis. Moreover, a number of variants also showed larger amounts of the shorter O-antigen chains, higher substrate level phosphorylation, and lower oxidative level phosphorylation.

Genomic Aspects of Resistance

Antimicrobial resistance is the finest illustration of fast adjustment of bacteria to a novel ecosystem. The capacity of bacteria to enlarge their ecological niche, inclusively when in contact with antibiotics, might be understood by the addition of specific mutations that ends in the alteration of existing genes and/or in the acquirement of resistance genes by horizontal gene transfer. Numerous *S. enterica* resistance genes have been reported (Table 2), and most of them are found in extra-chromosomal genetic elements or in segments inside the chromosome that come from other genomes. Nevertheless, an acquirement of a novel gene can take place, either by genetic transformation or conjugative transfer, this last case when resistance genes are situated on plasmids (self-replicating double-stranded rings of DNA). Moreover, conjugative transfer can happen at high rate and effectiveness, with the possibility of numerous resistance genes being incorporated at the same time [118]. Resistance genes fixed in plasmids are frequently positioned inside genetic elements named transposons, which comprise the transposase function that allows the transposon to recombine into the bacterial chromosome or plasmids. A resistance gene present in a plasmid positioned inside a transposon or an integron) can be relocated to other strains and species, which allows it to access niches that were not reachable to its original host strain [119]. The importance of plasmids for the propagation of antimicrobial resistance in *S. enterica* was reviewed by Carattoli [120], where it was highlighted the involvement of plasmid-mediated resistance against antimicrobials normally used in human treatment. In fact, genes such as *spvA*, *spvB* and *spvC* (salmonella plasmid virulence), and the *rck* (resistance to complement killing) - which are known to enhance colonization and resistance to complement killing [121] - are encoded in host-adapted virulence plasmids found in numerous *S. enterica* isolates.

Table 2. S. enterica genes involved in resistance against biocides and/or antibiotics

Gene or locus	Encoded protein / Putative function
rck	Involved in resistance to human complement
qepA	Quinolone efflux pump / Extrudes hydrophilic fluoroquinolones including ciprofloxacin from the bacterial cell
fabI	Enoyl-acyl carrier protein reductase/ Involved in fatty acid biosynthesis
acr	Multi-drug efflux pumps
fnr	Global regulator of virulence and anaerobic metabolism
soxS	Regulon / Direct activator of genes for resistance to both oxidants and antibiotics
tet	Tetracycline resistance
aadB	Gentamicin resistance
cat, floR	Chloramphenicol / florphenicol resistance
aac	Aminoglycoside acetyltransferase variant gene / Confers resistance to aminoglycosides
bla	β-lactam resistance
ompF	Outer membrane protein – Porin / Associated with reduced susceptibility to antimicrobial compounds
marA	The major regulator of the genetic cascade controlling multi-drug resistance / Resistance to several antibiotics ad superoxide-generating agents
tolC	Outer membrane efflux channel / Specific tolerance to colicin E1; segregation of daughter chromosomes; role in organic solvent tolerance
ramA	Transcriptional regulator / Implicated in resistance to multiple antibiotics
qnr	Plasmid-mediated quinolone resistance
spv	Operon common to all *Salmonella* virulence plasmids / Associated with multidrug-resistance

As mentioned, mobile genetic elements such as integrons, plasmids, and transposons can propagate antibiotic resistance genes by vertical or horizontal transmission, and revealed to have a significant part in the development and diffusion of multidrug resistance in Gram-negative bacteria [122, 123, 124]. Integrons are genetic elements with the capacity to detain gene cassettes from the environment and fit them in by through site-specific recombination. Mainly related with the components of the Tn21 or Tn402 transposon family, Class 1 integrons are the most extensively distributed ones between the elements of the family *Enterobacteriaceae* [125], with several of the *S. enterica* serovars included [126, 115]. Integrons of this class enclose a 50 conserved segment (50-CS) with the integrase gene intI1, the attI1 recombination site and the promoter, usually followed by a variable region corresponding to one or more resistance gene cassettes. Most of the class 1 integrons also include a 30 conserved segment (30-CS) of variable length that generally consists of qacED1 (which encodes minor resistance to a number of antiseptics), the sul1 gene (that encodes sulphonamide resistance), and two open reading frames - orf5 and orf6 [127]. On the other hand, class 2 integrons are related with the Tn7 transposon family and, until now, have just been found in *S. enterica* Typhimurium and *S. enterica* Paratyphi B [D-tartrate positive (dT+)] [128, 129]. A study performed by Miko *et al.* [130], where distinct serovars of *S. enterica* obtained from German foodstuffs were used, has corroborated the extensive variety of resistance mechanisms intervening in antimicrobial resistance. In this work, 75.5% of the examined multidrug-resistant (MDR) *Salmonella* isolates revealed to hold class 1 or class 2 integrons, which indicates the significant part of such genetic elements in the intricacy of antimicrobial resistance dynamics. Since class 1 integrons have turn out to be incorporated into the chromosome in MDR DT104 and its relatives, they can persevere even in the lack of antimicrobial selection and with no noticeable burden to the cell. In Germany, this has motivated a steady and broadly dispersion of MDR clones in farm animals and foodstuff [129, 131]. Miko *et al.* [130] have also pointed out that, although until now all gene cassettes within the non-SGI1 class 1 integrons have been related with resistance to chloramphenicol, 'older' aminoglycosides (as streptomycin/ spectinomycin and gentamicin), trimethoprim, and β-lactams, the incorporation of genes that allow resistance to antimicrobials of superior generations might just be a matter of time.

Resistance to fluoroquinolones is characteristically enhanced by alterations in drug uptake and efflux or by modifications in the target enzymes topoisomerase IV (ParE and ParC) DNA gyrase (GyrA and GyrB) [132]. A few years ago, plasmid-mediated quinolone resistance (PMQR) has associated to *Salmonella* and other *Enterobacteriaceae*, while the occurrence of PMQR is globally rising [133]. The initial PMQR determinant described was the *qnrA* gene [134], which was followed by *qnr* alleles (e.g., *qnrD, qnrB*, *qnrC*, and *qnrS*) [135, 136]. Additionally, two other PMQR genes have been identified: *aac(6')-Ib-cr* and *qepA*. The first one consists on an aminoglycoside acetyltransferase variant gene that promotes resistance to aminoglycosides and lower susceptibility to ciprofloxacin [133], while the second one is a quinolone efflux pump that expels hydrophilic fluoroquinolones from the bacterial cell, including ciprofloxacin [137]. Even though all these PMQR determinants contribute to just a low-level resistance to fluoroquinolones, it is likely that PMQR is accountable for the fast increase of fluoroquinolone resistance among *Enterobacteriaceae* [133, 138]. Moreover, it is worrying that there can be a connection between *qnr*-positive and extended-spectrum -lactamase-positive isolates [139, 140, 141]. Recently, Gunell *et al.* [142] had verified the rising of an extremely mobile *qnr* genotype that gives *S. enterica* isolates a non-classical quinolone resistance phenotype. These authors had also observed that, although the non-classical phenotype can in part be influenced by efflux, the *qnr* genes are sufficient to create isolates with low fluoroquinolone susceptibility. This is an alarming finding given that non-classical quinolone resistance is plasmid related and, thus, can be mobilized.

As mentioned many times before in this chapter, efflux pumps are proteins that expel a large variety of harmful chemicals from the cell (such as biocides, antibiotics, and dyes), and that can lead to a low-level MAR phenotype [143]. Moreover, in the last years it has been shown that the existence of the main efflux system AcrAB–TolC is a requirement for pathogenicity in *S. enterica*, and a prerequisite for selection of high-level resistance to some antibiotics [144, 145, 146, 147, 148]. Webber *et al.* [149] performed a study in which they selected and analyzed TLN-resistant mutants of *S. enterica* Typhimurium, examined the function of AcrAB–TolC in the expansion of TLN resistance, and ultimately investigated the condition of mutants in a significant animal model (chick). The authors found that there are three different phenotypes and mechanisms of TLN resistance in *Salmonella*, and that a several different genes are implicated in TLN resistance, such as *ramA*, *fabI*, *tolC*, and *acrB*. In this way, Webber *et al.* [149] demonstrated that TLN resistance is multi-factorial and that several resistance mechanisms take place in synergy to accomplish high-level resistance. Facing these results, the author also highlighted that, since contact with TLN might select for various resistance phenotypes, the ever-increasing employment of TLN in a growing sort of applications (including those in food processing), must be well thought-out.

CONCLUSIONS

Bacterial resistance is one of the major barriers as far as global public health is concerned, with *S. enterica* being one of the most dangerous pathogens involved in this subject matter. In fact, these bacteria are constantly confirming its ability to survive chemical challenges, towards both biocides and antibiotics. Several studies have shown that, in order to adapt to and survive the lethal effects of chemical compounds, *S. enterica* can employ an array of survival mechanisms, which encompass not only phenotypic/physiological aspects but also genetic adjustments. Taking into consideration these aspects, it became clear that application of biocidal agents can enhance the selective pressure on bacteria towards obtaining antibiotic and biocides resistance, not only concerning *S. enterica* but Gram-negative bacteria in general. In this manner, the growing attractiveness for biocide-containing home cleaning products corresponds to an actual danger for the promotion of bacterial resistance and, subsequently, cross-resistance. Nevertheless, in order to settle the most appropriate procedures and consequently impede or minimize the selection of bacterial resistance, it is yet necessary and important to perform additional studies. Such studies should concern the relations between bacterial resistance (against biocides and antibiotics) and virulence mechanisms, as well as epidemiological revisions that could allow verifying the role of distinct types of disinfectants to the development of antibiotic resistance.

REFERENCES

[1] European Food Safety Authority, European Centre for Disease Prevention and Control. The European Union Summary Report on Trends and Sources of Zoonoses, Zoonotic Agents and Food-borne Outbreaks in 2009. *EFSA Journal*, 2011 9(3), 2090.

[2] Helke, DM; Wong, ACL. Surviving and growth characteristics of *Listeria monocytogenes* and *Salmonella typhimurium* on stainless steel and bruna-N rubber. *Journal of Food Protection*, 1994 57, 963-968.

[3] Reij, MW; Den Aantrekker, ED. Recontamination as a source of pathogens in processed foods. *International Journal of Food Microbiology*, 2004 91, 1-11.

[4] Sasahara, K; Zottola, EA. Biofilm formation by *Listeria monocytogenes* utilizes a primary colonizing microorganism in flowing systems. *Journal of Food Protection*, 1993 56, 1022-1028.

[5] Costerton, JW; Lewandowski, Z; Caldwell, DE; Korber, DR; Lappin Scott, HM. Microbial biofilms. *Annual Review of Microbiology*, 1995 45, 711-735.

[6] Holah, JT. 2003. CEN/TC 216: its role in producing current and future European disinfectant testing standards. *International Biodeterioration and Biodegradation*, 51, 239-243.

[7] Whiteley, M; Bangera, MG; Bumgarner, RE; Parsek, MR; Teitzel, GM; Lory, S; Greenberg, EP. Gene expression in *Pseudomonas aeruginosa* biofilms. *Nature*, 2001 413, 860-864.

[8] Aarnisalo, K; Salo, S; Miettinen, H; Suihko, M-L; Wirtanen, G; Autio, T; Lúnden, J; Korkeala, H; Sjöberg, A-M.. Bactericidal efficiencies of commercial disinfectants against *Listeria monocytogenes* on surfaces. *Journal of Food Safety*, 2000 20, 237-250.

[9] Peng, JS; Tsai, WC; Chou, CC. Inactivation and removal of *Bacillus cereus* by sanitizer and detergent. *International Journal of Food Microbiology*, 2002 77, 11-18.

[10] Sallam, SS; Donnely, CW. Destruction, injury and repair of *Listeria* species exposed to sanitizing compounds. *Journal of Food Protection*, 1992 55, 771-776.

[11] Rodrigues, D; Teixeira, P; Oliveira, R; Azeredo, J. *Salmonella enterica* Enteritidis biofilm formation and viability on regular and triclosan incorporated bench cover materials. *Journal of Food Protection*, 2011 74, 32-37(6).

[12] Chmielewski, RAN; Frank, JF. Biofilm formation and control in food processing facilities. *Comprehensive Reviews in Food Science and Food Safety*, 2003 2, 22-32.

[13] Joseph, B; Otta, SK; Karunasagar, I; Karunasagar, I. Biofilm formation by *Salmonella* spp. on food contact surfaces and their sensitivity to sanitizers. *International Journal of Food Microbiology*, 2001 64, 367-372.

[14] Aarnisalo, K; Lundén, J; Korkeala, H; Wirtanen, G. Susceptibility of *Listeria monocytogenes* strains to disinfectants and chlorinated alkaline cleaners at cold temperatures. *LWT-Food Science and Technology*, 2007 40, 1041-1048.

[15] Alonso-Hernando, A; Capita, R; Prieto, M; Alonso-Calleja, C. Comparison of antibiotic resistance patterns in Listeria monocytogenes and *Salmonella enterica* strains pre-exposed and exposed to poultry decontaminants. *Food Control*, 2009 20, 1108-1111.

[16] Kastbjerg, VG; Nielsen, S; Aneborg, N; Gram, L. Response of *Listeria monocytogenes* to disinfection stress at the single-cell and population levels as monitored by intracellular pH measurements and viable-cell counts. *Applied and Environmental Microbiology*, 2009 75, 4550-4556.

[17] Ammor, S; Chevallier, I; Laguet, A; Labadie, J; Talon, R; Dufour, E. Investigation of the selective bactericidal effect of several decontaminating solutions on bacterial biofilms including useful, spoilage and/or pathogenic bacteria. *Food Microbiology*, 2004 21, 11-17.

[18] Pan, Y; Breidt, F; Kathariou S. Resistance of *Listeria monocytogenes* biofilms to sanitizing agents in a simulated food processing environment. *Applied and Environmental Microbiology*, 2006 72, 7711-7717.

[19] Ramesh, N; Joseph, SW; Carr, LE; Douglass, LW; Wheaton, FW. Evaluation of chemical disinfectants for the elimination of *Salmonella* biofilms from poultry transport containers. *Poultry Science Association Inc.*, 2002 904-910.

[20] Rodrigues, D; Cerca, N; Teixeira, P; Oliveira, R; Ceri, H; Azeredo, J. *Listeria monocytogenes* and *Salmonella enterica* Enteritidis biofilms susceptibility to different disinfectants and stress-response and virulence gene expression of surviving cells. *Microbial Drug Resistance*, 2011 17(2), 181-189.

[21] Cogan, TA; Humphrey, T.J. The rise and fall of *Salmonella* Enteritidis in the UK. *Journal of Applied Microbiology*, 2003 94, 114-119.

[22] Romanova, NA; Wolffs, PFG; Brovko, LY; Griffths, MW. Role of efflux pumps in adaptation and resistance of *Listeria monocytogenes* to benzalkonium chloride. *Applied and Environmental Microbiology*, 2006 72, 3498-3503.

[23] SCENIHR (Scientific Comittee on Emerging and Newly Identified Health Risks). Opinion on the effects of the active substances in biocidal products on antibiotic resistance. Version of 4 November 2008 for public consultation. Available at: http://ec.europa.eu/health/ph_risk/committees/04_scenihr/docs/scenihr_o_020.pdf

[24] SCHER/SCENIHR (Scientific Comittee on Health and Environmental Risks/ Scientific Comittee on Emerging and Newly Identified Health Risks). Scientific opinion on the environmental impact and effect of antimicrobial resistance of four substances used for the removal of microbial surface contamination of poultry carcasses. April 2008. Available at: http://ec.europa.eu/health/ph_risk/committees/04_scenihr/docs/scenihr_o_015.pdf

[25] Clark, GM; Kaufmann, AF; Gangarosa, EJ; Thompson, MA. Epidemiology of an international outbreak of *Salmonella* Agona. *Lancet*, 1973 2(7827), 490-493.

[26] CDC. Centers for Diseases Control and Prevention. Multiple outbreaks of salmonellosis associated with precooked roast beef- Pennsylvania, New York, Vermont. *Morbidity and Mortality Weekly Report*, 1981 30(46), 569-570.

[27] Spitalny, KC; Okowitz, EN; Vogt, RL. Salmonellosis outbreak at a Vermont hospital. *The Southern Medical Journal*, 1984 77(2), 168-172.

[28] Delpech, V; McAnulty, J; Morgan, K. A salmonellosis outbreak linked to internally contaminated pork meat. *Australian and New Zealand Journal of Public Health*, 1998 22(2), 243-246.

[29] Yousef, AE; Carlstrom, C. *Salmonella*. In Yousef, AE and Carstrom, C. (Eds.). *Food microbiology: A laboratory manual*, p. 167-205. New Jersey: John Wiley and Sons, Inc. 2003.

[30] Bhunia, AK. Foodborne microbial pathogens: Mechanisms and pathogenesis. United States of America: Springer Science + Business Media, LLC. 2008

[31] Newell, DG; Koopmans, M.; Verhoef, L; Duizer, E; Aidara-Kane, A; Sprong, H; Giessen, Jvd; Kruse, H. Food-borne diseases-the challenges of 20 years ago still persist while new ones continue to emerge. *International Journal of Food Microbiology*, 2010 139, S3-S15.

[32] Bouchrif, B; Paglietti, B; Murgia, M; Piana, A; Cohen, N; Ennaji, M; Rubino, S; Timinouni, M. Prevalence and antibiotic-resistance of Salmonella isolated from food in Morocco. *Journal of Infection in Developing Countries*, 2009 28(3), 35-40.

[33] Pui, CF; Wong, WC; Chai, LC; Nillian, E; Ghazali, FM; Cheah, YK; Nakaguchi, Y; Nishibuchi, M; Radu, S. Simultaneous detection of *Salmonella* spp., *Salmonella* Typhi and *Salmonella* Typhimurium in sliced fruits using multiplex PCR. *Food Control*, 2011 22, 337-342.

[34] Penteado, AL; Leitão, MFF. Growth of *Salmonella* Enteritidis in melon, watermelon and papaya pulp stored at different times and temperatures. *Food Control*, 2004 15(5), 369-373.

[35] Bordini, MEB; Asturiano Ristori, C; Jakabi, M; Gelli, DS. Incidence, internalization and behaviour of *Salmonella* in mangoes, var. Tommy Atkins. *Food Control*, 2007 18(8), 1002-1007.

[36] Jay, S; Grau, FH; Smith, K; Lightfoot, D; Murray, C; Davey, GR. *Salmonella.* In Hocking, A. D., Arnold, G., Jenson, I., Newton, K. and Sutherland, P. (Eds.). *Foodborne microorganisms of public health significance*, p. 169-229. Australia: Australian Institute of Food Science and Technology Inc. 1997.

[37] CDC. Centers for Diseases Control and Prevention. Multistate Outbreak of Human *Salmonella* Enteritidis Infections Associated with Shell Eggs. *Epi Trends*, 2010 15(9), 1-4.

[38] EFSA. European Food Safety Authority. The Community Summary Report on Food-borne Outbreaks in the European Union in 2007. *The EFSA Journal*, 2009 271.

[39] CDC. Centers for Diseases Control and Prevention. Outbreak of *Salmonella* serotype Typhimurium infection associated with eating raw ground beef-Wisconsin, 1994. *Morbidity and Mortality Weekly Report*, 1995 44(49), 905-909.

[40] Davies, A; O'Neill, P; Towers, L; Cooke, M. An outbreak of *Salmonella* Typhimurium DT104 food poisoning associated with eating beef. *Communicable Disease Report. CDR Review*, 1996 6(11), 159-162.

[41] Roels, TH; Frazak, PA; Kazmierczak, JJ; Mackenzie, WR; Proctor, ME; Kurzynski, TA; Davis, JP. Incomplete sanitation of a meat grinder and ingestion of raw ground beef: contributing factors to a large outbreak of *Salmonella* Typhimurium infection. *Epidemiology and Infection*, 1997 119(2), 127-134.

[42] Shapiro, R; Ackers, ML; Lance, S; Rabbani, M; Schaefer, L; Daugherty, J; Thelen, C; Swerdlow, D. *Salmonella* Thompson associated with improper handling of roast beef at a restaurant in Sioux Falls, South Dakota. *Journal of Food Protection*, 1999 62(2), 118-122.

[43] Haeghebaert, S; Duché, L; Gilles, C; Masini, B; Dubreuil, M; Minet, JC; Bouvet, P; Grimont, F; Delarocque Astagneau, E; Vaillant, V. Minced beef and human salmonellosis: review of the investigation of three outbreaks in France. *Euro Surveillance*, 2001 6(2), 21-26.

[44] Freitas Neto, OC; Penha Filho, RAC; Barrow, P; Berchieri Junior, A. Sources of human non-typhoid salmonellosis: a review. Revista *Brasileira de Ciência Avícola*, 2010 12, 01-11.

[45] Pastore, R; Schmid, H; Altpeter, E; Baumgartner, A; Hächler, H; Imhof, R; Sudre, P; Boubaker, K. Outbreak of *Salmonella* serovar Stanley infections in Switzerland linked to locally produced soft cheese, September 2006 - February 2007. *Euro Surveillance*, 2008 13(37), 18979.

[46] Wong, DMA; Hald, LF; Wolf, T; Swanenburg, M. Epidemiology and control measures for Salmonella in pigs and pork. *Livestock Production Science*, 2002 76(3), 215-222.

[47] McDonnell, G; Russell, AD. Antiseptics and disinfectants: activity, action and resistance. *Clinical Microbiology Reviews*, 1999 12, 147–79.

[48] McMurry, LM; Oethinger, M; Levy, S. Overexpression of *marA*, *soxS*, or *acrAB* produces resistance to triclosan in laboratory and clinical strains of *Escherichia coli. FEMS Microbiology Letters*, 1998 166, 305–9.

[49] Russell, AD. Introduction of biocides into clinical practice and the impact on antibiotic-resistant bacteria. *Journal of Applied Microbiology*, 2002 92, S121–35.

[50] Schweizer, HP. Triclosan: a widely used biocide and its link to antibiotics. *FEMS Microbiology Letters*, 2001 1, 1–7.

[51] Braoudaki, M; Hilton, AC. Adaptive resistance to biocides in *Salmonella enterica* and *Escherichia coli* O157 and cross-resistance to antimicrobial agents. *Journal of Clinical Microbiology*, 2004 42, 73–78.

[52] Russell, AD. Do biocides select for antibiotic resistance? *Journal of Pharmacy and Pharmacology*, 2000 52, 227–233.

[53] Russell, AD; Tattawajaet, U; Maillard, J-Y; Furr, JR. Possible link between bacterial resistance and use of antibiotics and biocides. *Antimicrobial Agents and Chemotherapy*, 1998 42, 2151.

[54] Jones, RD; Jampani, HB; Newman, JL; *et al.* Triclosan: a review of effectiveness and safety in health care settings. *American Journal of Infection Control*, 2000 28, 184–96.

[55] Brown, MRW; Gilbert, P. Sensitivity of biofilms to antimicrobial agents. *Journal of Applied Bacteriology - Symposium Supplement*, 1993 74, 87S–97S.

[56] Leriche, V; Carpentier, B. Viable but nonculturable *Salmonella* Typhimurium in single- and binary-species biofilms in response to chlorine treatment. *Journal of Food Protection*, 1995 58, 1186–1191.

[57] Szomolay, B; Klapper, I; Dockery, J; Stewart, PS. Adaptive responses to antimicrobial agents in biofilms. *Environmental Microbiology*, 2005 7, 1186– 1191.

[58] Gilbert, P.; Allison, D.G.; McBain, A.J. Biofilms in vitro and in vivo: do singular mechanisms imply cross-resistance? *Journal of Applied Microbiology*, 2002 92, 98S-110S.

[59] Sailer, F.C.; Meberg, B.M.; Young, K.D. *β*-Lactam induction of colonic acid gene expression in *Escherichia coli*. *FEMS Microbiology Letters*, 2003 226, 245-249.

[60] Bagge, N. *et al. Pseudomonas aeruginosa* biofilms exposed to imipenem exhibit changes in global gene expression and *β*-lactamase and alginate production. *Antimicrobial Agents and Chemotherapy*, 2004 48, 1175-1187.

[61] Brown, M.L.; Henry Aldrich, H.C.; Gauther, J.J. Relationship between glycocalyx and povidence-iodine resistance in *Pseudomonas aeruginosa* (ATCC 27853) biofilms. *Applied and Environmental Microbiology*, 1995 61, 187-193.

[62] Gilbert, P.; Allison, D.G.; Evans, D.J.; Handley, P.S.; Brown, M.R. Growth rate control of adherent bacterial populations. *Applied Environmental Microbiology*, 1989 55, 1308-1311.

[63] Huang, C.T.; Philip Yu, F.P.; McFeters, G.A.; Stewart, P.S. Nonuniform spatial patterns of respiratory activity within biofilms during disinfection. *Applied and Environmental Microbio*logy, 1995 61, 2252-2256.

[64] Gilbert, P.; Brown, M.R.W. Mechanisms of the protection of bacterial biofilms from antimicrobial agents. In: Lappin-Scott, H., Costerton, J.W. (Eds.), Microbial Biofilms. *Cambridge University Press*, Cambridge, 1995 pp. 118-130.

[65] Leid, J.G.; Shirtliff, M.E.; Costerton, J.W.; Stoodley, A.P. Human leukocytes adhere to, penetrate, and respond to *Staphylococcus aureus* biofilms. *Infection and Immunity*, 2002 70, 6339–6345.

[66] Mangalappalli-Illathu, AK; Korber, DR. Adaptive resistance and differential protein expression of *Salmonella enterica* serovar Enteritidis biofilms exposed to benzalkonium chloride. *Antimicrobial Agents and Chemotherapy*, 2006 50, 3588– 3596.

[67] Simões, M; Pereira, MO; Vieira, MJ. Action of a cationic surfactant on the activity and removal of bacterial biofilms formed under different flow regimes. *Water Research*, 2005 39, 478-486.
[68] Maxcy, RB; Tiwari, P; Sporey, PR. Changes in *Escherichia coli* associated with acquired tolerance for quaternary ammonium compounds. *Applied Microbiology*, 1971 22, 229-232.
[69] Mukhopadhyay, S; Schellhorn, HE. Identification and characterization of hydrogen peroxide-sensitive mutants of *Escherichia coli*: genes that require OxyR for expression. *Journal of Bacteriology*, 1997 179, 330–338.
[70] Langsrud, S; Sidhu, MS; Heir, E; Holck, AL. Bacterial disinfectant resistance—a challenge for the food industry. *International Biodeterioration and Biodegradation*, 2003 51, 283–290.
[71] Brown, M.R.W.; Williams, P. The influence of environment on envelope properties affecting survival of bacteria in infections. *Annual Review of Microbiology*, 1985 39, 527–556.
[72] Power, E.G.M. Aldehydes as biocides. *Progress in Medicinal Chemistry*, 1995 34, 149–201.
[73] Russell, A.D. Glutaraldehyde: current status and uses. *Infection Control and Hospital Epidemiology*, 1994 15, 724–733.
[74] Russell, A.D.; Chopra, I. Understanding antibacterial action and resistance, 2nd ed. *Ellis Horwood, Chichester*, England, 1996.
[75] Russell, A.D.; Russell, N.J. Biocides: activity, action and resistance. *Symposium of the Society for General Microbiology*, 1995 53, 327–365.
[76] Annous, B.A.; Becker, L.A.; Bayles, D.O.; Labeda, D.P.; Wilkinson, B.J. Critical role of anteiso-C15:0 fatty acid in the growth of Listeria monocytogenes at low temperatures. *Applied and Environmental Microbiology*, 1997 63, 3887–3894.
[77] Sakagami, Y.; Yokoyama, H.; Nishimura, H.; Ose, Y.; Tashima, T. Mechanism of resistance to benzalkonium chloride by *Pseudomonas aeruginosa*. *Applied and Environmental Microbiology*, 1989 55, 2036–2040.
[78] Scher, K.; Römling, U.; Yaron, S. Effect of heat, acidification, and chlorination on *Salmonella enterica* serovar Typhimurium cells in a biofilm formed at the air-liquid interface. *Applied and Environmental Microbiology*, 2005 71, 1163–1168.
[79] Bruinsma, G.M.; Rustema-Abbing, M.; van der Mei, H.C.; Lakkis, C.; Busscher, H.J. Resistance to a polyquaternium-1 lens care solution and isoelectric points of *Pseudomonas aeruginosa* strains. *Journal of Antimicrobial Chemotherapy*, 2006 57, 764-6.
[80] Russell, A.D.; Furr, J.R.; Maillard, J-Y. Microbial susceptibility and resistance to biocides: an understanding. *ASM News* 1997 63, 481 487.
[81] Mangalappalli-Illathu, A.K.; Vidović, S.; Korber, D.R. Differential adaptive response and survival of *Salmonella enterica* serovar Enteritidis planktonic and biofilm cells exposed to benzalkonium chloride. *Antimicrobial Agents and Chemotherapy*, 2008 52, 3669-2680.
[82] Braoudaki, M; Hilton, AC. Mechanisms of resistance in *Salmonella enterica* adapted to erythromycin, benzalkonium chloride and triclosan. *International Journal of Antimicrobial Agents*, 2005 25, 31–37.

[83] Levy, SB. Active efflux, a common mechanism for biocide and antibiotic resistance. *Journal of Applied Microbiology - Symposium Supplement*, 2002 92, 65S–71S.

[84] Paulsen, I.T.; Brown, M.H.; Skurray, R.A. Proton-dependent multidrug efflux systems. *Microbiological Reviews*, 1996 60, 575–608.

[85] Nikaido, H. Multiple antibiotic resistance and efflux. *Current Opinion in Microbiology*, 1998 1, 516–523.

[86] Poole, K. Efflux-mediated resistance to fluoroquinolones in Gram-negative bacteria. *Antimicrobial Agents and Chemotherapy*, 2000 44, 2233–2241.

[87] Poole, K. Efflux-mediated resistance to fluoroquinolones in gram-positive bacteria and the mycobacteria. *Antimicrobial Agents and Chemotherapy*, 2000 44, 2595–2599.

[88] Brown, M.H.; Paulsen, I.T.; Skurray, R.A. The multidrug efflux protein NorM is a prototype of a new family of transporters. *Molecular Microbiology*, 1999 31, 393–395.

[89] Chung, Y.J.; Saier, M.H. Jr SMR-type multidrug resistance pumps. *Current Opinion in Drug Discovery and Development*, 2001 4, 237– 245.

[90] Jack, D.L.; Yang, N.M.; Saier, M.H. The drug/metabolite transporter superfamily. *European Journal of Biochemistry*, 2001 268, 3620– 3639.

[91] Zgurskaya, H.I.; Nikaido, H. Multidrug resistance mechanisms: drug efflux across two membranes. *Molecular Microbiology*, 2000 37, 219–225.

[92] Pao, S.S.; Paulsen, I.T.; Saier, M.H. Jr Major facilitator superfamily. *Microbiology and Molecular Biology Reviews*, 1998 62, 1–34.

[93] van Veen, H.W.; Konings, W.N. The ABC family of multidrug transporters in microorganisms. *Biochimica Biophysica Acta*, 1998 1365, 31–36.

[94] Rouche, D. A.; Cram, D. S.; DiBernadino, D.T.; Littlejohn, G.; Skurray, R. A. Efflux-mediated antiseptic gene qacA from *Staphylococcus aureus*: common ancestry with tetracycline- and sugar-transport proteins. *Molecular Microbiology*, 1990 4, 2051–2062.

[95] Skurray, R. A.; Firth, N. Molecular evolution of multiply antibiotic-resistant staphylococci. *Ciba Foundation Symposium*, 1997 207, 167–191.

[96] Skurray, R. A.; Rouch, D.A.; Lyon, B.R.; Gillespie, M.T.; Tennent, J.M.; Byrne, M.E.; Messerotti, L.J.; May, J.W. Multiresistant *Staphylococcus aureus*: genetics and evolution of epidemic Australian strains. *Journal of Antimicrobial Chemotherapy*, 1988 21(Suppl. C), 19–39.

[97] Horiyama, T.; Yamaguchi, A.; Nishino, K. TolC dependency of multidrug efflux systems in *Salmonella enterica* serovar Typhimurium. *Journal of Antimicrobial Chemotherapy*, 2010 65, 1372–1376.

[98] Randall, LP.; Cooles, SW.; Coldham, N.G.; Penuela, E.G.; Mott, A.C.; *et al.* Commonly used farm disinfectants can select for mutant *Salmonella enterica* serovar Typhimurium with decreased susceptibility to biocides and antibiotics without compromising virulence. *Journal of Antimicrobial Chemotherapy*, 2007 60, 1273–1280.

[99] Karatzas, K.A.; Webber, M.A.; Jorgensen, F.; Woodward, M.J.; Piddock, L.J.; *et al.* Prolonged treatment of *Salmonella enterica* serovar Typhimurium with commercial disinfectants selects for multiple antibiotic resistance, increased efflux and reduced invasiveness. *Journal of Antimicrobial Chemotherapy*, 2007 60, 947–955.

[100] Eaves, D.J.; Ricci, V.; Piddock, L.J. Expression of *acrB*, *acrF*, *acrD*, *marA*, and *soxS* in *Salmonella enterica* serovar Typhimurium: role in multiple antibiotic resistance. *Antimicrobial Agents and Chemotherapy*, 2004 48, 1145–1150.

[101] Whitehead R.N.; Overton, T.W.; Kemp, C.L.; Webber, M.A. Exposure of *Salmonella enterica* serovar Typhimurium to high level biocide challenge can select multidrug resistant mutants in a single step. *PLoS ONE*, 2011 6(7), e22833.

[102] Smith, TL; Jarvis, WR. Antimicrobial resistance in *Staphylococcus aureus. Microbes and Infection*, 1999 1, 795–805.

[103] Beumer, R; Bloomfield, SF; Exner, M; Fara, GM; Nath, KJ; Scott, E. Microbial resistance and biocides. *International Scientific Forum on Home Hygiene, Geneva, Switzerland*, September 2000. [Online.] http://www.ifh-homehygiene.org/forum/antresFINAL.pdf.

[104] Maillard, J-Y. Bacterial target sites for biocide action. *Journal of Applied Microbiology - Symposium Supplement*, 2002 92, 16S–27S.

[105] Chaplin, CE. Bacterial resistance to quaternary ammonium disinfectants. *Journal of Bacteriology*, 1952 63, 453–458.

[106] Hoffmann, H-P; Geftic, SG; Gelzer, J; Haymann, H; Adair, FW. Ultrastructural alterations associated with the growth of resistant *Pseudomonas aeruginosa* in the presence of benzalkonium chloride. *Journal of Bacteriology*, 1973 113, 409–416.

[107] Loughlin, MF; Jones, MV; Lambert, PA. *Pseudomonas aeruginosa* cells adapted to benzalkonium chloride show resistance to other membrane- active agents but not to clinically relevant antibiotics. *Journal of Antimicrobial Chemotherapy*, 2002 49, 631–639.

[108] Mangalappalli-Illathu, AK; Korber DR. Unpublished data.

[109] Moreillon, P. Means of bacterial resistance. *Revue Medicale de la Suisse Romande*, 2000 120, 641–650.

[110] Nikaido, H. Multidrug efflux pumps of gram-negative bacteria. *Journal of Bacteriology*, 1996 178, 5853–5859.

[111] Braoudaki, M.; Hilton, A.C. Adaptive resistance to biocides in *Salmonella enterica* and *scherichia coli* O157 and cross-resistance to antimicrobial agents. *Journal of Clinical Microbiology*, 2004 42, 73-78.

[112] Alekshun, MN; Levy, SB. Regulation of chromosomally mediated multiple antibiotic resistance: the *mar* regulon. *Antimicrobial Agents and Chemotherapy*, 1997 41, 2067–75.

[113] Randall, LP; Cooles, SW; Sayers, AR; *et al*. Cyclohexane resistance in *Salmonella* of different serovars is associated with increased resistance to multiple antibiotics, disinfectants and dyes. *Journal of Medical Microbiology*, 2001 50, 1–6.

[114] Randall, LP; Woodward, MJ. The multiple antibiotic resistance (*mar*) locus and its significance. *Research in Veterinary Science*, 2002 72, 87–93.

[115] Randall, LP; Cooles, SW; Piddock, LJ; *et al*. Effect of triclosan or a phenolic farm disinfectant upon the selection of antibiotic resistant *Salmonella enterica. Journal of Antimicrobial Chemotherapy*, 2004 54, 621–7.

[116] Randall, LP; Clouting, CS; Gradel, KO; *et al*. Farm disinfectants select for cyclohexane resistance, a marker of multiple antibiotic resistance, in *Escherichia coli. Journal of Applied Microbiology*, 2005 98, 556–63.

[117] Karatzas, KAG; Randall, LP; Webber, M; *et al.* Phenotypic and proteomic characterization of multiply antibiotic-resistant variants of *Salmonella enterica* serovar Typhimurium selected following exposure to disinfectants. *Applied and Environmental Microbiology*, 2008 74, 1508–16.

[118] Waters, VL. Conjugative transfer in the dissemination of beta-lactam and aminoglycoside resistance. *Frontiers in Bioscience*, 1999 4, 416-439.

[119] O'Brien, TF. Emergence, spread, and environmental effects of antimicrobial resistance: how use of an antimicrobial anywhere can increase resistance to any antimicrobial anywhere else. *Clinical Infectious Disease*, 2002 34, S78- 84.

[120] Carattoli, A. Plasmid-mediated antimicrobial resistance in *Salmonella enterica. Current Molecular Biology*, 2003 5(4), 113-122.

[121] Guiney, DG; Fang, FC; Krause, M; Libby, S. Plasmid-mediated virulence genes in non-typhoidal *Salmonella* serovars. *FEMS Microbiology Letters*, 1994 124, 1-9.

[122] Hall, RM. Mobile gene cassettes and integrons: moving antibiotic resistance genes in gram-negative bacteria. *Ciba Foundation Symposium*, 1997 207, 192–202.

[123] Liebert, CA; Hall, RM; Summers, AO. Transposon Tn21, flagship of the floating genome. *Microbiology and Molecular Biology Reviews*, 1999 63, 507–22.

[124] Carattoli, A. Importance of integrons in the diffusion of resistance. *Veterinary Research*, 2001 32, 243–59.

[125] Leverstein-van Hall, MA; Blok, HEM; Donders, ART; *et al.* Multidrug resistance among *Enterobacteriaceae* is strongly associated with the presence of integrons and is independent of species or isolate origin. *Journal of Infectious Diseases*, 2003 187, 251–9.

[126] Guerra, B; Soto, S; Cal, S; *et al.* Antimicrobial resistance and spread of class 1 integrons among *Salmonella* serotypes. *Antimicrobial Agents and Chemotherapy*, 2000 44, 2166–9.

[127] Partridge, SR; Recchia, GD; Stokes, HW; *et al.* Family of class 1 integrons related to In4 from Tn*1696*. *Antimicrobial Agents and Chemotherapy*, 2001 45, 3014–20.

[128] Sundstrom, L; Roy, PH; Skold, O. Site-specific insertion of three structural gene cassettes in transposon Tn7. *Journal of Bacteriology*, 1991 173, 3025–8.

[129] Miko, A; Pries, K; Schroeter. A; *et al.* Multiple-drug resistance in D-tartrate-positive *Salmonella enterica* serovar Paratyphi B isolates from poultry is mediated by class 2 integrons inserted into the bacterial chromosome. *Antimicrobial Agents and Chemotherapy*, 2003 47, 3640–3.

[130] Miko, A; Pries, K; Schroeter, A; Helmuth, R. Molecular mechanisms of resistance in multidrug-resistant serovars of *Salmonella enterica* isolated from foods in Germany. *Journal of Antimicrobial Chemotherapy*, 2005 56, 1025–1033.

[131] Schroeter, A; Hoog, B; Helmuth, R. Resistance of *Salmonella* isolates in Germany. *Journal of Veterinary Medicine. B, Infectious Diseases and Veterinary Public Health*, 2004 51, 389–92.

[132] Jacoby, GA. Mechanisms of resistance to quinolones. *Clinical Infectious Diseases*, 2005 41(Suppl. 2), S120–S126.

[133] Robicsek, A; Jacoby, GA; Hooper, DC. The worldwide emergence of plasmid-mediated quinolone resistance. *The Lancet Infectious Diseases*, 2006 6, 629–640.

[134] Martinez-Martinez, L; Pascual, A; Jacoby, GA. Quinolone resistance from a transferable plasmid. *Lancet*, 1998 351, 797–799.

[135] Cavaco, L M; Hasman, H; Xia, S; Aarestrup, FM. *qnrD*, a novel gene conferring transferable quinolone resistance in *Salmonella enterica* serovar Kentucky and Bovismorbificans strains of human origin. *Antimicrobial Agents and Chemotherapy*, 2009 53, 603–608.

[136] Martinez-Martinez, L; Eliecer Cano, M; Manuel Rodriguez-Martinez, J; Calvo, J; Pascual, A. Plasmid-mediated quinolone resistance. *Expert Review of Anti-Infective Therapy*, 2008 6, 685–711.

[137] Yamane, K; Wachino, J; Suzuki, S; Kimura, K; Shibata, N; Kato, H; Shibayama, K; Konda, T; Arakawa, Y. New plasmid-mediated fluoroquinolone efflux pump, QepA, found in an *Escherichia coli* clinical isolate. *Antimicrobial Agents and Chemotherapy*, 2007 51, 3354–3360.

[138] Strahilevitz, J; Engelstein, D; Adler, A; Temper, V; Moses, AE; Block, C; Robicsek, A. Changes in qnr prevalence and fluoroquinolone resistance in clinical isolates of *Klebsiella pneumoniae* and *Enterobacter* spp. collected from 1990 to 2005. *Antimicrobial Agents and Chemotherapy*, 2007 51, 3001–3003.

[139] Poirel, L; Pitout, JD; Calvo, L; Rodriguez-Martinez, JM; Church. D; Nordmann, P. In vivo selection of fluoroquinolone-resistant *Escherichia coli* isolates expressing plasmid-mediated quinolone resistance and expanded-spectrum -lactamase. *Antimicrobial Agents and Chemotherapy*, 2006 50, 1525– 1527.

[140] Cattoir, V; Poirel, L; Rotimi, V; Soussy, CJ; Nordmann, P. Multiplex PCR for detection of plasmid-mediated quinolone resistance *qnr* genes in ESBL-producing enterobacterial isolates. *Journal of Antimicrobial Chemotherapy*, 2007 60, 394–397.

[141] Murray, A; Mather, H; Coia, JE; Brown DJ. Plasmid-mediated quinolone resistance in nalidixic-acid-susceptible strains of *Salmonella enterica* isolated in Scotland. *Journal of Antimicrobial Chemotherapy*, 2008 62, 1153–1155.

[142] Gunell, M; Webber, MA; Kotilainen, P; Lilly, AJ; Caddick, JM; Jalava, J; Huovinen, P; Siitonen, A; Hakanen, AJ; Piddock, LJ. Mechanisms of resistance in nontyphoidal *Salmonella enterica* strains exhibiting a nonclassical quinolone resistance phenotype. *Antimicrobial Agents and Chemotherapy*, 2009 53, 3832–3836.

[143] Piddock, LJ. Multidrug-resistance efflux pumps—not just for resistance. *Nature Reviews Microbiology*, 2006 4, 629–36.

[144] Giraud, E; Cloeckaert, A; Kerboeuf, D; *et al.* Evidence for active efflux as the primary mechanism of resistance to ciprofloxacin in *Salmonella enterica* serovar Typhimurium. *Antimicrobial Agents and Chemotherapy*, 2000 44, 1223–8.

[145] Baucheron, S; Imberechts, H; Chaslus-Dancla, E; *et al.* The AcrB multidrug transporter plays a major role in high-level fluoroquinolone resistance in *Salmonella enterica* serovar Typhimurium phage type DT204. *Microbial Drug Resistance*, 2002 8, 281–9.

[146] Baucheron, S; Mouline, C; Praud, K; *et al.* TolC but not AcrB is essential for multidrug-resistant *Salmonella enterica* serotype Typhimurium colonization of chicks. *Journal of Antimicrobial Chemotherapy*, 2005 55, 707–12.

[147] Buckley, AM; Webber, MA; Cooles, S; *et al.* The AcrAB-TolC efflux system of *Salmonella enterica* serovar Typhimurium plays a role in pathogenesis. *Cellular Microbiology*, 2006; 8: 847–56.

[148] Ricci, V; Tzakas, P; Buckley, A; *et al.* Ciprofloxacin-resistant *Salmonella enterica* serovar Typhimurium strains are difficult to select in the absence of AcrB and TolC. *Antimicrobial Agents and Chemotherapy*, 2006 50, 38–42.

[149] Webber, MA; Randall, LP; Cooles, S; *et al*. Triclosan resistance in *Salmonella enterica* serovar Typhimurium. *Journal of Antimicrobial Chemotherapy*, 2008 62(1), 83-91.

In: Salmonella: Classification, Genetics and Disease Outbreaks ISBN: 978-1-61942-928-4
Editors: Adelaide S. Monte, Paulo Eduardo De Santos

Chapter 5

ALTERNATIVE METHODS FOR RAPID WHOLE-CELL DETECTION OF *SALMONELLA* SPP.

Bledar Bishaand Lawrence D. Goodridge*
Department of Animal Sciences, Colorado State University, Colorado, US

ABSTRACT

Culture-based methods for detection of *Salmonella* spp. in food demand the performance of several steps in stages (preenrichment, enrichment, selective plating, identification, and confirmation). This results in significant time-to-detection, media and reagents and labor needed. As a consequence of the need for rapid and specific detection techniques, molecular-based rapid detection methods such as real time polymerase chain reaction (RT-PCR), nucleic acid sequence based amplification (NASBA) or immunoassays have been developed. These methods, however, may still be negatively affected by interference from inhibitors, may be qualitative in nature or require extraction of target molecules (DNA, rRNA, mRNA) prior to analysis allowing for possible contamination or amplification of target sequences from non-viable cells. Alternative rapid detection techniques for *Salmonella* spp. in food have been developed which accomplish identification and enumeration of whole-cell targets. Fluorescence *in situ* hybridization (FISH) employs sequence-specific rRNA-targeted fluorescently-labeled oligonucleotide probes to specifically hybridize whole permeabilized bacterial cells. FISH can be coupled with fluorescence microscopy, flow cytometry or capillary electrophoresis to achieve detection and enumeration. Bacteriophage-based detection techniques for *Salmonella* spp. which make use of the inherent specificity of phages for their target bacterial host have also been described. In addition, biosensor-based detection may offer simplicity and high throughput capability for whole-cell detection of *Salmonella* spp. in food. These alternative methods for whole-cell detection of *Salmonella* spp. have shown potential as sensitive, specific, and quantitative methods for detection and identification of this pathogen in foods. The advantages and disadvantages of these methods as well as the current status of development and future directions are discussed here.

---

* Corresponding author. Mailing Address: 1171 Campus Delivery, 350 W. Pitkin Street, Department of Animal Sciences, Colorado State University, Fort Collins, CO, 80523. Tel: (970)-491-6271. Fax: (970) 491–5326. E-mail: Lawrence.Goodridge@colostate.edu.

Introduction

Overview of Salmonella spp. Salmonella spp. are rod-shaped, Gram negative and facultatively anaerobic bacteria. Except for *Salmonella* ser. Pullorum and ser. Gallinarum, all other members of the genus are motile by means of peritrichous flagella. Salmonellae are chemorganotrophic, grow best at 37°C and produce gas and acid when they ferment glucose and other carbohydrates. Furthermore, they are oxidase negative, catalase positive, grow on citrate as a sole carbon source, can generate hydrogen sulfide, and do not hydrolyze urea and decarboxylate lysine and ornithine (D'Aoust and Maurer, 2007). While the optimum pH for growth of *Salmonella* is 6.5-7.5, it has been shown that these pathogens can grow over a wide range of pH, from 4.5 to 9.5 (D'Aoust and Maurer, 2007). Optimal growth temperature is established as 35°C-37°C at neutral pH (Andrews and Bäumler, 2005), though *Salmonella* has been shown to possess the ability to grow at low temperatures in foods stored at 2-4°C, and they have been shown to adapt to such low temperatures if previously exposed (D'Aoust et al., 1975; Airoldi and Zotola, 1988). While information on the upper temperature limit of growth remains to be elucidated, it has been shown that *Salmonella enterica* serovar Typhimurium can develop mutations that can allow it to grow at temperatures as high as 54°C (Droffner and Yamamoto, 1992; D'Aoust and Maurer, 2007). Generally it is recognized that *Salmonella* does not grow at water activities lower than 0.93. Anaerobic conditions and increases in temperature have been shown to induce tolerance to high salt concentrations (Anonymous, 1986; D'Aoust, 1989; D'Aoust and Maurer, 2007).

Salmonella serovars are found in a great number of vertebrates, from reptiles to mammals and birds, with S. *enterica* subs. I mainly isolated from birds and mammals. It has been suggested that the reason that subspecies I is found more often in the food supply is also the reason why it is isolated more often from foods and clinical specimens and is associated with foodborne disease. *Salmonella* serovars can cause disease in food animals, who are often asymptomatic carriers, shedding salmonellae via the fecal route, allowing for transmission of the disease from animal to animal, or via contamination of feed, water, and equipment (Aleksic et al., 1996; Olsen et al., 2000; Hurd et al., 2001; Crump et al., 2002; Andrews and Bäumler, 2005).

The taxonomy of the genus *Salmonella* has undergone many changes over the years, and the current classification recognizes two species within the genus,*Salmonella enterica* and *Salmonella bongori* (former subgroup V). Most serovars are included in the species *Salmonella enterica* with only a few serovars included in the other species. *S. enterica* is grouped into six subspecies based on genomic relatedness and biochemical tests. These subspecies are delineated by names or roman numerals as subs. *enterica* (I), subs. *salamae* (II), subs. *arizonae* (IIIa), subs. *diarizonae* (IIIb), subs. *houtenae* (IV), and subs. *indica* (VI). Serological identification is performed using antisera for somatic (O) lipopolysaccharides (LPS) on the surface of the outer membrane, flagellar (H) antigens and in the case of serovars Typhi, Paratyphi C, and Dublin the capsular (Vi) antigen (Brenner et al., 2000; Andrews and Bäumler, 2005; D'Aoust and Maurer, 2007). For epidemiological analysis, phage typing can be used to further differentiate between isolates within serovars allowing determination of epidemic clones (Anderson et al., 1978).

Cultural methods for detection of Salmonella spp.: *Salmonella* spp. is commonly detected using the US Department of Agriculture-Food Safety and Inspection Service (USDA-FSIS) method (Rose, 2001) and the Federal Drug Administration (FDA) method (Andrews and Hammack, 2011). The FDA method involves preenrichment in lactose broth followed by selective enrichment in Tetrathionate (TT) broth and Rappaport-Vassiliadis (RV) medium. Selective plating is performed on Bismuth Sulfite (BS) agar, Xylose Lysine Desoxycholate (XLD) agar, and Hektoen Enteric (HE) agar. Biochemical screening is performed by stabs in Triple Sugar Iron (TSI) agar and Lysine Iron Agar (LIA), followed by an array of biochemical tests for identification and confirmation. Some of these tests include motility testing, Methyl-Red, Vogues-Proskauer (MR-VP Test), Lysine Decarboxylase test, and the ability to ferment sugars. Serological testing is performed using antisera for the O and H antigens. While the USDA-FSIS method uses the same scheme for biochemical screening, identification, confirmation, and serological typing, it differs in the choice of media for preenrichment and selective plating. In the USDA-FSIS method Buffered Peptone Water (BPW) is used for preenrichment and Xylose Lactose Tergitol™ 4 (XLT4) agar or Double Modified Lysine Iron agar (DMLIA) and Brilliant Green Sulfa (BGS) agar is utilized for selective plating.

While cultural-based methods are widely accepted and used for isolation, detection and confirmation of *Salmonella* spp., it takes between 5-7 days to obtain results which limits control over distribution of contaminated food products.

*Rapid methods for detection of Salmonella spp.:*In light of the current fast-paced production and distribution practices in the food industry, the development and application of alternative rapid methods for detection of *Salmonella* spp. is needed to assure effective and timely detection before foodcan reach the consumer. There is a continued need in food microbiological analysis for methods that can provide comparable results to traditional methods, while permitting the possibility of more rapid analysis with fewer preparation steps. This has led to extensive research in development of rapid tests (Feng, 2007). Rapid methods should impart rapidity, high accuracy with high specificity and sensitivity, be reproducible, easy to perform, be validated against standard methods preferably in real life scenarios and naturally contaminated samples, and be capable of being automated, minimally perturbed by the sample matrix and cost effective. While it is clear that such 'ideal' detection methods do not yet exist, many of the rapid methods fulfill some of these desired characteristics.

*Immunological-based methods.:*Immunological methods are built upon the premise of the specific binding of an antigen on a bacterial cell to monoclonal or polyclonal antibodies specific for those antigens. Several types of immunoassays that facilitate detection of foodborne pathogens have been developed including latex agglutination assays, gel immunodiffusion assays, immunomagnetic separation, the Enzyme-Linked Immunosorbent Assay (ELISA) and immunoprecipitation methods (Feng, 2007). The direct fluorescent antibody assay is another form of immunoassay which can be combined with fluorescence microscopy for detection of bacterial pathogens (Feng, 2007).

There are several potential advantages and disadvantages associated with the use of immunological-based methods. Immunological-based methods are amenable to semi-automation and full automation as is the case of the commercially available VIDAS system, which reduces hands-on time, increases sample throughput and decreases time needed to release the product. Another clear advantage is the relatively short assay time, which for ELISA can be two to three hours (Baylis, 2003; McCarthy, 2003). Among disadvantages, the low sensitivity (10^5 cells/ml for ELISA) is one of the most important. This increases the total assay time, because rapid immunological-based techniques need to be coupled with enrichment steps that can take between 24-48 hours to perform. Specificity is limited by potential cross-reactivity of antibodies with non-target microbiota, which when closely-related to the target cells might express the same antigens targeted by the specific monoclonal or polyclonal antibodies. Food components can interfere with the assay, as is the example of peroxidases present in food, which might cause a positive reaction even in absence of the target, when peroxidase based ELISA assays are employed. Lastly, the cost of immunoassays is still higher than that of cultural methods, and results obtained by immunological-based test methods are regarded as presumptive and not confirmatory (McCarthy, 2003).

*Nucleic acid-based methods:*Nucleic acid methods employ techniques to specifically recognize and amplify unique nucleic acid sequences (DNA, rRNA, mRNA) in target cells. The most widely nucleic acid-based methods are polymerase chain reaction (PCR) and its real-time variations, nucleic acid sequence-based amplification (NASBA), DNA hybridization and fluorescence *in situ*hybridization (FISH).

For *Salmonella* spp., the most common diagnostic target employed has been the *invA* gene, which is highly conserved within the genus (Rahn et al, 1992). For specific serovars, diagnostic targets have included sequences encoding antibiotic resistance (Carlson et al., 1999) or phage proteins (Hermans et al, 2005), as well as genes or sequences encoding surface antigens (Luk et al., 1993; Herrera-León, 2004).

One example of the nucleic acid-based detection techniques is the GeneTrack commercial kit (DNA hybridization), which uses a dipstick with a capture probe specifically targeting rRNA encoding genes and is available for detection of *Salmonella*, *Listeria,Campylobacter* and *E. coli* O157:H7 (Fung, 2002). Another example would be the NASBA method exemplified by the NucliSens kit to detect *S. enterica* in meat, poultry and other foods by targeting mRNA transcribed from the *dnaK* gene (Simpkins et al., 2000; D'Souza and Jaykus, 2003).

There are several potential advantages and disadvantages associated with use of nucleic acid-based methods. Among advantages, speed of analysis can be listed as the major benefit, allowing for a significant decrease in the sample analysis time. Theoretically, methods such as PCR are able to logarithmically amplify even one target sequence to a detectable number of copies. One disadvantage is the need for enrichment prior to the PCR reaction, which cannot be completely overcome. Also, the inability to distinguish between live and dead cells has been listed as a potential disadvantage of nucleic acid-based methods such as PCR and NASBA, where target nucleic acids have been shown to persist for 30 hours following cell death by heat inactivation (Birch et al., 2001; Sanderson and Nichols, 2003), though this pitfall has been overcome with the use of RT-PCR, which uses RNA as the diagnostic target. Other known disadvantages include the fact that PCR is prone to interference from inhibitors such as glycogen, calcium ions, phenolics, fat and other organic compounds which are abundant in food. This requires careful and effective sample preparation which can remove interfering inhibitors from samples prior to analysis. Several steps are needed to perform these procedures, as nucleic acids need to be extracted before running PCR reactions, forming grounds for possible contamination.

Need for approaches involving whole-cell rapid detection for Salmonella spp.:Molecular-based rapid methods can present a valid alternative to conventional detection methods, allowing for fast and sensitive detection of bacterial foodborne pathogens. However, these methods are still hindered by problems that prevent them from fully replacing traditional culture methods. While these methods have advantages, it is clear that detection of whole cells without need for analyte extraction can simplify the procedures and allow for reduced sample preparation steps. The possibility for cross-contamination or degradation of assay targets is reduced if the target can be assayed directly. Automation becomes a more attainable option as a result of reduction in sample preparation steps and the obviation of the need for analyte extraction.

Some alternative rapid detection methods employing approaches involving detection of whole-cells are:

1. *Fluorescence in situ hybridization (FISH),*which targets specific nucleic acid sequences inside whole intact cells.
2. *Phage-based detection,* employing the natural affinity, specificity and ability of bacteriophages (phages) to infect their host bacteria.
3. *Biosensors,*which couple biological recognition components with transducers of non-biological nature (primarily electronic or electrical).

While biosensors are also designed to detect analytes such as nucleic acids, this chapter will focus on biosensors dedicated to detection of whole cells. It must be said that a clear separation between these approaches cannot be made due to the fact that two or moreapproaches are often used in conjunction. An example is given by the use of phages or phage-derived molecules as biorecognition molecules for use with biosensors, or the combination of FISH with flow cytometry.

FLUORESCENCE *IN SITU* HYBRIDIZATION

Overview: The fundamental principle in FISH is the specific hybridization of complementary nucleic acid sequences within whole permeabilized cells via fluorescently labeled probes for detection. Oligonucleotide probes are designed *in silico* by aligning them with known target sequences in databases by using the probe matching tools in resources such as the ARB database (Ludwig et al., 2004) or the Ribosomal Database Project II (RDP-II) (Maidak et al., 2001). For direct fluorescent labeling, probes are chemically labeled with fluorochromes at the 5' end via an aminolinker or less often labeled at the 3' end enzymatically using a terminal transferase. Fluorochromes used for probe labeling are fluorescein-derivatives (e.g. fluorescein isothiocyanate or FITC), rhodamine dyes (e.g. Texas Red) or cyanine dyes like Cy3, Cy5 and Cy7, which typically produce brighter staining (Zimmer and Vähnert, 1986; Moter and Göbel, 2000).

FISH assays are usually performed by using rRNA as a target. This diagnostic target is desired because it is genetically stable, contains both highly conserved and variable regions, and it is present in a high number of copies in each target cell (Woese, 1987; Moter and Göbel, 2000). The fact that rRNA contains both variable and conserved regions allows for development of probes that can differentiate target cells at different taxonomic levels. Probes can discriminate between large taxonomic groups (Archea, Bacteria, and Eukarya) or down to the specific genus or species (Moter and Göbel, 2000; Amann and Fuchs, 2008). FISH-based assays are performed by completion of several discrete steps. Fixation, the first step, is performed in order to permeabilize the cells allowing for the entry of the probes as well as to prevent nucleic acids from degradation. This procedure is carried on using cross-linking fixatives like aldehydes (e.g. formaldehyde or paraformaldehyde) or precipitating fixatives such as methanol or ethanol, to fix the sample (usually on a microscope slide) prior to analysis. The second step, preparation, may involve treatment bacteria with compounds which improve the permeability of cells to probes (e.g. lysozyme or lysostaphin) (Schönhuber et al., 1997; Wagner et al., 1998; Moter and Göbel, 2000), and also includes coating the slides with gelatin (Amann et al., 1990) or other coating agents, ethanol dehydration of samples air-dried onto slides or de-waxing of samples that were paraffin-embedded (Boye et al., 1998). The third step is hybridization, which basically involves annealing of the probe to its target sequence in the cell rRNA. Washing is performed in order to mediate removal of the unbound probe. Visualization can be performed by either fluorescence microscopy or following mounting of the samples in a mounting medium with or without added agents which prevent fading of the fluorochromes under intense illumination or by cytometry.

Several variations to FISH have been described, which utilize hybridization with differing probes and probe chemistries including monolabeled oligonucleotides targeted to different sequences (Glöckner et al., 1996), oligonucleotides labeled with horseradish peroxidase followed by catalyzed reported deposition of fluorescently-labeled tyramide (CARD-FISH) (Schönhuber et al., 1997; Pernthaler et al., 2002), using molecular beacons (MBs) (Tyagi et al., 1996; Xi et al., 2003; Lenaerts et al., 2007), and peptide nucleic acids (PNA) (molecules that mimic DNA, but instead are in possession of an uncharged, achiral backbone consisting of repetitive units of *N*-(2-aminoethyl) glycine)(Egholm et al., 1993; Demidov et al., 1994; Perry O'Keefe et al., 2001; Stender et al., 2002; Brehm-Stecher et al., 2005; Almeida et al., 2010).

Application of FISH for detection of Salmonella spp.: Nordentoft et al. (1997) designed a an 18-mer oligonucleotide probe named Sal3 directed against 23S rRNA sequences of *Salmonella* by using available 23S rRNA sequences of *S. enterica and S. bongori.* The probe hybridized specifically with 49 of 55 *Salmonella* serovars tested (subspecies I, II, IIb, IV and VI), but not with representatives of subspecies IIIa *(S.* Arizonae*)* or *S. bongori*. Further testing of the developed FISH probe was performed by on-slide hybridizations of paraffin-fixed and formalin-embedded tissue sections from mice experimentally inoculated with *Salmonella* or from naturally infected animals. Rapid detection was not the scope of this work; however hybridization at 45°C could be performed within 3 hours with a brief washing step for 20 minutes. The authors concluded that the probe was able to specifically hybridize with single cells even within fixed tissue sections and that it could serve as a powerful tool for detection and identification of *S. enterica*. Another DNA-oligonucleotide for use with FISH was introduced by Kutter et al. (2006), who used FISH as a tool to characterize colonization of barley with *S. enterica* in a study that also involved *Listeria* spp. The probe Salm63, which also cross-hybridized with *Plesiomonas shigelloides* was designed to successfully evaluate *in situ* the colonization of barley roots by *S. enterica*. Fang et al. (2003) employed FISH using the previously developed Sal3 and Salm63 probes as well as the newly designed DNA probe Sal544 to detect *Salmonella* spp. in food. The procedure involved a 16 hour preenrichment protocol prior to processing for FISH and comparison with standard culture methods. When FISH was used to detect *Salmonella* spp. in naturally contaminated food samples, Sal-1 detected 52, Sal-3 detected 56 and Sal-544 detected 35 positives out of 225 samples analyzed, in comparison to cultural methods which detected *Salmonella* in 30 samples out of 225. Lantz et al. (2008) coupled FISH with capillary electrophoresis for single cell detection of *S.*

Typhimurium in mixed cultures. As few as 3 cells of hybridized *S.* Typhimurium could be detected following 15-20 minutes run time by capillary electrophoresis against 100-fold concentration of background microorganisms, with the authors concluding that single cell detection is possible by using this technique. Bisha and Brehm-Stecher (2009a) used FISH combined with an adhesive-tape based cell extraction method to detect *Salmonella* spp. on tomato surfaces. On tape hybridizations (slide hybridizations) visualized by epifluorescence microscopy, and liquid hybridizations ultimately detected by flow cytometry were performed. A detection limit of approximately10^3 CFU/cm^2 was reported and the combined procedures, including sample preparation, fixation, hybridization and visualization could be performed within approximately two hours when direct detection was performed. The approach was later extended to other types of produce, including jalapeño peppers and cilantro (Bisha and Brehm-Stecher, 2010). FISH using a combination of the Sal3 and Salm63 probes was also employed to investigate interactions of *Salmonella* spp. in alfalfa sprouts with sprout material and other background microbiota. The use of these two methods in conjunction provided information beyond simple detection as valuable information on the spatial arrangement of target cells could be obtained at very high speeds(Bisha and Brehm-Stecher, 2009b). FISH based PNA probes have also been used to effect detection of *Salmonella*. For example, Perry O'Keefe et al. (2001) introduced the genus-specific PNA probe for *Salmonella,* Sal23S10, targeted at specific 23S rRNA sequences of *Salmonella* spp. The probe was also complementary to *Actinobacillus actinomycetemcomitans*, *Buchnera aphidicola* and *Haemophilus influenzae* and cross-reacted with *Serratia marcescens*, *Yersinia pseudotuberculosis,*and *Escherichia hermanii*, whose sequences were not available during the process of designing the probe. Another PNA oligonucleotide suitable for FISH was introduced by Almeida et al. (2010). The probe SalPNA1873 was reported by the authors to impart 100% sensitivity and specificity, thus being an improvement to the previous PNA probe described in the literature. FISH using the newly developed PNA probe was applied to a number of samples spiked with *Salmonella*, including blood, water, powdered infant formula and feces. Following a preenrichment step (12-20h), low levels of the spiked pathogen could be detected. For example the reported sensitivity of detection of *Salmonella* from blood was 1 CFU/10 ml of blood after 10 hours of preenrichment, while the sensitivity of detection in powdered infant formula was also 1 CFU/g following only 12 hours of preenrichment, demonstrating good potential of the method for rapid detection of this pathogen in various matrices. FISH-based detection technology for detection of *Salmonella* is also available in the form of a commercially available kit (VIT®-Salmonella, Vermicon, Munich, Germany).

The scientific literature shows that FISH is a sensitive and robust molecular method that uses sequence-specific rRNA-targeted fluorescently-labeled oligonucleotide probes to specifically hybridize whole permeabilized bacterial cells. FISH protocols are easy to perform, extraction of nucleic acids is not required and probes and reagents needed to conduct this procedure are not costly. The natural abundance of ribosomes in an actively growing bacterial cell makes rRNA an attractive diagnostic target, assuring acceptable fluorescence signals which facilitate detection even against naturally autofluorescent backgrounds. Recent developments in probe technology, such as peptide nucleic acid (PNA) probes or self-ligating (molecular beacons) probes have further improved the hybridization kinetics and decreased the number of preparatory steps needed to perform hybridizations, ultimately allowing for better signal-to-noise ratios and faster hybridizations. Potential problems with FISH might arise from the fact that the ribosomes might not be found in abundance in starved or injured cells, however this problem can be overcome with short preenrichments and still deliver faster test results than cultural detection methods. However, while FISH has become an indispensable tool in the study of microbial communities in microbial ecology, it has not yet attracted considerable attention as an alternative foodborne pathogen detection approach to nucleic acid amplification-based detection methods which are instead finding widespread use for detection of *Salmonella* sp. in food and environment.

PHAGE-BASED DETECTION

Overview: Bacteriophages (phages) are viruses that infect bacteria and contain genetic material in the form of ssDNA, dsDNA, ssRNA, or dsRNA. They are considered the most abundant species on earth with numbers estimated at 10^{32}, serving as the primary regulator of microbial balance on earth (Kutter and Sulakvelidze, 2005; Zourob and Ripp, 2010). More than 5,000 bacteriophages have been characterized morphologically and they provide intriguing possibilities for use as recognition agents for bacteria (Ripp, 2010). Phages display specificity for the bacteria they infect (hosts), down to the species or serovar level, or they can infect an entire genus as is the case for *Listeria* phage A511 (Zink and Loessner, 1992; Hagens and Loessner 2007). The ability of a phage to bind to its host is largely dependent on number of factors such asphage tail-associated proteins, and bacterial surface receptors, which include pili, polysaccharides, and surface or membrane associated proteins (Hagens and Loessner, 2007; Ripp, 2010). Phages remain dependent on the host's metabolic machinery as they are not capable of multiplying without the aid of their hosts. It is very well known that upon recognition of the host cell, phages will initiate infection and can exhibit either a temperate lifestyle, in which they conduct a lysogenic cycle, incorporating their genome into the genome of the host or a phage can be virulent and conduct a lytic cycle, ultimately lysing the infected bacteria with subsequent release of the progeny phage. While virulent phages which infect the host and ultimately destroy the cell they are infecting may be candidates for use as diagnostic tools, they are exclusively useful for biocontrol (Hagens and Loessner, 2007). One use of phages for detection of bacteria is employment of reporter bacteriophages. DNA carrying a reporter gene is introduced in the host bacteria by means of a bacteriophage, which will only replicate in the presence of the target bacteria, allowing for the reporter gene to be expressed (Goodridge and Griffiths, 2002). Reporter genes from both prokaryotic and eukaryotic microorganisms have been used, including genes encoding luciferase (*lux* and *luc* genes), ice nucleation (*inaW*) and *E. colilacZ* (Ulitzur and Kuhn, 1987; Wolber and Green, 1990; Goodridge and Griffiths, 2002, Willford and Goodridge, 2008). The use of phages as bacterial cell wall recognition elements during separation and detection of target bacteria has also been described (Kretzer et al., 2007).

Application of phages for detection of Salmonella spp. in food: Early work from Fey et al. (1978) proposed the use of phage Felix O1 as a diagnostic approach for salmonellae and found that from a large pool of *Salmonella* serovars, 96.1% were phage sensitive. Even though very successful in their approach, the authors used phage as a confirmatory test, since it followed culturing and was done on bacterial colonies. Hirsh and Martin (1983) applied the Felix O1 bacteriophage in conjunction with high pressure liquid chromatography for detection of *Salmonella* in milk. They were able to detect as few as 5 CFU/ml at 24 hours after the samples were collected, and were able to detect *Salmonella enterica* serovars Typhimurium, Dublin, Anatum, Krefeld, Saintpaul, Agona, and Enteritidis. However, the assay could not detect 1 of 3 *S.* Agona isolates and 3 of 7 *S.* Enteritidis isolates (Hirsh and Martin, 1983). The *Salmonella* specific phage P22 was genetically modified to carry the *lux* genes of *V. fischeri* by Chen and Griffiths (1996) to detect groups B and D and some isolates from group C of *Salmonella.* Upon infection of the target bacteria, resulting luminescence was detected via x-ray film or a photon-counting charge coupled device (CCD) camera. The assay detected all 57 *Salmonella* strains tested and none of the 22 non-*Salmonella* isolates included in the assay. Following 6 h of preincubation, the assay was able to detect 10 CFU/ml salmonellae in pure culture, while detection of the same contamination level in a food system (eggs) required 24 hours of incubation. Time to detection, defined as the time needed to detect 10^8 CFU/ml was reported to be 1 to 3 hours without the needfor preincubation(Chen and Griffiths, 1996). A modified bacterial ice nucleation assay (BIND) which makes use of the *ina* genes conferring ice nucleation ability was described by Irwin et al. (2000). Phages were genetically modified to encode ice nucleation protein, which causes the infected host to express the protein on the outer membrane. The assay involved a supercooling step which allowed for infected salmonellae to freeze which was detectable by the color change of a phase-sensitive dye. Quantitative detection was achieved and in combination with an immunomagnetic separation protocol, a detection limit of 4.5 cells per ml of *S.* Enteritidis was reported(Irwin et al, 2000). Prior work using the BIND assay with phage P22 carrying the *inaW* gene had also been conducted by Wolber and Green (1990) who were able to detect as few as 10 CFU/ml of *S.* Dublin against a background of 10^7 background microorganisms when applied to the detection of *Salmonella* in broth and raw eggs. The *Salmonella* BIND assay was commercialized by IDEXX (Westbrook, ME) but is no longer available (Irwin et al. 2000). Also, Thouand et al. (2008) used the genetically modified P22::*luxAB* to detect *S.* Typhimurium in poultry, feed and environmental samples. A luminometer was used for detection of luminescence ensuring specific detection of *S.* Typhimurium LT2, with direct detection limits in culture reported as ~10^2 CFU/ml and ~10^4 CFU/ml in food. Following preenrichment for up to 16 hours, the target could be detected in all samples.

Blasco et al. (1998) utilized the ability of lytic phage to lyse their bacterial hosts to develop a phage-specific lysis assay for detection of *S.* Newport followed by measurement of released adenylate kinase to detect the target at a level of 10^3 CFU/ml within two hours of assay time. Phage SJ2 was used in conjunction with the bioluminescence assay of adenylate kinase released by lysed host bacteria (Wu et al., 2001) to detect *S.* Enteritidis in broth. It was determined that the largest increase in released adenylate kinase was achieved at a multiplicity of infection (MOI) of 10-100, and a detection limit of 10^3 CFU/ml was reported following two hours of assay performance.

Stewart et al. (1998) developed the phage amplification assay which makes use of the natural ability of phages to amplify themselves upon infection of their host bacteria. In this assay, exogenous phage are added to the sample to be tested and phages that infect target bacteria replicate within the bacteria, while exogenous phages which have not infected bacteria are destroyed by the use of a virucidal agent consisting of pomegranate rind extract in combination with ferrous sulfate. The authors reported a detection limit of 600 CFU/ml for *S.* Typhimurium within 4 hours of assay time. Following up on this work, Favrin and colleagues (2001) used phage SJ2 to detect *S.* Enteritidis in broth with a detection sensitivity of 10^4 CFU/ml with the assay requiring 4-5 hours for its performance. The assay was comprised of an immunomagnetic separation step, infection of target bacteria, amplification and recovery of progeny phages, and then detection of the progeny phages on fresh host cells, allowing for coupling with a turbidity or fluorescence end-point detection step.

The studies discussed above described the use of genetically modified phages for detection of target bacteria, or alternatively, took advantage of the natural ability of phages to either lyse the host cell or amplify themselves during infection to develop detection strategies for bacteria. Another approach to the use of phage in detection of bacteria is to label them with fluorophores and use them to tag the target bacteria cells in a manner analogous to antibodies. Goodridge and colleagues (1999 a, b) were the first to demonstrate this technique for detection of foodborne pathogens. More recently, Mosier-Boss et al. (2003) were able to visualize phage P22 infecting *S.* Typhimurium LT2 by epifluorescence microscopy following labeling of the phage DNA with the nucleic acid stain SYBR gold. The technique exploited the affinity of the phage for the host as well as the affinity of the dye for dsDNA of the P22 phage, allowing for discrimination of the target cells from non-target microorganisms via an optical method.

Others have combined the use of phage with ELISA based methods to effect rapid detection of *Salmonella*. Guan's group (2006) described detection of the antibiotic resistant *S.* Typhimurium DT104 via a phage replication-competitive enzyme-linked immunosorbent assay (PR-cELISA). This work employed phage BP1 to infect the host cells, and then observed the replication of the phages by cELISA using competitive binding of BP1 and biotinylated BP1 to *S.* Typhimurium smooth LPS. Using this assay, 39 of 40 *S.* Typhimurium strains and 27 of 27 DT104 strains tested could be detected, however 2 of 10 non-Typhimurium and 5 of 18 *Salmonella* somatic group D1 strains were also detected. In addition, Galikowska et al. (2011) substituted antibodies with bacteriophages for specific detection of *S. enterica* in an ELISA format, which achieved comparable levels of detection with conventional ELISA at 10^6 CFU/ml. The authors however argue that there are distinct benefits to using phages instead of antibodies in an ELISA assay, including cost, availability and simplicity of the assay. Phage recombinant technology has also found use in commercial assays for detection of *Salmonella* from food as exemplified by the product Vidas® SPT assay for *Salmonella* (Biomerieux, Marcy l'Etoile, France), which uses phage tail proteins that are specific for *Salmonella* to capture whole bacteria from enrichments prior to detection by enzyme linked antibodies.

Finally, a non direct approach for aiding detection of *Salmonella* against background microorganisms was proposed by (Muldoon et al., 2007). The method involved the use of phages specific for bacteria such as *Citrobacter* spp. and *E. coli* which may out-compete *Salmonella* growth during enrichment. Use of the phage cocktail in primary enrichment from artificially and naturally contaminated meat and poultry samples significantly improved detection of *Salmonella* by reducing the number of false positive samples. Against a background of more than 10^5 competing microorganisms, from 32 of 115 samples which previously tested false positive, the number of false positive samples was reduced to none following employment of the phage cocktail in enrichment as confirmed by detection via lateral flow immunochromatography.

The use of phage technology to detect foodborne pathogenic bacteria including *Salmonella* spp. offers the advantageous of rapidity, reliability and sensitivity. Despite this, the technology as a whole has not been commercialized, with the exception of the now defunct *Salmonella* BIND assay, and the Vidas SPT assay. One reason for this situation may be the fact that, until recently it was expensive to sequence the genomes of phages, in order to obtain the necessary genetic information needed to modify the phages, or identify components of the phages (phage tail proteins) useful for a diagnostic assay. Hopefully, as more and more genetic sequences of diverse phages are published, the use of phages as diagnostic agents will be fully recognized. The potential for a revolution in microbial testing can be realized through the near on-line detection of foodborne pathogens such as *Salmonella*. By using phages to define the pathogens present within a food in a rapid manner, it should be possible to quickly determine the safety of foods prior to their shipment to retail.

BIOSENSORS

Overview:Biosensors are analytical instruments which translate biological inputs into electrical signals, and are comprised of two basic components: a biorecognition component (tissue, antibody, nucleic acid, cell, bacteriophage, enzyme, etc) and a transducer which converts this signal into an electrical signal (piezoelectric, electrochemical, thermal, magnetic, mechanical and combinations thereof) which can be analyzed (Velusamy et al., 2010). Biosensors can be classified based on the types of transducers used (optical, electrochemical) or alternatively based on the types of biorecognition elements. For the purposes of this chapter, biosensors employed in detection of whole cells of *Salmonella* spp. will be broadly grouped based on the biorecognition elements they employ.

Immunosensors:Brookset al. (1992) described an immunosensor specific for *Salmonella* employing alkaline phosphatase as the reporter, using both direct detection and detection following enzyme amplification. The authors reported short assay times (4 hours) and detection limits of 10^4-10^5 CFU/ml in pure cultures and food systems. When applied to spiked foods, detection limits of 1-5 CFU/ml or g were achieved following non-selective or selective enrichments with false positive results eliminated when the enrichment time was optimized (Brooks et al., 1992). Seo et al. (1999) proposed an approach involving a combination of anti-*Salmonella* antibodies with an integrated optic interferometer and tested it against *S.* Typhimurium in mixed culture and a food system. In a sandwich assay format with a second antibody or gold-conjugated antibodies, the method allowed for a detection sensitivity of 10^5 CFU/ml within 10 minutes assay time; the use of the direct reductive amination method for immobilization of capture antibodies allowed for further enhancement of the limit of detection to 10^4 CFU/ml. Following non-selective enrichment for 12 hours, spiked *S.* Typhimurium could be detected from chicken carcass fluid at levels of 20 CFU/ml (Seo et al., 1999). Dill et al. (1999) was able to detect as few as 119 CFU of *S.* Typhimurium in chicken carcass water by using a light addressable potentiometric biosensor on a silicon chip following capture of the target by filtration on an antibody-functionalized nitrocellulose membrane. Also in chicken carcass wash water, Che et al. (2000) were able to detect *S.* Typhimurium at 10^3 CFU/ml using a combination of immunomagnetic separation and an immunoelectrochemical method involving a reaction of alkaline phosphatase and measurements performed using an amperometric tyrosinase carbon paste electrode. The commercial surface plasmon resonance biosensor Biacore 3000 (GE Healthcare) was employed to correctly detect 53 different *Salmonella* serovars at high levels in pure culture using antibodies to *Salmonella* groups A, B, D, and E (Kauffmann-White scheme), while no cross reactivity was observed with 30 non-*Salmonella* strains (Bokken et al., 2003). Groups C, G, L, and P were not detected as previously predicted. Detection of *S.* Typhimurium in pure culture was achieved at levels as low as 10^3 CFU/ml. Mazumdar et al. (2007) applied SPR using polyclonal antibodies against *Salmonella* in a sandwich-type assay for both capture and detection of *S.* Typhimurium in spiked milk samples. The authors reported detection of the target microorganism at levels of 10^5 CFU/ml within 1 hour, with no differences observed in pure culture from spiked milk samples. SPR has also been successfully used to assess infection status with *Salmonella* in slaughter pigs (Mazumdar et al., 2008). LPS extracted from *S.* Typhimurium was used as a biorecognition molecule by coating of an SPR chip. This method was able to differentiate between low, medium and high *Salmonella* infection rates when applied to sera from slaughter pigs. In addition, it displayed very good correlation with a commercial ELISA kit (r=0.90), but it did not require extensive sample preparation and could be performed in about 45 minutes. No cross-reactivity with *S.* Cholerasuis or *E. coli* antibodies was observed (Mazumdar et al., 2008).

Besides SPR, other sensors have also been employed to detect *Salmonella*. Guntupalli et al. (2007) used polyclonal antibodies as biorecognition molecules for detection in combination with a magnetoelastic biosensor. Fu et al. (2008) coated silicon/gold nanorods with anti-*Salmonella* antibodies and organic dye for detection of *Salmonella*. An enhancement in fluorescence was achieved upon binding of the target analytes to antibodies on the functionalized nanorods. Pournaras et al. (2008) coated electropolymerized polytyramine films with polyclonal antibodies and employed impedance measurements to detect *S.* Typhimurium, observing signal alterations of 33% and 88% following 3 and 8 hours incubation, respectively. The method was also applied to successfully detect the target in milk samples spiked at approximately 10^4 CFU/ml. Immunosensors were applied in a food system (milk) for detection of *Salmonella* (Liébana et al., 2009). This assay involved capture and preconcentration of target cells from milk via immunomagnetic separation, followed by detection with peroxidase labeled polyclonal antibodies and detection with a magneto-electrode (electrochemical). Following preenrichment of skimmed milk for 6 hours, highly sensitive detection of 2.7 CFU/25 g of milk was achieved, as well as discrimination of target salmonellae from non-target *E. coli*. Yang et al. (2009) used monoclonal antibodies as biorecognition molecules attached to gold nanoparticles in an assay format that comprised ultimate detection by electrochemical impedance spectroscopy. This assay was able to detect *Salmonella* spp. at a level of ~10^2 CFU/ml in pure cultures while preliminary steps towards application of the method in pork samples were also undertaken in this work.

Label-free biosensors: Mid-infrared (mid-IR) spectroscopy was employed by Ravindranath et al. (2009) for detection of *S.* Typhimurium in pure culture as well as spinach and 2% fat milk within 30 minutes. However, label-free spectroscopy fingerprinting was only performed following a form of immunomagnetic separation of target microorganism with biofunctionalized nanoparticles from the food matrices, which was reported to enhance mid-IR fingerprinting, and achieved limits of detection in the 10^4-10^5 CFU/2 ml sample (Ravindranath et al., 2009). Banada et al. (2009) reported the use of label free detection of *Salmonella* spp. colonies among other pathogens with an accuracy of 90-99%. This was based on the forward scattering 'fingerprint' of colonies originating from one single cell. Forward-scatter phenotyping (FSP) was evaluated by Rajwa et al (2010) for detection of colonies of *Salmonella*using the label-free pathogen recognition technology termed BARDOT (Bacteria

Rapid Detection using Optical scattering Technology). The authors stated that recognition and differentiation was possible down to the serovar level, if growth and sample handling conditions are maintained constant. The method has the advantage of being able to identify colonies rapidly without need to destroy the sample allowing for further identification and confirmation methods to be applied. A disadvantage is the fact that the development of a database which will encompass all possible recognition patterns seems crucial for the successful completion of the approach. Also it remains to be seen whether it is possible to maintain growth conditions constant at a satisfactory level to allow for reproducible results to be obtained.

Aptamers were evaluated as biorecognition molecules for *S.* Typhimurium for use with biosensors by Book et al. (2011). The authors used two aptamers previously constructed by Joshi et al. (2009) with affinity for outer membrane proteins of *S.* Typhimurium, and evaluated them on live single cells by fluorescence correlation spectroscopy (FCS). The authors concluded that these aptamers displayed high affinity for the target surface proteins, which in turn were found to be abundant on target cells. As a result, it was shown that aptamers have very good potential for use in a biosensor setting.

The potential of biosensors to meet the demands for speed, sensitivity, specificity, high throughput analysis and versatile real-time microbiological detection methods has led to their development and evaluation of their use to rapidly detect food and waterborne pathogens. Still, a great deal of research is needed before biosensors can become a viable alternative to current detection methods. Furthermore, in order to become more attractive, they must be able to obtain detection levels comparable to more acceptable methods, with a high level of reproducibility. Additionally, in the food safety arena, there is still a lack of portable, integrated biosensor systems (Palchetti and Mascini, 2008).

Conclusions and Future Directions

In conclusion, rapid detection methods for whole *Salmonella* cells provide a valuable alternative to established cultural and molecular detection methods. As with all detection assays, there advantages and disadvantages to the detection of whole bacterial cells. The methods described here offer the advantages of rapidity, capability for automation, and simplicity. Still, there are several disadvantages that are associated with whole cell detection methods. In order to fully assess their usefulness, more studies are needed which are applied to complex food matrices as the whole cell methods described are often tested using pure cultures with unrealistic contamination levels. Sample preparation methods that could increase the sensitivity of whole cell detection methods have not progressed beyond the use of enrichment to increase bacterial concentration. Such methods should be developed and be designed in combination with the whole cell detection assays to provide an integrated solution to the detection of foodborne pathogens. Finally, the labor intensiveness and cost effectiveness of whole cell detection methods such as biosensors must be scrutinized. Even though there are disadvantages associated with the use of these methods for detection of *Salmonella* spp. in food, the potential impact that the refinement and application of these methods can have on the food supply cannot be ignored and warrants more attention and future research.

REFERENCES

Airoldi AA, Zottola EA. 1988. Growth and Survival of *Salmonella typhimurium* at low temperature in nutrient deficient media. *J. Food Sci.* 53(5):1511-3.

Aleksic S, Heinzerling F, Bockemuhl J. 1996. Human infection caused by Salmonellae of subspecies II to VI in Germany, 1977-1992. *Zentralbl. Bakteriol.* 283(3):391-8.

Almeida C, Azevedo NF, Fernandes RM, Keevil CW, Vieira MJ. 2010. Fluorescence in situ hybridization method using a peptide nucleic acid probe for identification of *Salmonella* spp. in a broad spectrum of samples. *Appl. Environ. Microbiol.* 76(13):4476-85.

Amann R, Fuchs BM. 2008. Single-cell identification in microbial communities by improved fluorescence in situ hybridization techniques. *Nat. Rev. Microbiol.* 6(5):339-48.

Amann RI, Krumholz L, Stahl DA. 1990. Fluorescent-oligonucleotide probing of whole cells for determinative, phylogenetic, and environmental studies in microbiology. *J. Bacteriol.* 172(2):762-70.

Anderson ES, Ward LR, De Saxe MJ, Old DC, Barker R, Duguid JP. 1978. Correlation of phaga type, biotype and source in strains of *Salmonella typhimurium*. *J. Hyg.* (Lond). 81(2):203-17.

Andrews WH, Hammack TS. 2011. *Salmonella*, In *Bacteriological Analytical Manual Online*, Chapter 5. http://www.fda.gov/Food/ScienceResearch/LaboratoryMethods/BacteriologicalAnalyticalManualBAM/ucm070149.htm. Accessed December 21, 2011.

Andrews HL, Bäumler AJ. 2005. *Salmonella* species, In Fratamico PM, Bhunia AK, Smith JL (Eds.), *Foodborne Pathogens*, Caister Academic Press, Norfolk, UK.

Anonymous. 1986. Microbiological safety of vacuum-packed, high salt foods questioned. *Food Chem. News.* 28:30-1.

Banada PP, Huff K, Bae E, Rajwa B, Aroonnual A, Bayraktar B, Adil A, Robinson JP, Hirleman ED, Bhunia AK. 2009. Label-free detection of multiple bacterial pathogens using light-scattering sensor. *Biosens. Bioelectron.* 24(6):1685-92.

Baylis CL. 2003. Immunological techniques: immunochromotography enzyme-linked immunofluorescent assays and agglutination techniques, In McMeekin TA (Ed.),*Detecting pathogens in food*, Woodhead Publishing Limited and CRC Press LLC.

Birch L, Dawson CE, Cornett JH, Keer JT. 2001. A comparison of nucleic acid amplification techniques for the assessment of bacterial viability. *Lett. Appl. Microbiol.* 33(4):296-301.

Bisha B, Brehm-Stecher BF. 2009a. Simple adhesive-tape-based sampling of tomato surfaces combined with rapid fluorescence in situ hybridization for *Salmonella* detection. *Appl. Environ. Microbiol.* 75(5):1450-5.

Bisha B, Brehm-Stecher BF. 2009b. Flow-through imaging cytometry for characterization of *Salmonella* subpopulations in alfalfa sprouts, a complex food system. *Biotechnol. J.* 4(6):880-7.

Bisha B, Brehm-Stecher BF. 2010. Combination of adhesive-tape-based sampling and fluorescence in situ hybridization for rapid detection of *Salmonella* on fresh produce. *J. Vis. Exp.* (44). pii: 2308.

Blasco R, Murphy MJ, Sanders MF, Squirrell DJ. 1998. Specific assays for bacteria using phage mediated release of adenylate kinase. *J. Appl. Microbiol.* 84(4):661-6.

Bokken GC, Corbee RJ, van Knapen F, Bergwerff AA. 2003. Immunochemical detection of *Salmonella* group B, D and E using an optical surface plasmon resonance biosensor. *FEMS Microbiol. Lett.* 222(1):75-82.

Book B, Chen J, Irudayaraj J. 2011. Quantification of receptor targeting aptamer binding characteristics using single-molecule spectroscopy. *Biotechnol. Bioeng.* 108(5):1222-7.

Boye M, Jensen TK, Møller K, Leser TD, Jorsal SE. 1998. Specific detection of the genus *Serpulina, S. hyodysenteriae* and *S. pilosicoli* in porcine intestines by fluorescent rRNA in situ hybridization. *Mol. Cell Probes.* 12(5):323-30.

Brehm-Stecher BF, Hyldig-Nielsen JJ, Johnson EA. 2005. Design and evaluation of 16S rRNA-targeted peptide nucleic acid probes for whole-cell detection of members of the genus *Listeria. Appl. Environ. Microbiol.* 71(9):5451-7.

Brenner FW, Villar RG, Angulo FJ, Tauxe R, Swaminathan B. 2000. *Salmonella* nomenclature. *J. Clin. Microbiol.* 38(7):2465-7.

Brooks JL, Mirhabibollahi B, Kroll RG. 1992. Experimental enzyme-linked amperometric immunosensors for the detection of salmonellas in foods. *J. Appl. Bacteriol.* 73(3):189-96.

Carlson SA, Bolton LF, Briggs CE, Hurd HS, Sharma VK, Fedorka-Cray PJ, Jones BD. 1999. Detection of multiresistant *Salmonella typhimurium* DT104 using multiplex and fluorogenic PCR. *Mol. Cell Probes.* 13(3):213-22.

Che YH, Li Y, Slavik M, Paul D. 2000. Rapid detection of *Salmonella typhimurium* in chicken carcass wash water using an immunoelectrochemical method. *J. Food Prot.* 63(8):1043-8.

Chen J, Griffiths MW. 1996. *Salmonella* detection in eggs using *lux*+ bacteriophages. *J. Food Prot.* 59:908–14.

Crump JA, Griffin PM, Angulo FJ. 2002. Bacterial contamination of animal feed and its relationship to human foodborne illness. *Clin. Infect. Dis.* 35(7):859-65.

D'Aoust JY, MaurerJ. 2007. *Salmonella* species, In Doyle MP, Beuchat LR (Eds.), *Food Microbiology: Fundamentals and Frontiers*, 3d Ed., ASM Press, Washington D.C.

D'Aoust JY. 1989. *Salmonella*, In Doyle MP (Ed.), *Foodborne Bacterial Pathogens*, Marcel Dekker, New York, N.Y.

D'Aoust JY, Aris BJ, Thisdale A, Durante N, Brisson D, Dragon G, Lachapelle M, Johnston M, Laidley R. 1975. *Salmonella eastbourne* outbreak associated with chocolate. *Can. Inst. Food Sci. Technol. J.* 8:181–4.

Demidov VV, Potaman VN, Frank-Kamenetskii MD, Egholm M, Buchard O, Sönnichsen SH, Nielsen PE. 1994. Stability of peptide nucleic acids in human serum and cellular extracts. *Biochem. Pharmacol.* 48(6):1310-3.

Dill K, Stanker LH, Young CR. 1999. Detection of salmonella in poultry using a silicon chip-based biosensor. *J Biochem Biophys Methods*. 41(1):61-7.

Droffner ML, Yamamoto N. 1992. Procedure for isolation of *Escherichia*, *Salmonella*, and *Pseudomonas* mutants capable of growth at the refractory temperature of 54°C. *J. Microbiol. Methods*. 14:201-6.

D'Souza DH, Jaykus LA. 2003. Nucleic acid sequence based amplification for the rapid and sensitive detection of *Salmonella enterica* from foods. *J. Appl. Microbiol.* 95(6):1343-50.

Egholm M, Buchardt O, Christensen L, Behrens C, Freier SM, Driver DA, Berg RH, Kim SK, Norden B, Nielsen PE. 1993. PNA hybridizes to complementary oligonucleotides obeying the Watson-Crick hydrogen-bonding rules. *Nature.* 365(6446):566-8.

Fang Q, Brockmann S, Botzenhart K, Wiedenmann A. 2003. Improved detection of *Salmonella* spp. in foods by fluorescent in situ hybridization with 23S rRNA probes: a comparison with conventional culture methods. *J. Food Prot.* 66(5):723-31.

Favrin SJ, Jassim SA, Griffiths MW. 2001. Development and optimization of a novel immunomagnetic separation- bacteriophage assay for detection of *Salmonella enterica* serovar Enteritidis in broth. *Appl. Environ. Microbiol.* 67(1):217-24.

Feng P. 2007. Rapid methods for the detection of foodborne pathogens: current and next generation technologies, In Doyle MP, Beuchat LR (Eds.), *Food Microbiology: Fundamentals and Frontiers*, 3d Ed., ASM Press, Washington D.C.

Fey H, Bürgi E, Margadant A, Boller E. 1978. An economic and rapid diagnostic procedure for the detection of salmonella/shigella using the polyvalent salmonella phage O-1. *Zentralbl. Bakteriol. Orig.* A. 240(1):7-15.

Fu J, Park B, Siragusa G, Jones L, Tripp R, Zhao Y, Cho YJ. 2008. An Au/Si hetero-nanorod-based biosensor for *Salmonella* detection. *Nanotechnology.* 19(15):155502.

Fung DYC. 2002. Rapid methods and automation in microbiology. *Compr. Rev. Food Sci. Food Saf.* 1:3-22.

Galikowska E, Kunikowska D, Tokarska-Pietrzak E, Dziadziuszko H, Łoś JM, Golec P, Węgrzyn G, Łoś M. 2011. Specific detection of *Salmonella enterica* and *Escherichia coli* strains by using ELISA with bacteriophages as recognition agents. *Eur. J. Clin. Microbiol. Infect. Dis.* 30(9):1067-73.

Glöckner FO, Amann R, Alfreider A, Pernhaler J, Psenner R, Trebesius K, Schleifer K-H. 1996. An in situ hybridization protocol for detection and identification of planktonic bacteria. *Syst. Appl. Microbiol.* 19:403–6.

Goodridge L, Chen J, Griffiths M. 1999a. Development and characterization of a fluorescent-bacteriophage assay for detection of *Escherichia coli* O157:H7. *Appl. Environ. Microbiol.* 65(4):1397-404.

Goodridge L, Chen J, Griffiths M. 1999b. The use of a fluorescent bacteriophage assay for detection of *Escherichia coli* O157:H7 in inoculated ground beef and raw milk *Int. J. Food Microbiol.* 47(1-2):43-50.

Goodridge L, Griffiths M. 2002. Reporter bacteriophage assays as a means to detect foodborne pathogenic bacteria. *Food Res. Int.* 35(9):863-70.

Guan J, Chan M, Allain B, Mandeville R, Brooks BW. 2006. Detection of multiple antibiotic-resistant *Salmonella enterica* serovar Typhimurium DT104 by phage replication-competitive enzyme-linked immunosorbent assay. *J. Food Prot.* 69(4):739-42.

Guntupalli R, Hu J, Lakshmanan RS, Huang TS, Barbaree JM, Chin BA. 2007. A magnetoelastic resonance biosensor immobilized with polyclonal antibody for the detection of *Salmonella typhimurium*. *Biosens. Bioelectron.* 22(7):1474-9.

Hagens S, Loessner MJ. 2007. Application of bacteriophages for detection and control of foodborne pathogens. *Appl. Microbiol. Biotechnol.* 76(3):513-9.

Hermans AP, Abee T, Zwietering MH, Aarts HJ. 2005. Identification of novel *Salmonella enterica* serovar Typhimurium DT104-specific prophage and nonprophage chromosomal sequences among serovar Typhimurium isolates by genomic subtractive hybridization. *Appl. Environ. Microbiol.* 71(9):4979-85.

Herrera-León S, McQuiston JR, Usera MA, Fields PI, Garaizar J, Echeita MA. 2004. Multiplex PCR for distinguishing the most common phase-1 flagellar antigens of *Salmonella* spp. *J. Clin. Microbiol.* 42(6):2581-6.

Hirsh DC, Martin LD. 1983. Detection of *Salmonella* spp. in milk by using Felix-O1 bacteriophage and high-pressure liquid chromatography. *Appl. Environ. Microbiol.* 46(5):1243-5.

Hurd HS, Gailey JK, McKean JD, Rostagno MH. 2001. Rapid infection in market-weight swine following exposure to a *Salmonella typhimurium*-contaminated environment. *Am. J. Vet. Res.* 62(8):1194-7.

Irwin P, Gehring A, Tu SI, Brewster J, Fanelli J, Ehrenfeld E. 2000. Minimum detectable level of Salmonellae using a binomial-based bacterial ice nucleation detection assay (BIND). *J. AOAC Int.* 83(5):1087-95.

Joshi R, Janagama H, Dwivedi HP, Senthil Kumar TM, Jaykus LA, Schefers J, Sreevatsan S. 2009. Selection, characterization, and application of DNA aptamers for the capture and detection of *Salmonella enterica* serovars. *Mol. Cell Probes.* 23(1):20-8.

Kretzer JW, Lehmann R, Schmelcher M, Banz M, Kim KP, Korn C, Loessner MJ. 2007. Use of high-affinity cell wall-binding domains of bacteriophage endolysins for immobilization and separation of bacterial cells. *Appl. Environ. Microbiol.* 73(6):1992-2000.

Kutter E, Sulakvelidze A. 2005. *Bacteriophages: biology and applications,* CRC Press, Boca Raton, FL.

Kutter S, Hartmann A, Schmid M. 2006. Colonization of barley (*Hordeum vulgare*) with *Salmonella enterica* and *Listeria* spp. *FEMS Microbiol. Ecol.* 56(2):262-71.

Lantz AW, Brehm-Stecher BF, Armstrong DW. 2008. Combined capillary electrophoresis and DNA-fluorescence in situ hybridization for rapid molecular identification of *Salmonella* Typhimurium in mixed culture. *Electrophoresis.* 29(12):2477-84.

Lenaerts J, Lappin-Scott HM, Porter J. 2007. Improved fluorescent in situ hybridization method for detection of bacteria from activated sludge and river water by using DNA molecular beacons and flow cytometry. *Appl. Environ. Microbiol.* 73(6):2020-3.

Liébana S, Lermo A, Campoy S, Cortés MP, Alegret S, Pividori MI. 2009. Rapid detection of *Salmonella* in milk by electrochemical magneto-immunosensing. *Biosens. Bioelectron.* 25(2):510-3.

Ludwig W, Strunk O, Westram R, Richter L, Meier H, Yadhukumar, et al. 2004. ARB: a software environment for sequence data. *Nucleic AcidsRes.* 32(4):1363-71.

Luk JM, Kongmuang U, Reeves PR, Lindberg AA. 1993. Selective amplification of abequose and paratose synthase genes (*rfb*) by polymerase chain reaction for identification of *Salmonella* major serogroups (A, B, C2, and D).*J. Clin. Microbiol.* 31(8):2118-23.

Maidak BL, Cole JR, Lilburn TG, Parker CT Jr, Saxman PR, Farris RJ, Garrity GM, Olsen GJ, Schmidt TM, Tiedje JM. 2001. The RDP-II (Ribosomal Database Project). *Nucleic Acids Res.* 29(1):173-4.

Mazumdar SD, Barlen B, Kramer T, Keusgen M. 2008. A rapid serological assay for prediction of *Salmonella* infection status in slaughter pigs using surface plasmon resonance. *J. Microbiol. Methods.* 75(3):545-50.

Mazumdar SD, Hartmann M, Kämpfer P, Keusgen M. 2007. Rapid method for detection of *Salmonella* in milk by surface plasmon resonance (SPR). *Biosens. Bioelectron.* 22(9-10):2040-6.

McCarthy J. 2003. Immunological techniques: ELISA, In McMeekin TA (Ed.), *Detecting pathogens in food.* Woodhead Publishing Limited and CRC Press LLC.

Mosier-Boss PA, Lieberman SH, Andrews JM, Rohwer FL, Wegley LE, Breitbart M. 2003. Use of fluorescently labeled phage in the detection and identification of bacterial species. *Appl. Spectrosc*. 57(9):1138-44.

Moter A, Göbel UB. 2000. Fluorescence in situ hybridization (FISH) for direct visualization of microorganisms. *J. Microbiol. Methods*. 41(2):85-112.

Muldoon MT, Teaney G, Li J, Onisk DV, Stave JW.2007. Bacteriophage-based enrichment coupled to immunochromatographic strip-based detection for the determination of *Salmonella* in meat and poultry. *J. Food Prot.* 70(10):2235-42.

Nordentoft S, Christensen H, Wegener HC. 1997. Evaluation of a fluorescence-labelled oligonucleotide probe targeting 23S rRNA for in situ detection of *Salmonella* serovars in paraffin-embedded tissue sections and their rapid identification in bacterial smears. *J. Clin. Microbiol.* 35(10):2642-8.

Olsen SJ, MacKinnon LC, Goulding JS, Bean NH, Slutsker L. 2000. Surveillance for foodborne-disease outbreaks--United States, 1993-1997. *MMWR CDC Surveill. Summ.* 49(1):1-62.

Palchetti I, Mascini M. 2008. Electroanalytical biosensors and their potential for food pathogen and toxin detection. *Anal. Bioanal. Chem*. 391(2):455-71.

Pernthaler A, Pernthaler J, Amann R. 2002. Fluorescence in situ hybridization and catalyzed reporter deposition for the identification of marine bacteria. *Appl. Environ. Microbiol.* 68(6):3094-101.

Perry-O'Keefe H, Rigby S, Oliveira K, Sørensen D, Stender H, Coull J, Hyldig-Nielsen JJ. 2001. Identification of indicator microorganisms using a standardized PNA FISH method. *J. Microbiol. Methods*. 47(3):281-92.

Pournaras AV, Koraki T, Prodromidis MI. 2008. Development of an impedimetric immunosensor based on electropolymerized polytyramine films for the direct detection of *Salmonella typhimurium* in pure cultures of type strains and inoculated real samples. *Anal. Chim. Acta*. 624(2):301-7.

Rahn K, De Grandis SA, Clarke RC, McEwen SA, Galán JE, Ginocchio C, Curtiss R 3rd, Gyles CL. 1992. Amplification of an *invA* gene sequence of *Salmonella typhimurium* by polymerase chain reaction as a specific method of detection of *Salmonella*. *Mol. Cell Probes*. 6(4):271-9.

Rajwa B, Dundar MM, Akova F, Bettasso A, Patsekin V, Hirleman ED, Bhunia AK, Robinson JP. 2010. Discovering the unknown: detection of emerging pathogens using a label-free light-scattering system. *Cytometry* A. 77(12):1103-12.

Ravindranath SP, Mauer LJ, Deb-Roy C, Irudayaraj J. 2009. Biofunctionalized magnetic nanoparticle integrated mid-infrared pathogen sensor for food matrixes. *Anal. Chem.* 81(8):2840-6.

Ripp S. 2010. Bacteriophage-based pathogen detection. *Adv. Biochem. Eng. Biotechnol.* 118:65-83.

Rose BE. 2001. Isolation and identification of *Salmonella* from meat, poultry and egg products, *Microbiology laboratory guidebook*, 3rd ed., rev. 1, Food Safety and Inspection Service, U.S. Department of Agriculture, Washington, D.C.

Sanderson K, Nichols D. 2003. Genetic techniques: PCR, NASBA, hybridisation and microarrays, In McMeekin TA (Ed.), *Detecting pathogens in food,* Woodhead Publishing Limited and CRC Press LLC.

Schönhuber W, Fuchs B, Juretschko S, Amann R. 1997. Improved sensitivity of whole-cell hybridization by the combination of horseradish peroxidase-labeled oligonucleotides and tyramide signal amplification. *Appl. Environ. Microbiol.* 63(8):3268-73.

Seo KH, Brackett RE, Hartman NF, Campbell DP. 1999. Development of a rapid response biosensor for detection of *Salmonella typhimurium*. *J. Food Prot.* 62(5):431-7.

Simpkins SA, Chan AB, Hays J, Pöpping B, Cook N. 2000. An RNA transcription-based amplification technique (NASBA) for the detection of viable *Salmonella enterica*. *Lett. Appl. Microbiol.* 30(1):75-9.

Stender H, Fiandaca M, Hyldig-Nielsen JJ, Coull J. 2002. PNA for rapid microbiology. *J. Microbiol. Methods*. 48(1):1-17.

Stewart GS, Jassim SA, Denyer SP, Newby P, Linley K, Dhir VK. 1998. The specific and sensitive detection of bacterial pathogens within 4 h using bacteriophage amplification. *J. Appl. Microbiol.* 84(5):777-83.

Thouand G, Vachon P, Liu S, Dayre M, Griffiths MW. 2008. Optimization and validation of a simple method using P22::*luxAB* bacteriophage for rapid detection of *Salmonella enterica* serotypes A, B, and D in poultry samples. *J. Food Prot.* 71(2):380-5.

Tyagi S, Kramer FR. 1996. Molecular beacons: probes that fluoresce upon hybridization. *Nat. Biotechnol.* 14(3):303-8.

Ulitzur S, Kuhn J, 1987. Introduction of *lux* genes into bacteria, a new approach for specific determination of bacteria and their antibiotic susceptibility, In Schölmerich J, Anreesen R, Kapp A, Ernst M, Woods WG, (Eds.), *Bioluminescence new perspectives,* John Wiley, New York.

Velusamy V, Arshak K, Korostynska O, Oliwa K, Adley C. 2010. An overview of foodborne pathogen detection: in the perspective of biosensors. *Biotechnol. Adv.* 28(2):232-54.

Wagner M, Schmid M, Juretschko S, Trebesius KH, Bubert A, Goebel W, Schleifer KH. 1998. In situ detection of a virulence factor mRNA and 16S rRNA in *Listeria monocytogenes*. *FEMS Microbiol. Lett.* 160(1):159-68.

Willford J, Goodridge LD. 2008. An integrated assay for rapid detection of *Escherichia coli* O157:H7 on beef samples. *Food Prot. Trends*. 28(7):468-72.

Woese CR. 1987. Bacterial evolution. *Microbiol. Rev*. 51:221-71.

Wolber PK, Green RL. 1990. Detection of bacteria by transduction of ice nucleation genes. *Trends Biotechnol.* 8(10):276–9.

Wu Y, Brovko L, Griffiths MW. 2001. Influence of phage population on the phage-mediated bioluminescent adenylate kinase (AK) assay for detection of bacteria. *Lett. Appl. Microbiol.* 33(4):311-5.

Xi C, Balberg M, Boppart SA, Raskin L. 2003. Use of DNA and peptide nucleic acid molecular beacons for detection and quantification of rRNA in solution and in whole cells. *Appl. Environ. Microbiol.* 69(9):5673-8.

Yang GJ, Huang JL, Meng WJ, Shen M, Jiao XA. 2009. A reusable capacitive immunosensor for detection of *Salmonella* spp. based on grafted ethylene diamine and self-assembled gold nanoparticle monolayers. *Anal. Chim. Acta.* 647(2):159-66.

Zimmer C, Wähnert U. 1986. Nonintercalating DNA-binding ligands: specificity of the interaction and their use as tools in biophysical, biochemical and biological investigations of the genetic material. *Prog. Biophys. Mol. Biol.* 47(1):31-112.

Zink R, Loessner MJ. 1992. Classification of virulent and temperate bacteriophages of *Listeria* spp. on the basis of morphology and protein analysis. *Appl. Environ. Microbiol.* 58(1):296-302.

Zourob M, Ripp S. 2010. Bacteriophage-based biosensors, In Zourob M (Ed.), *Recognition Receptors in Biosensors*, Springer Science+Business Media, LLC.

In: Salmonella: Classification, Genetics and Disease Outbreaks ISBN: 978-1-61942-928-4
Editors: Adelaide S. Monte, Paulo Eduardo De Santos

Chapter 6

SALMONELLA NEWPORT CONTAMINATION OF PRODUCE: ECOLOGICAL, GENETIC AND EPIDEMIOLOGICAL ASPECTS

Rebecca L. Bell[1], Guojie Cao[2], Jianghong Meng[2], Marc W. Allard[1], Christine Keys[1], Thomas Hill[1], Andrea Ottesen[1] and Eric W. Brown[1]

[1]Center for Food Safety and Applied Nutrition, Baltimore, MD, US
U.S. Food and Drug Administration, College Park
[2]Joint Institute for Food Safety and Applied Nutrition,
University of Maryland, College Park, Baltimore, MD, US

ABSTRACT

Salmonella enterica is the most frequent source of bacterial foodborne illness in the U.S., causing an estimated 1.4 million cases of salmonellosis annually. Historically, infection by *Salmonella* occurs after eating undercooked meats, poultry and eggs. However, over the past decade, the consumption of raw ready-to-eat produce has been implicated in several severe and widespread outbreaks within the U. S. Most notably, an *S. enterica* Saintpaul outbreak associated with jalapeño and Serrano peppers sickened over 1400 individuals during the summer of 2008. One *Salmonella* serovar in particular, *Salmonella enterica* Newport, has been associated perennially with contamination events involving fresh tomatoes and prepared fresh foods containing tomatoes. *S.* Newport is a non-typhoidal salmonellae classified taxonomically as subspecies (i.e. "group") I *Salmonella enterica enterica*. Prior to its emergence in produce and in produce growing environments, *S.* Newport was found predominantly in swine, cattle and other livestock commodities. *S.* Newport association with tomatoes retains a geographically skewed distribution. Metagenomic analyses of tomato phyllopsheres, based on 16S rDNA sequences and deep genome sequencing of tomato microbial communities, point to resident colonization on tomatoes from the Mid-Atlantic growing regions but not other predominant fresh tomato growing regions such as Florida or California, signaling niche adaptation of *S.* Newport in some growing environments but not others. Genetic analysis of *S.* Newport has revealed specific differences among strains from disparate locales.

Pulsed-field gel electrophoresis, for example, has yielded several pulsotypes of environmental *S.* Newport primarily associated with the Virginia eastern shore, a prominent fresh tomato production region of the county. Whole-genome sequencing affirmed these phylo-geographic differences within the serovar. Surprisingly, certain genotypes of *S.* Newport have been isolated from this region that genetically match previous outbreaks where tomatoes were a suspected vehicle. *S.* Newport can be readily detected in the environment of the Virginian eastern shore growing region using both molecular (i.e. PCR) and microbiological (i.e. FDA-BAM) screening methods. Taken together, these issues highlight the important intersection of microbiological, genetic, and ecological investigation for fully understanding the complex life cycle of this dangerous foodborne pathogen.

I. Introduction

An estimated 48 million illnesses due to the consumption of contaminated food occur annually in the United States. The most common causative agent of these infections is *Salmonella sp.* In 2010, U.S. FoodNet [1] attributed over 40% of the reported cases to salmonellae, far exceeding all other pathogens tracked. Typically infection occurs after eating undercooked meat, poultry and eggs that have been exposed to *Salmonella* [2]. In recent years, however, several outbreaks have occurred where fresh, ready-to-eat produce was identified as the food vehicle. In fact 14% of all foodborne outbreak cases reported in North America can be attributed to consumption of raw or minimally-processed fruits and vegetables [3]. With more awareness by the American population to eat a healthy diet, produce consumption has increased in the U.S. As more people are looking for fresh fruits and vegetable to replace unhealthy, highly-processed foods, there is more of a chance for infection due to *Salmonella* contamination. Outbreaks of salmonellosis have been associated with melons, sprouts, tomatoes, peppers, mangoes and leafy greens [4]. While food vehicles can be identified it is much harder to pin point the source of contamination. Experimental studies have suggested many possible pre-harvest routes of contamination of the produce commodities, such as internalization through the roots, surface contamination of leaves and blossoms, and co-infection with common plant pathogens [5-9]. To compound matters, *Salmonella* is a hardy enteric organism capable of prolonged survival outside of the animal host. Several studies have demonstrated its ability to survive in soil used for planting and fresh water sources used for irrigation and/or pesticide application [4, 6, 10-12]. Post-harvest practices have also been implicated in the spread of contaminants on fresh produce. Dirty equipment, inadequate disinfection of wash water and poor temperature controls are just a few areas identified that can lead to cross-contamination and enhancement of *Salmonella* growth in/on produce [4, 7]. Point-of-sale surveillance studies have shown that the incidence of contamination of produce is quite low [7, 13]. However, the fact that fresh fruits and vegetables are not always cooked before ingestion leads to huge consequences in terms of the number of individuals sickened by *Salmonella* contamination.

Prior to the early 1990's, tomatoes were not considered a typical vehicle for the transmission of *Salmonella* into the human populace. However, a series of outbreaks in the 2000's have propelled tomatoes to one of the most common non-animal food commodities associated with salmonellosis [14-17]. With approximately five billion pounds of fresh market tomatoes eaten in the U.S. annually, the potential for large outbreaks of salmonellosis is cause for concern. Between 1990 and 2007, at least 12 multistate outbreaks of salmonellosis traced to various types of tomatoes (e.g. red round, Roma and grape) have been reported, accounting for approximately 1,990 culture-confirmed infections. However, an estimated 97.5% of *Salmonella* infections are not culture-confirmed, signifying that as many as 79,600 illnesses may have occurred during these outbreaks [16]. These outbreaks tended to be widely dispersed, with cases in multiple states, indicating that contamination occurred early in the distribution chain, such as on the farm or at the packinghouse, rather than at the point of use. How tomatoes naturally become contaminated with *Salmonella* is still not known. Many hypotheses abound but none have been demonstrated in the farm environment. Experimentally it has been shown that planting seeds in *Salmonella* contaminated soil led to the surface contamination of the tomato plants [6]. *Salmonella* has also been shown to internalize into tomato plants through the roots of hydroponically grown tomatoes [18]. It is possible that *Salmonella* cells on the surface of the plants or internalized into the roots may migrate to and contaminate the developing tomato fruit. Guo et. al. [19] demonstrated that inoculation of the tomato flowers leads to the internalization of *Salmonella* into the developing fruit. Fruit may also be surface contaminated by contact with soil or water containing *Salmonella*. These cells are then capable of internalizing into the fruit through the stem scar [20]. Field contaminated fruit can then spread the bacteria during subsequent washing, packing and processing steps. After harvest tomatoes from several fields are mixed in one large dump tank for washing, sorting and packing. Any *Salmonella* that may be present on the fruits can then pass into the wash solution and adhere to other uncontaminated tomatoes. Even after packing *Salmonella* is able to survive for extended periods of time in the tomato fruit as demonstrated by Beuchat [21] who showed that artificially inoculated tomatoes held at 21°C and 12°C were able to support the growth of *Salmonella* over 14 and 27 day period, respectively. *Salmonella* was also able to survive in diced tomatoes over a 10 day period at 21°C and 12°C [21]. Taken together these studies highlight the fact that tomatoes and tomato plants are perfectly suitable environments for *Salmonella* to survive and grow.

One particular serotype of *Salmonella*, *Salmonella enterica* subsp. *enterica* serovar Newport, has been named one of the top 3 serovars for the last decade. In 2010, *S*. Newport was the second most commonly identified serovar. Also, alarmingly, *S*. Newport infections have been on the rise since 1996 [1]. In produce, *S*. Newport is considered to be a prominent and rising serotype responsible for foodborne illnesses and outbreaks. One main concern is that many strains of *S*. Newport are resistant to one and in some cases multiple antibiotics rendering treatment of these infections difficult to impossible [22]. Phylogenetic analysis of *S*. Newport suggests that this serovar is polyphyletic meaning that all the strains within the serogroup do not all cluster together in a dendogram. This was first suggested after MLEE analysis of eight different serotypes [23]. Here it was found that the 72 isolates of *S*. Newport analyzed separated into two distinct groups- division I and division II. Also it was noted that these two groups were associated with different hosts where most of the isolates from division I were recovered from humans and most of the isolates form division II were recovered from swine and other domestic animals [23]. The polyphyletic nature was also found using multilocus sequence tying (MLST) analyses using different gene sets. In one analysis using three housekeeping genes, *manB*, *fimA* and *mdh*, *S*. Newport grouped into two distinct lineages each having a different host origin, one avian associated and one bovine associated [24, 25]. Interestingly these two groups were also associated with different antibiotic resistance profiles. Group A, consisting mainly of strains isolated from a bovine source, were found to be multidrug resistance (MDR) while isolates in group B, comprised of avian associated isolates, were found to be pan-sensitive to the antibiotics tested [25]. Population analysis using seven housekeeping genes, *aroC*, *dnaN*, *hemD*, *hisD*, *purE*, *sucA* and *thrA*, also showed two populations of *S.* Newport among strains isolated from clinically ill animals, animal-derived foods and human infections [26]. These two groups also differed in their susceptibility to antibiotics with the poultry associated group showing more susceptibility and the bovine associated group showing more MDR [26]. More recently it has been suggested that, globally, there are three lineages of *S.* Newport, I, II and III [27]. These lineages show a geographical distribution with most of the Newport I isolates coming from Europe and most of the Newport II and III isolates coming from North America. Interestingly, Newport I may be a newer lineage, not seen before 1960, which may have arisen recently from a horizontal transfer event of the genes encoding serotype determinants [27]. Even on the global scale these lineages differ in their antibiotic susceptibility patterns. Here 59% of the MDR isolates and all of the MDR-AmpC isolates were found within Newport II. Meanwhile 87% of the isolates in Newport III were pan-susceptible [27].

As mentioned above *S.* Newport is an emerging pathogen associated with produce outbreaks, and of particular importance to this chapter, tomato outbreaks. The following sections will discuss the endemic nature of *S.* Newport in the Delmarva Peninsula, the biodiversity associated with this region, whole-genomic insights to these strains isolated from this area and implications for the future of tomato safety.

II. *SALMONELLA* NEWPORT ASSOCIATED WITH THE VIRGINIAN EASTERN SHORE

Tomatoes are the fourth most popular fresh market vegetable in the U.S. Of the fresh market producers of tomatoes, Virginia ranks third, behind California and Florida [28]. Approximately 80% of the vegetables grown in Virginia are grown along the Virginian Eastern Shore (VES), located on the Delmarva Peninsula. Half of the vegetables grown here are tomatoes with roughly 6,000 acres devoted to tomato production making this one of the largest industries along the VES. Several varieties of tomatoes are grown here including red round, Roma and grape/cherry. The majority of these tomatoes are intended for the fresh, ready-to-eat market and supply all states east of the Mississippi river during the growing season.

Almost yearly, since 2002, an outbreak or incident of *S.* Newport associated with tomatoes grown on the VES has been documented in PulseNet, the Center for Disease Control's molecular subtyping network for bacterial foodborne diseases [29]. Of note, one particular pulsotype, *S.* Newport XbaI pattern JJPX01.0061, has recurred in 2002, 2005, 2006 and 2010 (Figure 1; 16, 17, this report). Trace-back investigations of these outbreaks implicated tomatoes grown along the eastern shore of VA. Inspection of the packinghouses did not result in the discovery of the pathogen or source of contamination for these outbreaks. On the other hand, environmental assessments of the growing fields resulted in the isolation of *S.* Newport, with the same PFGE pattern. This strain was isolated from an irrigation pond used to water tomato fields and mix pesticides for direct application to tomato fruits, implying that the tomatoes were contaminated on the field, pre-harvest [17]. Unfortunately the ultimate source of contamination in this environment is not known and only speculative hypotheses are available. The ecological and epidemiological complexities of this recurrent contamination of tomatoes by *Salmonella* mandate (i) a thorough investigation and identification of the potential natural source reservoirs of these *S.* Newport outbreaks; (ii) an evaluation to gain a better understanding of the endemic prevalence of *Salmonella* in various VES microcosms; and (iii) a greater understanding of precisely how *Salmonella* can persist both on or in a tomato, as well as in adjacent potential reservoirs such as drainage ponds, creeks and streams, wells and indigenous wildlife.

Prevalence studies in the local Delmarva growing areas may answer questions as to the distribution and pervasiveness of *Salmonella* in the U.S. tomato supply and may aid in accounting for infection rates in the mid-Atlantic regions and in other areas of the U.S. that rely on tomatoes cultivated on the VES. To this end, a large environmental study of the tomato-growing environment was conducted during the summer of 2010 on Virginia Tech's Agricultural Research Extension Center (AREC) located in the heart of the tomato industry of the VES.

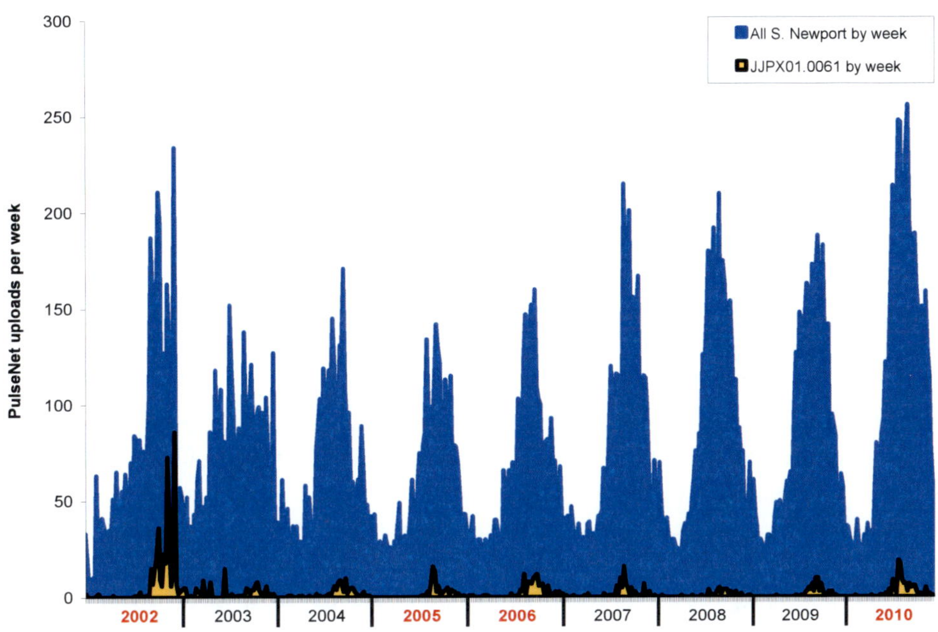

Figure 1. Frequency of *S.* Newport, PFGE XbaI pattern JJPX01.0061. The frequency of *S.* Newport, JJPX01.0061, in PulseNet for 2002 to 2010 by week compared to all *S.* Newport . Years of recurrent JJPX01.0061-associated outbreaks linked to the VES are highlighted in red.

The location of AREC allows it access to the same wildlife, insects, native vegetation and water sources as the commercial tomato fields that surround it making it the ideal model for a commercial growing field. Four sampling trips were made over a 4-month period (one per month) just before and during the height of the growing season (i.e. June - September). Over the four month period almost 900 samples were collected from the farm and surrounding areas. Samples collected included tomatoes (leaves, stems, flowers and fruit) other produce commodities (melons, cucumbers, squashes, soybeans- stems/leaves, flowers and fruits), native vegetation adjacent to the field, farm soil, irrigation water and insects. In addition, water from the irrigation pond, as well as water and sediment from a creek downstream of the pond was collected. Finally blinded tomato fruit samples from the surrounding commercial fields or roadside produce stands were collected. All of these samples were tested for the presence of *Salmonella* using real-time PCR (qPCR) methods specific for *Salmonella.* Moreover, a pre-determined set of samples, along with any that were positive from the qPCR assay, were cultured using a modified FDA-BAM [30] method for the isolation of *Salmonella* from tomatoes.

The qPCR assays used to screen for the presence of *Salmonella* were 3-target, multiplex assays. Two of the targets were specific for *Salmonella* and third target was an internal amplification control (IAC) [31]. The *Salmonella* specific gene targets were *invA* and *tsaA* (June and July) or *invA* and the *ttrRS* gene region (August and September) [32, 33]. Unfortunately in both of these multiplex assays the second *Salmonella* gene target typically failed to amplify so positive results were based on the amplification of the *invA* gene only. Also several samples tended to be problematic for the qPCR reactions causing a failure of the IAC to amplify. These samples were typically soils/sediments, water, avian feces and certain weeds. All of these samples are problematic for any PCR reaction, real-time or not, due to the high concentration of inhibitors in them [34]. The soils/sediments, water and fecal samples were pre-chosen to be cultured so that a failure in the qPCR screen would not permit the presence of any *Salmonella* microbes to be missed.

The results of the molecular screen are summarized in Figure 2. Here the highest number of qPCR positive samples was obtained in June and decrease each month with no molecular positives in September. Of the samples that were cultured three were positive in June, five in July, three in August and one in September. Disappointingly, the qPCR method missed detecting *Salmonella* in the majority of the culture positive samples (66% of culture positive samples were qPCR negative). The qPCR also gave a high false positive rate. Collectively these results indicate that the molecular procedures used for this study were not robust enough to reliably indicate when a sample contained *Salmonella* and when it did not. Of the 12 culture-positive samples 24 *Salmonella* isolates were obtained (see Table 1). The majority of the isolates were *S.* Newport, followed by *S.* Javiana, *S. enterica* subsp. *salamae*, and *S.* [1]4,5,12:i:-. Interestingly the *S.* Newport isolates were recovered from creek water and/or sediment and from goose feces collected next to the irrigation pond. However more in-depth analyses are needed to tell if the bodies of water contaminated the goose or if the goose contaminated the water. Geese are known to carry *Salmonella* in their intestinal tracts and *Salmonella* is capable of long-term survival in sediments [10, 12, 35]. Finding *S.* Newport in both is significant. While the creek water is not used to irrigate the tomato fields, its source is the pond that does irrigate the fields. It stands to reason that the creek, which is seeded by the contents of the pond, would be an indicator of what may be present in the pond. The presence of *Salmonella* in migratory fowl, such as geese, would enable the spread of this organism all along the VES including other bodies of water and tomato fields that they may land in.

The finding of *S.* Javiana and *S. salamae* is also quite interesting. *S.* Javiana has caused outbreaks linked to tomatoes before [15]. Discovery of this pathogen in this environment may be a predictor of future tomato-related outbreaks linked to this region. *S. enterica* subsp.

salamae (subspecies II) is not typically seen in human disease. While it is still capable of causing human illness it is typically found in amphibians and reptiles.

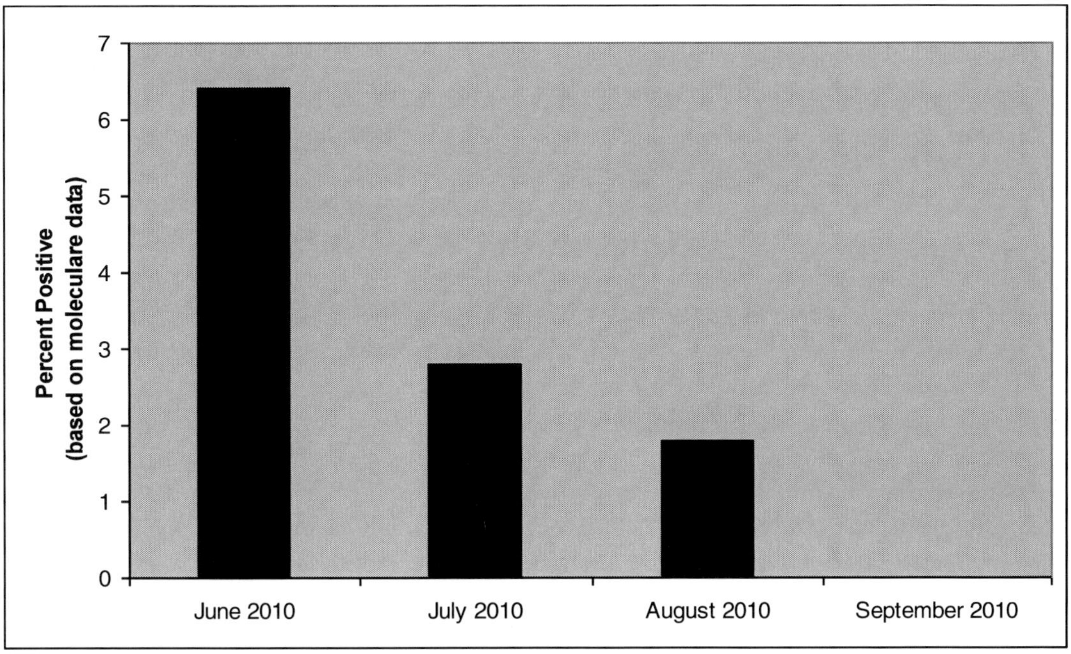

Figure 2. Percent positive samples based on molecular screening assays. All samples collected from AREC during the summer of 2010 were screened for the presence of *Salmonella* using qPCR. The highest incidence of positive samples was in June 2010 and decreased each month thereafter.

Table 1. Salmonella isolated from AREC, summer 2010

Type	Source(s)	Number of isolates
S. Newport	creek water, creek sediment, goose feces	16
S. Javiana	creek water, creek sediment	5
S. enterica subsp. *salamae*	tomato leaves	2
S. [1]4,5,12:i:-	creek sediment	1

Collectively these results reveal environmental water sources as a potential reservoir for *S*. Newport in the VES ecosystem. *S*. Newport was isolated from creek water, creek sediment and waterfowl throughout the summer of 2010. The ultimate source of this contamination was not uncovered during this survey. Also, the vector of transmission from the bodies of water to the tomato plants can still only be hypothesized. However it is reasonable to imagine that the use of contaminated water to irrigate the tomato fields, or to mix pesticides for direct application to tomato plants could lead to contaminated fruit. Especially in light of the fact that *S*. Newport contaminated irrigation water has been shown to contaminate tomato roots, stems and fruits [36] and that direct inoculation of tomato flowers leads to internalized *Salmonella* contamination of tomato fruits [19]. Future studies will focus on waterways throughout the VES to get a better understanding of the true prevalence of this endemic pathogen. Finally the results of this study and others like it will lead to improvements in tomato safety and good agricultural practices (discussed later in this chapter).

III. Understanding the Ecological Interplay of Salmonella in the Tomato Growing Environment: The Role of Metagenomics

Microbial ecology has become a critical component to the investigation and understanding of bacterial contamination of a food source by pathogenic species and strains. Such studies hold the potential for elucidating bacterial outbreaks to their points of origin including unsuspected food commodities and unprocessed food constituents. The information gleaned from understanding the ecologic microcosms in which these pathogens persist is key to understanding the link between a pathogen and a food source as well as to developing stop-gap measures to deter future outbreak events. Why *Salmonella* Newport predominates among salmonellae associated with Eastern Shore tomatoes and persists over years in this microcosm remains unclear. One explanation is that *S.* Newport strains enjoy a genetic and/or ecological fitness advantage over other salmonellae in this environment. It maybe that *S.* Newport enjoys a growth advantage over other subtypes. Clearly, ecological studies are well positioned to explore these hypotheses. Additionally, focused studies in local tomato growing areas may answer questions as to the distribution and prevalence of *Salmonella* in the U.S. tomato supply and may explain unusual infection rates in certain mid-Atlantic regions. In an ideal scenario, ecological research may lead us ever closer to a kill-step against *Salmonella* infestation of Eastern shore tomatoes and provide important intervention steps by exploiting naturally-occurring epiphytic microflora endemic to the tomato growing environment.

The association of *Salmonella* with tomatoes is ecologically complex and not yet fully understood. Nonetheless, the regularity of outbreaks associated with *Salmonella*, *S.* Newport in particular, in certain growing regions predicates a need for more in-depth surveillance of the tomato production environment along with the surrounding ecosystems for the presence of *Salmonella* endemic to this environment. Such studies serve to reveal natural reservoirs of *Salmonella* that may be responsible for reoccurring contamination of tomatoes. In addition, the outcome of such work should provide a better understanding of the environmental factors that contribute to the colonization of tomato plants and/or fruit surfaces with this deadly pathogen. Equally important is the need for a real-time examination of the tomato growing environs. If we are to stay in step with the need for more effective tomato-safety through good agricultural practices, then information concerning the presence, the extent, and the kind of *Salmonella* contamination will be invaluable. Metagenomic analysis proffers one such solution.

Metagenomics focuses on the examination of environmental assemblages of organisms. It is the study of genetic material collected directly from plant, farm, or other samples without the use of culturing methods. The discipline of metagenomics has been referred to as environmental genomics, eco-genomics or community genomics [37]. The great power of metagenomic analysis lies in its ability to gain access to the total physiological and genetic potential of an environment. Traditional microbiology and microbial genome sequencing are dependent upon purified bacterial cultures. Most organisms cannot be grown with traditional culturing methods and in the past, this precluded their study. Access to these previously unstudied organisms and their functional processes via their genetic code has spearheaded a deeper understanding of the entire microbial world [38]. This approach has become even more powerfully descriptive as next generation sequencing technologies, databases and bioinformatic pipelines continue to improve. Preliminary "metagenomics" relied on specific conserved genes, such as 5S and 16S rRNA genes, to ascribe diversity in an environmental sample [39]. While these approaches propelled a paradigm shift in our understanding of the breath of consortia associated with environmental samples, the use of shotgun sequencing of total environmental DNA, has provided a much more functionally informative snapshot of diverse environments.

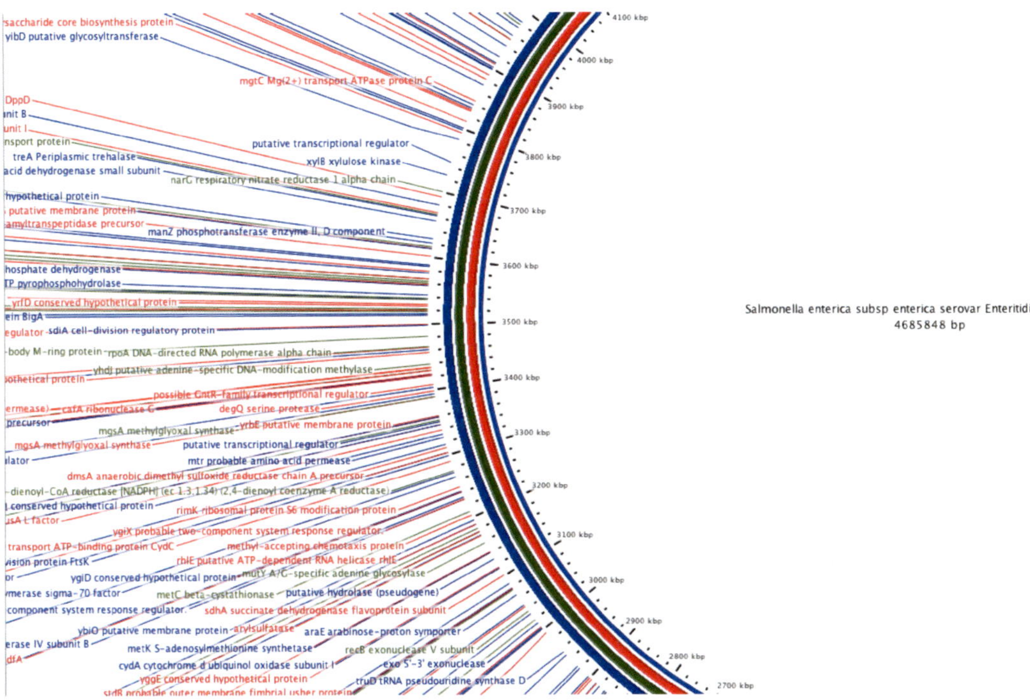

Figure 3. Biogeographical phyllosphere metagenomes aligned to *Salmonella enterica* subsp. *enterica* Enteritidis. *Salmonella* reference genome (Accession #NC_011294) was used to examine gene fragments from metagenomic tomato phyllosphere datasets that map to *Salmonella*. Using reference genomes, we can evaluate individual hits of diverse genes from metagenomes that may provide diagnostic verification of the presence or absence of *Salmonella* in environmental samples.

Application of metagenomics to study of foodborne diseases such as endemic salmonellae in tomato-growing environments provides a new approach to epidemiology. Increased understanding of microflora associated with fresh produce and agricultural environments is paving the way for a new era of surveillance. As an example, metagenomic analysis based on shotgun sequences of phyllosphere samples from tomatoes collected in California and Florida provided evidence for the persistence of *S. enterica* in these tomato growing environments (Figure 3). As databases grow more robust and gene annotations improve, gene homologies will continue to improve, providing even more resolution in the identification of *S. enterica* and serovars within specific environments. Nonetheless, this approach is now allowing for a detailed genetic and ecologic examination of environmental fingerprints and strain diversity. Moreover, this technology is providing valuable information regarding the kinds (i.e., serovars) of *Salmonella* that dominate in distinct tomato growing environments. Genome databases are growing daily with a variety of *Salmonella* serovars allowing for assessments of the taxonomic structure and relative fitness of *Salmonella* in disparate high-production tomato growing regions (Figure 4).

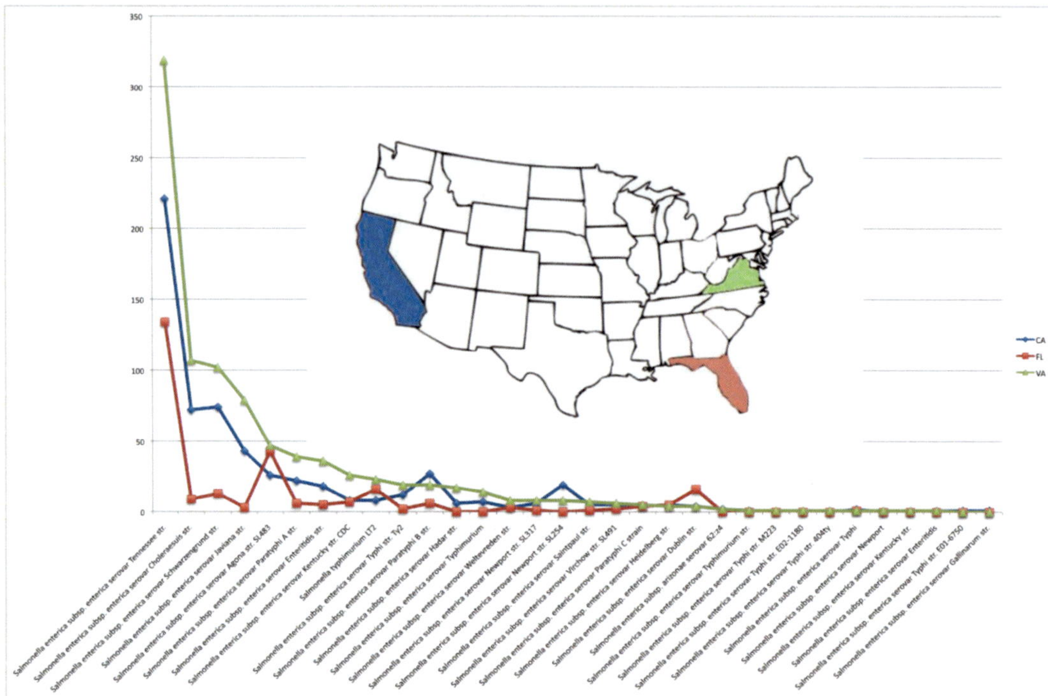

Figure 4. Hits to diverse *Salmonella* serotypes by geographic region (VA, CA and FL). Tomato phyllosphere metagenomes were blasted against FDA in house databases of *Salmonella* genomes to develop preliminary hypotheses to describe geographic incidence of particular serovars. More complete databases of *Salmonella* serovars in combination with deeper metagenomic sequencing of phyllosphere microflora will enhance the ability of this of approach to describe ecological patterns associated with *Salmonella* serovar biogeography.

Geographical differences in tomato-borne outbreaks trace back to different tomato growing locales. Metagenomics may provide clues as to why. It appears that *S.* Newport association with tomatoes retains a somewhat geographically skewed distribution. Metagenomic analyses of tomato phyllopsheres, based on 16S rDNA sequences and deep genome sequencing of tomato microbial communities, point to resident colonization on tomatoes in some growing regions but not other predominant fresh tomato growing regions such as Florida or California, signaling niche adaptation of *S.* Newport in some growing environments but not others. The interesting phenomenon that *Salmonella*–tomato outbreaks seem to be predominantly associated with tomatoes grown in the eastern United States provides an intriguing geographical question in terms of *Salmonella* persistence and fitness in different environments associated with tomato production. Certainly, epiphytic microbial ecology of the tomato phyllosphere may be unique in different parts of the world and thereby contribute to *Salmonella*'s ability to persist in these niches in very different ways. Pest pressures, atmospheric pressures, water sources and local flora will all influence the bacterial and fungal species present on the surfaces of tomato plants.

Thus, examination of agricultural microbial ecology of high-risk crops like tomato provides an epidemiological focus for research that will eventually provide ecological markers to predict risk. Numerous culture independent studies have begun to characterize phyllosphere microflora associated with food plants and native ecosystems [40]. Recent work has also shown that bacterial flora can be significantly altered by diverse agricultural management practices (i.e. custom pesticides, etc.) [41].

Metagenomic analysis affords a high-resolution look at the microbial biodiversity that comprises geographically diverse growing regions, and their associated environmental parameters. This is important for two reasons: (i) metagenomic analysis can potentially detect and recognize unique signatures of biogeographic microbial diversity associated with high risk crops such as tomatoes; and (ii) it has the potential to provide epidemiological source tracking through agricultural phyllosphere microcosms. Improved understanding of eco-types of foodborne pathogens greatly enhances the opportunity for intervention and control of *Salmonella* in the tomato growing environment. The control of *Salmonella* by application of naturally occurring microorganisms that may serve to exclude *Salmonella* from a particular niche has been noted previously and represents a biologically sound intervention strategy [42].

One of the most interesting differences between microflora associated with California and Virginia grown tomatoes (observed in cloned sequences of 16S rRNA genes from tomato phyllosphere microflora) has been the differentially abundant incidence of Firmicutes in California samples when compared to Virginia samples. *Weisella* spp. are members of *Leuconostocaceae*, a family of lactic acid producing heterofermentative Gram positive Lactobacillales. This genus was the second most abundant group of bacteria in California 16S rRNA gene libraries. Lactic acid bacteria and *Weisella spp.* in particular demonstrate strong antibiotic activity against Gram negative bacteria including certain human pathogens and uropathogens such as *Escherichia coli, Pseudomonas aeruginaosa*, *Enterobacter cloaceae, Citrobacter freundii* and *Proteus mirabilis* [43]. One species of *Weisella*, *Weisella cibaria*, has been shown to disrupt oral biofilms so the possibility exists that *Weisella* species found in California tomato fields may actually have the ability to disrupt biofilms that occur in that environment thereby functioning as a natural bio-control of potentially pathogenic species.

Because of the vast complexity of the phyllosphere environment of food plants and tomatoes in particular, increased sequencing depth combined with greater temporal and geographic replication will provide a more complete understanding of the phylloplane microbiology of eastern and western grown tomatoes and exactly what factors may or may not be contributing to *Salmonella*'s ability to persist in one environment or another. Understanding the ecology and environmental factors that contribute to contamination of tomatoes by *Salmonella*, through the use of metagenomic methods will support the development of critical control point intervention strategies.

IV. Genomic Analysis of Produce-Associated *Salmonella* Newport Strains

Microbial source tracking has become a critical component to the investigation and understanding of bacterial contamination of food sources by pathogenic species and strains. The traceback of foodborne bacterial outbreaks to the point of origin is key to understanding the underlying causes of the link between a pathogen and a food source as well as to developing preventative stop-gap measures to deter future outbreak events [44]. Most source tracking methods rely upon genotypic (i.e. molecular genetic-based) methods that can distinguish the subtle genetic nuances separating closely related strains. In fact, largely due to natural selective processes, genotypic differences have been identified that can distinguish host sources of enteric bacterial strains such as *E. coli* and other pathogenic species [44]. Moreover, microbial source typing methods can provide answers to questions pertaining to the microbial ecology, evolution, population structures, and diversity of pathogens known to be endemic problems to the food supply.

Recent outbreaks of *Salmonella* associated with VES tomatoes have underscored the need for more detailed source tracking of feral *Salmonella* strains isolated from numerous distinct ecological niches on the Delmarva Peninsula. Outbreak investigations typically involve screening of suspected sources for a single strain of a pathogen that are difficult or impossible to distinguish using conventional typing and detection methods. This is due, in part, to the rapid diversification of the pathogens allowing little to no time for phenotypic differences to develop between closely related strains and serovars. However, differences present in the genomes of these strains can be detected and used to identify and discriminate closely related isolates. Given the significance of *S.* Newport, as the third ranking serotype of *Salmonella* associated with foodborne outbreaks in the United States, a better understanding of its ecology and evolutionary history will play critical roles during epidemiological investigations of outbreaks.

As mentioned above, several isolates of *S.* Newport were recovered from AREC during the summer of 2010. Interestingly, at the same time as the environmental survey, a cluster of illnesses, due to *S.* Newport infection, occurred in the Washington D.C. area, which were associated with the consumption of raw tomatoes from one particular establishment. This cluster was distinctive in the fact that there were three different *S.* Newport PFGE patterns, namely JJPX01.0061, JJPX01.0011 and JJPX01.0030. The *S.* Newport isolates from AREC had the same PFGE, pattern JJPX01.0011, to some of the clinical strains associated with the D.C. cluster. In order to determine the relatedness of these environmental isolates to the clinical isolates and to perhaps glean some information about the possible source of the tomato contamination event whole genome sequencing (WGS) was applied. WGS was highly sensitive in its ability to further subdivide these *S.* Newport strains. The method holds great promise in providing more comprehensive information for a deeper understanding of genomics, evolution, ecology and pathogenicity of bacteria. The speed of newer sequencing technologies enhances the usefulness of WGS during epidemiological investigations. The combination of WGS with phylogenetic analysis greatly enhances the power of this tool to differentiate the subtle genomic variations among isolates being studied [45-48]. For example, during the investigation of one multi-state outbreak associated with *S.* Montevideo that infected approximately 300 people from 44 states and Washington D.C., FDA investigators utilized whole genome sequencing retrospectively to demonstrate the extraordinary power of the method to delimit the scope of a highly clonal contamination event [45]. This methodology was also able to parse-out strains not associated with the outbreak even though these strains had an identical PFGE pattern to the outbreak-associated isolates and were originally considered part of the outbreak [45].

In the phylogenetic analysis, along with the clinical isolates from the D.C. cluster and AREC isolates, several historical *S.* Newport isolated from VES tomato farms (FDA 72, 117, 118, 431, 432 and 434-437) and *S.* Newport reference genomes from other host sources and geographic locations (FDA 180-185, 189) were included. The four isolates (FDA309, FDA519, FDA520 and FDA521) from the AREC farm clustered together in 2 related subgroups B2 and B3 (Figure 5).

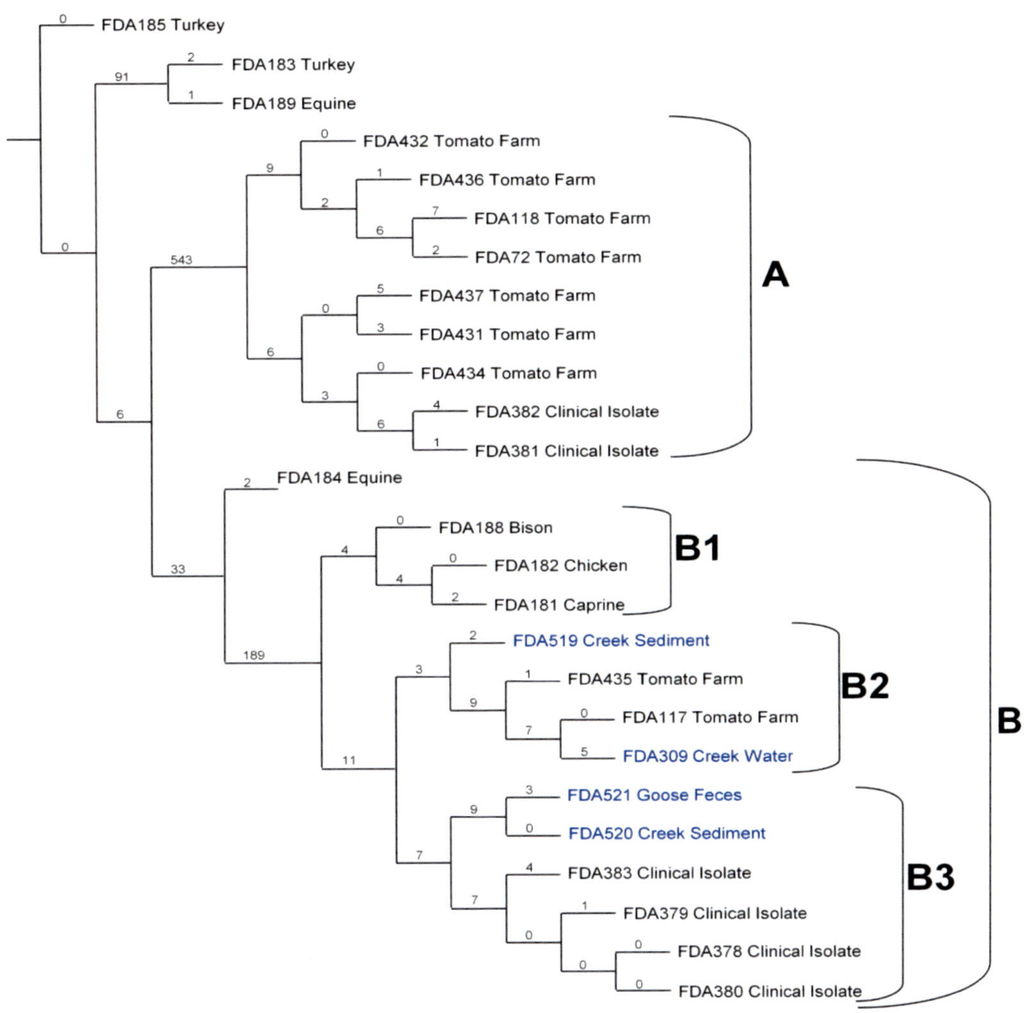

Figure 5. Whole-genome sequencing tree. Isolates obtained from AREC in 2010 along with clinical isolates associated with the "D.C. Cluster" were subjected to whole genome sequencing. The resulting tree shows the relationship of these strains to background *S.* Newport strains unrelated to the outbreak or 2010 environmental sampling. Numbers on the lines indicate the number of nucleotide changes found between the strains.

Furthermore FDA520 and FDA521 grouped together with four of the clinical isolates, associate with the D.C. cluster, within subgroup B3 indicating that these two strains are the most closely related to the clinical isolates. This information, along with the fact that FDA520 was isolated from creek sediment and FDA521 was isolated from goose feces near a pond from this farm suggests several possible routes of contamination of the tomato plants. One possibility is that the plants may have been irrigated with contaminated water, since the presence of salmonellae in the sediment indicates contamination of the water, or perhaps contaminated water was used to mix pesticides, which would have been directly added to the plant surfaces. Another possibility is that geese, infected with *S.* Newport, may have contaminated the tomato plants by defecating in the fields. Unfortunately there was still not enough evidence from the WGS to indicate whether the geese contaminated the water or the water contaminated the geese. However it is quite clear from the phylogenetic tree that both water and geese contributed to the contamination of the tomatoes. Several reference genomes were also included in the analysis. Each was isolated from various host sources and geographic locations, namely, from FDA180 (bison, Tennessee), FDA181 (caprine, Tennessee), FDA182 (chicken, Missouri), FDA183 (turkey, Maryland), FDA184 (equine, Tennessee), FDA185 (turkey, Colorado) and FDA189 (equine, Tennessee). FDA180, FDA181, FDA182 and FDA184 grouped within Cluster B indicating a closer evolutionary relatedness with the four outbreak isolates and the AREC isolates. The use of these reference genomes may indicate other possible sources of contamination from domestic farm animals in this environment. To answer this question more *S.* Newport strains need to be included in the analysis.

Collectively, WGS data differentiated between *S.* Newport isolates, providing detailed information about their evolutionary relatedness. From this data, inferences about the ecology of these strains and their possible route(s) of tomato plant contamination could be made. The power of this method will only improve as more strains are analyzed giving investigators even more information about *S.* Newport's complex ecology along the VES.

V. Tomato Safety and Good Agricultural Practices for Fresh-Cut Tomato Farming

From 1996 to 2008, 14 foodborne outbreaks were linked to the consumption of tomatoes. Out of these 14 outbreaks, five were traced to the consumption of fresh-cut tomatoes. Disturbingly, these tomato-associated outbreaks resulted in 1,927 illnesses and 3 deaths [49], and all were found to be due to bacterial agents. Federal regulators, such as the U.S. Food and Drug Administration, and the tomato industry have a vested interest in improving tomato safety. To this end the FDA and tomato industry have both introduced guidance for tomato growers, packers and retailers to improve production practices and reduce the risk of bacterial contamination of tomatoes.

Beginning in 1998, when the Good Agricultural Practices (GAPs) Guide was first introduced to industry, FDA took several steps to improve the safety of fresh produce for consumers. The Good Agricultural Practices (GAPs) Guide provided general guidance on the production and packing of fresh produce specifically at crucial production steps where food safety may be compromised. Additionally the GAPs Guide alerted the produce industry to critical points of potential microbial contamination associated with the whole produce production chain including previous land use of areas where produce is grown, water quality for irrigation and application of pesticides/herbicides, worker hygiene, and equipment sanitation [49]. Then in 2004, FDA introduced the Produce Safety Action Plan, to help further reduce the incidence of microbial contamination of produce. This plan consisted of four key objectives: 1) to prevent further contamination of fresh produce, 2) to minimize the impact on public health when a contamination event occurs, 3) to improve communication and 4) to support research on produce contamination [50]. As part of the Action Plan and to specifically address the recurrent outbreaks associated with tomatoes grown along the east coast, FDA initiated the Tomato Safety Initiative [51]. For this multi-year initiative, FDA along with Virginia's Department of Agriculture and Consumer Services, began visiting Virginia based tomato farms and packing facilities to assess their food safety practices and to what extent they had implemented GAPs and Good Manufacturing Practices (GMPs). Environmental assessments of tomato farms, including irrigation water sources, well quality, procedures for mixing chemicals, the occurrence of drought and flooding events, and the proximity of animals, both wild and domestic, to growing fields, were conducted [51]. The results of these studies were then incorporated into updated tomato specific guidance to industry [49]. Recently, FDA announced it would introduce a new regulation, the Produce Safety Regulation, which will establish science-based, mandatory, minimum standards for the safe growing, harvesting, sorting, packing, and storage of fresh fruits and vegetables [52]. Unlike the earlier GAPs Guide, which was simply a suggested guideline for industry to follow, industry will have to implement this new regulation in their production flow as a matter of enforceable law [52].

The implementation of GAPs is in the best interest of the tomato industry, as well, because consumers will not purchase produce if they fear it is unsafe. To this end, the tomato industry, with input from federal partners, FDA and USDA, created the Food Safety Programs and Auditing Protocol for the Fresh Tomato Supply Chain [53]. This guidance, agreed upon by industry, sets a minimum set of operation standards along with specific guidelines to implement these standards. The difference between these guidelines and the federal guidelines is the agreement of the tomato-growers and packers to one set of standards at all production facilities instead of many different protocols and procedures that many not be effective at reducing the risk of contamination. Retail suppliers have also adopted these standards as a way to check the quality of the product they are selling to consumers [53].

CONCLUSIONS

Unfortunately, even with GAPs in place, tomatoes continue to become contaminated with *Salmonella*. This clearly highlights the need for more research into the areas of possible contamination route(s), possible environmental reservoirs of *Salmonella* and new intervention steps. There is also a need for faster methods of detecting *Salmonella* contamination of tomatoes efficiently and accurately in order to quickly eliminate tainted tomatoes from the fresh market. These are not small tasks. Active research is ongoing to identify factors that are permitting *Salmonella* to persist in the tomato-growing environment and on ways to prevent contamination event(s). As highlighted in this chapter, newer methodologies, such as whole-genome sequencing and metagenomics, are paving the way to answer some very profound questions that have plagued researchers for years. The use of these techniques, along with traditional microbiological methods, has already lead to many new hypotheses concerning the survival of *Salmonella* in the VES environment (i.e. in the local waterways), the ultimate source of the environmental contamination and natural ways to control *Salmonella* contamination (i.e. natural bacterial antagonists). Collectively the results of the current studies, discussed here, and other ongoing and future work will lead to more effective and refined GAPs for the tomato industry to ensure that safe tomatoes are reaching the American consumer.

REFERENCES

[1] CDC. Vital signs: incidence and trends of infection with pathogens transmitted commonly through food--foodborne diseases active surveillance network, 10 U.S. sites, 1996-2010. *MMWR Morb. Mortal. Wkly. Rep. 2011* Jun 10;60(22):749-55.

[2] CDC. Preliminary FoodNet data on the incidence of infection with pathogens transmitted commonly through food--10 states, 2006. *MMWR Morb. Mortal. Wkly Rep. 2007* Apr 13;56(14):336-9.

[3] Beuchat LR. Ecological factors influencing survival and growth of human pathogens on raw fruits and vegetables. *Microbes and Infection2002* Apr;4(4):413-23.

[4] Hanning IB, Nutt JD, Ricke SC. Salmonellosis outbreaks in the United States due to fresh produce: sources and potential intervention measures. *Foodborne Pathog. Dis. 2009* Jul-Aug;6(6):635-48.

[5] Barak JD, Liang A, Narm KE. Differential attachment to and subsequent contamination of agricultural crops by Salmonella enterica. *Appl. Environ. Microbiol. 2008* Sep;74(17):5568-70.

[6] Barak JD, Liang AS. Role of soil, crop debris, and a plant pathogen in Salmonella enterica contamination of tomato plants. *PLoS One2008*;3(2):e1657.

[7] Doyle MP, Erickson MC. Summer meeting 2007 - the problems with fresh produce: an overview. *Journal of Applied Microbiology2008* Aug;105(2):317-30.

[8] Wells JM, Butterfield JE. Incidence of Salmonella on fresh fruits and vegetables affected by fungal rots or physical injury. *Plant Disease1999* Aug;83(8):722-6.

[9] Wells JM, Butterfield JE. Salmonella contamination associated with bacterial soft rot of fresh fruits and vegetables in the marketplace. *Plant Disease1997* Aug;81(8):867-72.

[10] Fish JT, Pettibone GW. Influence of freshwater sediment on the survival of Escherichia coli and Salmonella sp. as measured by three methods of enumeration. *Lett. Appl. Microbiol. 1995* May;20(5):277-81.

[11] Garcia R, Baelum J, Fredslund L, Santorum P, Jacobsen CS. Influence of Temperature and Predation on Survival of Salmonella enterica Serovar Typhimurium and Expression of invA in Soil and Manure-Amended Soil. *Applied and Environmental Microbiology2010* Aug;76(15):5025-31.

[12] Winfield MD, Groisman EA. Role of nonhost environments in the lifestyles of Salmonella and Escherichia coli. *Applied and Environmental Microbiology2003* Jul;69(7):3687-94.

[13] Heaton JC, Jones K. Microbial contamination of fruit and vegetables and the behaviour of enteropathogens in the phyllosphere: a review. *J. Appl. Microbiol. 2008* Mar;104(3):613-26.

[14] Hedberg CW, Angulo FJ, White KE, Langkop CW, Schell WL, Stobierski MG, et al. Outbreaks of salmonellosis associated with eating uncooked tomatoes: implications for public health. The Investigation Team. *Epidemiol. Infect. 1999* Jun;122(3):385-93.

[15] CDC. Outbreaks of Salmonella Infectons Associated with Eating Roma Tomatoes--United States and Canada, 2004. *Morbidity and Mortality Weekly Reports2005*; 54(13):325-8.

[16] CDC. Multistate Outbreaks of Salmonella Infections Associated with Raw Tomatoes Eaten in Restaurants--United States, 2005-2006. *Morbidity and Mortality Weekly Reports2007*;56(35):909-11.

[17] Greene SK, Daly ER, Talbot EA, Demma LJ, Holzbauer S, Patel NJ, et al. Recurrent multistate outbreak of Salmonella Newport associated with tomatoes from contaminated fields, 2005. *Epidemiol. Infect. 2008* Feb;136(2):157-65.

[18] Guo XA, van Iersel MW, Chen JR, Brackett RE, Beuchat LR. Evidence of association of salmonellae with tomato plants grown hydroponically in inoculated nutrient solution. *Applied and Environmental Microbiology2002* Jul;68(7):3639-43.

[19] Guo X, Chen JR, Brackett RE, Beuchat LR. Survival of Salmonellae on and in tomato plants from the time of inoculation at flowering and early stages of fruit development through fruit ripening. *Applied and Environmental Microbiology2001* Oct;67(10):4760-4.

[20] Guo X, Chen JR, Brackett RE, Beuchat LR. Survival of Salmonella on tomatoes stored at high relative humidity, in soil, and on tomatoes in contact with soil. *Journal of Food Protection2002* Feb;65(2):274-9.

[21] Beuchat LR, Mann DA. Survival and growth of acid-adapted and unadapted Salmonella in and on raw tomatoes as affected by variety, stage of ripeness, and storage temperature. *Journal of Food Protection2008* Aug;71(8):1572-9.

[22] Devasia RA, Varma JK, Whichard J, Gettner S, Cronquist AB, Hurd S, et al. Antimicrobial use and outcomes in patients with multidrug-resistant and pansusceptible Salmonella Newport infections, 2002-2003. *Microbial Drug Resistance-Mechanisms Epidemiology and Disease2005* Win;11(4):371-7.

[23] Beltran P, Musser JM, Helmuth R, Farmer JJ, Frerichs WM, Wachsmuth IK, et al. Toward a Population Genetic-Analysis of Salmonella - Genetic Diversity and Relationships among Strains of Serotypes S-Choleraesuis, S-Derby, S-Dublin, S-Enteritidis, S-Heidelberg, S-Infantis, S-Newport, and S-Typhimurium. *Proceedings of the National Academy of Sciences of the United States of America1988* Oct;85(20):7753-7.

[24] Sukhnanand S, Alcaine S, Warnick LD, Su WL, Hof J, Craver MP, et al. DNA sequence-based subtyping and evolutionary analysis of selected *Salmonella enterica* serotypes. *J. Clin. Microbiol 2005* Aug;43(8):3688-98.

[25] Alcaine SD, Soyer Y, Warnick LD, Su WL, Sukhnanand S, Richards J, et al. Multilocus sequence typing supports the hypothesis that cow- and human-associated *Salmonella* isolates represent distinct and overlapping populations. *Appl. Environ. Microbiol. 2006* Dec;72(12):7575-85.

[26] Harbottle H, White DG, McDermott PF, Walker RD, Zhao S. Comparison of multilocus sequence typing, pulsed-field gel electrophoresis, and antimicrobial susceptibility typing for characterization of *Salmonella enterica* serotype Newport isolates. *J. Clin. Microbiol. 2006* Jul;44(7):2449-57.

[27] Sangal V, Harbottle H, Mazzoni CJ, Helmuth R, Guerra B, Didelot X, et al. Evolution and Population Structure of Salmonella enterica Serovar Newport. *Journal of Bacteriology2010* Dec;192(24):6465-76.

[28] USDA ERS. Vegetables and Melons: Tomatoes. USDA, Economic Research Service; 2009 [updated 10-5-2009; cited 2011 11/2011]; Available from: http://www.ers.usda.gov/Briefing/Vegetables/ tomatoes.htm.

[29] Swaminathan B, Barrett TJ, Hunter SB, Tauxe RV. PulseNet: the molecular subtyping network for foodborne bacterial disease surveillance, United States. *Emerg Infect Dis2001* May-Jun;7(3):382-9.

[30] Andrews WH, Hammack TS. *Salmonella*: U.S. Food and Drug Administration; 2011. Available from: http://www.fda.gov/Food/ ScienceResearch/LaboratoryMethods /Bacteriological AnalyticalManualBAM/ucm070149.htm.

[31] Deer DM, Lampel KA, Gonzalez-Escalona N. A versatile internal control for use as DNA in real-time PCR and as RNA in real-time reverse transcription PCR assays. *Letters in Applied Microbiology2010* Apr;50(4):366-72.

[32] Hebrard M, Viala JPM, Meresse P, Barras F, Aussel L. Redundant Hydrogen Peroxide Scavengers Contribute to Salmonella Virulence and Oxidative Stress Resistance. *Journal of Bacteriology2009* Jul 15;191(14):4605-14.

[33] Malorny B, Paccassoni E, Fach P, Bunge C, Martin A, Helmuth R. Diagnostic real-time PCR for detection of Salmonella in food. *Applied and Environmental Microbiology2004* Dec;70(12):7046-52.

[34] Wilson IG. Inhibition and facilitation of nucleic acid amplification. *Applied and Environmental Microbiology1997* Oct;63(10):3741-51.

[35] Feare CJ, Sanders MF, Blasco R, Bishop JD. Canada goose (Branta canadensis) droppings as a potential source of pathogenic bacteria. *Journal of the Royal Society for the Promotion of Health1999* Sep;119(3):146-55.

[36] Hintz LD, Boyer RR, Ponder MA, Williams RC, Rideout SL. Recovery of Salmonella enterica Newport Introduced through Irrigation Water from Tomato (Lycopersicum esculentum) Fruit, Roots, Stems, and Leaves. *Hortscience*2010 Apr;45(4):675-8.

[37] Handelsman J, Rondon MR, Brady SF, Clardy J, Goodman RM. Molecular biological access to the chemistry of unknown soil microbes: A new frontier for natural products. *Chemistry and Biology1998* Oct;5(10):R245-R9.

[38] Handelsman J. Metagenomics: Application of genomics to uncultured microorganisms. *Microbiology and Molecular Biology Reviews2004* Dec;68(4):669-+.

[39] Pace NR, Stahl DA, Lane DJ, Olsen GJ. Analyzing natural microbial populations by rRNA sequences. *ASM News1985*;51:4-12.

[40] Redford AJ, Bowers RM, Knight R, Linhart Y, Fierer N. The ecology of the phyllosphere: geographic and phylogenetic variability in the distribution of bacteria on tree leaves. *Environmental Microbiology2010* Nov;12(11):2885-93.

[41] Ottesen AR, White JR, Skaltsas DN, Newell MJ, Walsh CS. Impact of Organic and Conventional Management on the Phyllosphere Microbial Ecology of an Apple Crop. *Journal of Food Protection2009* Nov;72(11):2321-5.

[42] Andrews JH. Biological control in the phyllosphere. *Annu. Rev. Phytopathol. 1992*;30:603-35.

[43] Ayeni FA, Adeniyi BA, Ogunbanwo ST, Tabasco R, Paarup T, Pelaez C, et al. Inhibition of uropathogens by lactic acid bacteria isolated from dairy foods and cow's intestine in western Nigeria. *Arch. Microbiol. 2009* Aug;191(8):639-48.

[44] Santo Domingo JW, Sadowsky MJ, editors. Microbial Source Tracking. Washington D.C.: ASM Press; 2007.

[45] Lienau EK, Strain E, Wang C, Zheng J, Ottesen AR, Keys CE, et al. Identification of a salmonellosis outbreak by means of molecular sequencing. *N. Engl. J. Med. 2011* Mar 10;364(10):981-2.

[46] Maki DG. Coming to grips with foodborne infection--peanut butter, peppers, and nationwide salmonella outbreaks. *N. Engl. J. Med. 2009* Mar 5;360(10):949-53.

[47] Harris SR, Feil EJ, Holden MTG, Quail MA, Nickerson EK, Chantratita N, et al. Evolution of MRSA During Hospital Transmission and Intercontinental Spread. *Science2010* Jan 22;327(5964):469-74.

[48] Chin CS, Sorenson J, Harris JB, Robins WP, Charles RC, Jean-Charles RR, et al. The Origin of the Haitian Cholera Outbreak Strain. *New England Journal of Medicine2011* Jan 6;364(1):33-42.

[49] FDA. Guidance for Industry: Guide to Minimize Microbial Food Safety Hazards of Tomatoes; Draft Guidance. U.S. Food and Drug Administration; 2009 [updated 8/25/2011; cited 2011 12-12-2011]; Available from: http://www.fda.gov/Food/ GuidanceCompliance RegulatoryInformation/GuidanceDocuments/ProduceandPlan Products/ucm173902.htm.

[50] FDA. Produce Safety From Production to Consumption: 2004 Action Plan to Minimize Foodborne Illness Associated with Fresh Produce Consumption. U.S. Food and Drug Administration; 2004 [updated 5-27-2009; cited 2011 12-12-2011]; Available from: http://www.fda.gov/Food/FoodSafety/Product-SpecificInformation/FruitsVegetablesJuices/FDAProduceSafetyActivities/ProduceSafetyActionPlan/ucm129487.htm.

[51] FDA. Tomato Safety Initiative. U.S. Food and Drug Administration; 2007 [updated 5-19-2009; cited 2011 12-12-2011]; Available from: http://www.fda.gov/Food/ FoodSafety/Product-SpecificInformation/FruitsVegetablesJuices/FDAProduceSafety Activities/ucm115334.htm.

[52] FDA. Safer Fruits and Vegetables: FDA Aims to Set Production Standards. U.S. Food and Drug Administration; 2011 [updated 12-8-2011; cited 2011 12-12-2011]; Available from: http://www.fda.gov/ForConsumers/ConsumerUpdates/ucm262031. htm.

[53] United Fresh. Food Safety Programs and Auditing Protocol for the Fresh Tomato Supply Chain Washington D.C.: United Fresh Produce Association; 2011 [cited 2011 12-12-2011]; Available from: http://www.unitedfresh.org/newsviews/ food_safety_ resource_center/fresh_tomato_supply_chain.

In: Salmonella: Classification, Genetics and Disease Outbreaks ISBN: 978-1-61942-928-4
Editors: Adelaide S. Monte, Paulo Eduardo De Santos

Chapter 7

SALMONELLA AND SALMONELLOSIS IN SOUTHERN BRAZIL: A REVIEW OF THE LAST DECADE

E. C. Tondo and A. C. Ritter
Food Science and Technology Institute,
Federal University of Rio Grande do Sul - ICTA/UFRGS, Brazil

ABSTRACT

Salmonella was identified as the first cause of food-borne diseases in the last decade in Brazil. Currently, Brazil is an important producer of pork and is the major poultry and beef exporter in the world. Brazilian animal products have been recognized worldwide, and to attend international standards the Brazilian food industries have been putting considerable effort in order to prevent food contamination, especially by *Salmonella*. A representative part of the Brazilian eggs, beef, poultry, and pork meats is produced in the State of Rio Grande do Sul (RS), in southern Brazil, where *Salmonella* was pointed out as the first cause of food-borne diseases for almost two decades. In this region, homemade mayonnaise was identified as the food preparation mostly involved with salmonellosis, and both meat and meat products were also identified as frequent vehicles for salmonellosis. A specific strain of *Salmonella* Enteritidis (named SE86) was identified as the responsible agent in more than 95 % of investigated food-borne diseases throughout the last decade. SE86 strains isolated from several outbreaks demonstrated the same DNA banding patterns when typed by PCR-methods and PFGE, suggesting that it is spread out through RS. SE86 demonstrated high percentages of sensitivity to many antibiotics; however, an increasing resistance to nalidixic acid and ampicillin has been identified. After exposure to sub-letal pHs, SE86 demonstrated a greater acid adaptation and also to be more acid-and-thermal-resistant than *S.* Typhimurium and *S.* Bredeney also isolated in RS State. Acid-adapted SE86 presents higher virulence than non-acid-adapted SE86 and acid-adapted *S.* Typhimurium in germ-free mice. This strain has shown to be able to form biofilms on stainless steel and polypropylene, and was more resistant to 200 and 400 ppm sodium hypochlorite than others *Salmonella* serovars, but was not more resistant than other *S.* Enteritidis isolated in countries such as Albania, Morocco, Pakistan and Zimbabwe. SE86 mutants (*dps, rpoS*) were constructed in order to investigate the involvement of these genes with oxidative stress caused by sodium hypochlorite exposure. The results demonstrated that both genes are expressed during such exposure;

however, *dps* was expressed in much higher amounts, increasing survival rates of SE86. Poultry meat produced in RS State demonstrated *Salmonella* prevalence of 4.4 % to 15 %, whilst expressively higher percentages of *Salmonella* were found in pork meat samples. Strains isolated from poultry and pork belonged to diverse serovars and, in general, demonstrated different patterns and higher antimicrobial resistance than SE86 isolated from salmonellosis.

INTRODUCTION

Brazil and General Data Concerning Food-Borne Outbreaks

Brazil is the biggest country in South America and the fifth biggest country in the world, with a population of approximately 190 million people distributed in 27 States. The southern region of Brazil is composed by three States called Paraná, Santa Catarina, and Rio Grande do Sul. This region is expressively industrialized and presents high standards of life quality. The southernmost State of Brazil is Rio Grande do Sul, a 10.7-million-people State, composed of 496 cities and presenting an area of 268,781.896 Km^2, bordering Argentina and Uruguay. According to data of the Ministry of Health, during the period from 2000 to 2011, *Salmonella* sp. was identified as the major cause of reported food-borne diseases in Brazil [1]. The most common food vehicles were identified as being mixed food preparations, as well as eggs and egg-based products, respectively. Beef and poultry meat were the fifth and seventh foods most frequent involved in salmonellosis. Private residences were the places where the largest number of outbreaks occurred, followed by restaurants, pastry shops and schools [1]. Among the 3,487 etiologic agents identified in food-borne diseases, *Salmonella* sp. was identified in 42.27 % do the outbreaks, followed by *Staphylococcus aureus* (20.34 %) and *Escherichia coli* (10.46 %) [1].

Salmonella and Salmonellosis in Southern Brazil

Based on the official data of the Division of Sanitary Surveillance of the RS State (DVS/RS), since 1993, *Salmonella* spp. became the major cause of reported food-borne diseases in RS State [2]. Official data also demonstrated that during the period of 1887 to 1993 *S. aureus* was the agent most identified in food-borne diseases in RS; however, *Salmonella* overcame *S. aureus*, probably as a consequence of mandatory good manufacturing practices, as well as training courses, implemented as an obligation for all people working in food services in the city of Porto Alegre, the capital of RS State. According to the same regulation body, the training course was responsible for the decrease of contamination originated from food handlers, justifying the reductions of outbreaks caused by *S. aureus*.

Epidemiological data on salmonellosis occurred in RS State in the periods from 1997 to 1999, 2000 to 2001, and 2002 to 2004, are summarized in Table 1. Data were published elsewhere [3, 4, 5] after analysing official data of DVS/RS. The following factors were analysed: total number of confirmed outbreaks, number of people involved, number of people hospitalized, incidence of outbreaks according to the period of the year, age and sex of the involved people, food vehicle, food storage conditions, local where the disease occurred, and possible causes of the *Salmonella* outbreaks. Salmonollosis data indicated that more than 8,200, 14,200, and 23,700 people were involved, and approximately 1,500, 1,900 and 1,800 had to be hospitalized during the three periods analysed, respectively. The highest number of salmonellosis occurred in springtime, and this fact could be explained by inadequate food refrigeration during this season presenting mild temperatures. The higher incidence of outbreaks in springtime also occurred with other etiological agents of food-borne diseases, confirming the negligence regarding control of temperature. Such carelessness is frequently observed during winter and is prolonged into spring when temperature in RS State is frequently lower than 10 °C [3].

The most affected age groups were those comprised in between 16- and 50-years old, and the most common food vehicle was potato salad made with homemade mayonnaise prepared with raw eggs. The second food vehicle was the group of meat and meat products. The principal causes for salmonellosis was the usage of raw materials not submitted to regulatory inspection (22.92 %, from 1997 to 1999), mainly eggs and foods maintained at room temperature for more than 2 hours (1997 to 2004).

The majority of the outbreaks took place in private homes, and in second place came food services. In the years of 2000 and 2001 two persons died, and in the period from 2002 to 2004 one person died. The incidence of male and female was practically the same, during all periods observed.

Table 1. Characteristics of salmonellosis occurred in Rio Grande do Sul State, southern Brazil, during 1999 to 2004

Period	**Involved people**	**Hospitalized people**	**Age group affected (years old)**	The most common food vehicle	Local of occurrence	Reference
1997-1999	8,217	1,557	16 - 50	Home-made mayonnaise (42.45%)	Private home (43.70%) and commercial food establishments (25.21%)	Costalunga and Tondo (2002)
2000-2001	14,253	1,938	20-49	Home-made mayonnaise (48.1%)	private homes (61.5%), and commercial food establishments (13.7%)	Silveira and Tondo (2006)
2002-2004	23,725	1,878	20-49	Home-made mayonnaise (53.51 %)	private homes (55.81%) and commercial food establishments (12.1%)	Wagner et al. (submitted)

Salmonellosis Caused by *S.* Enteritidis

Geimba et al. [6], when analyzing *Salmonella* strains (n=75), isolated from foods involved with food-borne outbreaks occurred in RS from 1999 to 2000 and found 98% of *S. enterica* serovar Enteritidis. Only two isolates were serotyped as *S.* Derby and *S.* Typhimurium. Among the strains of S. Enteritidis, 83 % were positive for the presence of the *Salmonella* Plasmid Virulence (*spv*R) regulatory gene, and a positive correlation (*P* <0.05) between *S.* Enteritidis and the presence of *spv*R gene was demonstrated. Oliveira et al. [7] investigated 85 *Salmonella* isolated from foods responsible for salmonellosis in RS in the period of 2001-2002, and observed that 93 % were also *S.* Enteritidis. Only six isolates were serotyped as *S.* Javiana (1), *S.* Infantis (1), *S.* Agona (1), *S.* Typhimurium (1), and *S. enterica* subspecies enterica 1, 4, 5 [7]. Comparing to other *Salmonella* serotypes involved in cases of salmonellosis in RS in 1990, *S.* Typhimurium was isolated from 86 % of the foods involved in salmonellosis, while *S.* Enteritidis was not found. However, in the year of 1993, *S.* Enteritidis was isolated from 64 % of the suspected foods, surpassing *S.* Typhimurium, which was isolated from only 4% of the analysed food [*3*]. Similar findings were verified by Usera et al. (*8*) describing the surpassing of *S.* Typhimurium by *S.* Enteritidis in 1990, becoming the most common *Salmonella* serotype reported in the United States.

Asymptomatic infections in poultry flocks were first noticed in the late 1970s, and in the 1980s they spread rapidly throughout the United Kingdom, the United States, South America and other regions of the world [9]. During this period the proportion of salmonellosis cases attributed to *S.* Enteritidis increased substantially, becoming the predominant cause of gastroenteritis in many countries. It is suggested that this rapid increase of the prevalence of *S.* Enteritidis may have been due to the successful campaign to eradicate *S.* Gallinarum and *S.* Pullorum, which are the causative agents of fowl typhoid and pullorum disease in chickens [*10*]. These campaigns may have opened an ecological niche that has since been occupied by *S.* Enteritidis [6].

Clonal Relationship of *S.* Enteritidis in the RS State

Using PCR-ribotyping, Oliveira et al. [7] demonstrated that isolates of *S.* Enteritidis responsible for several cases of salmonellosis in RS during 2001-2002, which were grouped in only two banding profiles (R1 and R2), being that profile R1 comprised 92.4 % of the strains. The same isolates were typed by RAPD and demonstrated four banding patterns (A to D), and the result was that profile A comprised 81 % of the strains. Later Oliveira et al. [11] investigated the clonal relationship of 152 isolates of *S.* Enteritidis involved in food-borne outbreaks isolated in the same State from 1999 to 2002, and concluded that a specific strain of *S.* Enteritidis was involved in the majority of the investigated cases. The DNA typing methods used were PCR ribotyping, Pulsed Field Gel Eletrophoresis (PFGE) and DNA sequencing.

The amount of *Salmonella* sp. present in different foods implicated in salmonellosis occurred in 2005 in RS was studied. After that, the isolates of *Salmonella* were characterized by means of phenotypic and genotypic methods. Food samples (n=19) involved with cases of salmonellosis were analysed by the Central Laboratory of the Department of Health of RS

State (FEPPS/LACEN/RS), demonstrating to be positive for *Salmonella*. Food samples were submitted to estimation of *Salmonella* using the Most Probable Number (MPN) technique. Higher counts (>10^7 MPN.g^{-1}) of *Salmonella* were detected mostly in foods containing mayonnaise. All strains were identified as *S.* Enteritidis, and presented a unique macrorestriction profile, demonstrating the predominance of one clonal group in foods involved in the salmonellosis outbreaks. A low frequency of antimicrobial resistant *S.* Enteritidis strains was observed and nalidixic acid was the only resistance marker detected [12].

During the period from 1999 to 2006, the Official Laboratory of RS (FEPPS/ LACEN/RS) isolated 931 *S.* Enteritidis isolates in 190 outbreaks officially investigated. Among them, S. Enteritidis isolates from 80 different outbreaks were randomly chosen to be analysed - the researchers picked ten isolates from each year of the period comprised from 1999 to 2006. The 80 *S.* Enteritidis samples were isolated from blood (n=12) and feces (n=68) of salmonellosis victims in RS, and were analysed by means of PCR ribotyping and XbaI macrorestriction PFGE. Results identified only three closely related PCR ribotyping patterns (R1, R2, and R3) and just one PFGE profile - this last one, however, grouped 97 % of the strains [13]. These findings confirmed the occurrence of the same DNA banding profile among *S.* Enteritidis isolated from foods, blood and feces of the victims of salmonellosis from 1999 to 2006 in RS, suggesting that a specific strain of *S.* Enteritidis was responsible for the majority of the cases of salmonellosis in this Brazilian State in the last years; this strain has been named *S.* Enteritidis SE86.

Acid and Thermal Resistance of S. Enteritidis SE86

After identifying the involvement of a specific strain of *S.* Enteritidis (SE86) in more than 95 % of the salmonellosis outbreaks investigated in RS between 1999 and 2006, the characteristics of this food pathogen were investigated. Malheiros et al. [14] have compared the growth kinetics, as well as the acid and the thermal resistance of the SE86 strain, with those of the *S.* Typhimurium and *S.* Bredeney strains; these last ones were not involved in foodborne outbreaks, but have also been isolated in RS. Each serovar was inoculated separately in nutrient broth (CN) and in potato salad prepared with homemade mayonnaise (SMC), and then incubated at 30 °C and 9.5 °C. In CN at 30 °C, similar growing characteristics were found for all serovars. However, when growing in homemade mayonnaise, SE86 demonstrated higher counts at the first 6 hours. These results are interesting because SMC has been identified as the major food vehicle responsible for salmonellosis in RS [3, 4]. In CN and in SMC at 9.5 °C, there was no detectable growth of any *Salmonella* serovars during the first 24 hours, suggesting that such temperature was adequate to control the multiplication of these microorganisms.

The acid and thermal resistances of *Salmonella* serovars were evaluated. The three serovars were cultivated separately in Nutrient Broth (NB), as well as Nutrient Broth supplemented with 1 % glucose (NBG) - the later medium was used in order to induce acid-adapted cells. Thus, the three serovars were exposed to different pH (3.5, 4.0 and 4.5) and temperatures (52, 56 and 60 °C). Results indicated that *S.* Bredeney demonstrated higher resistance to pH 3.5 and 4.0; nevertheless, SE86 presented a better capacity for acid adaptation than *S.* Typhimurium and *S.* Bredeney. At pH 4.5, all serovars demonstrated a similar behavior, remaining at the same levels of viable cells for 300 minutes. At 52 ºC, *S.* Bredeney presented higher survivor rates, even though acid adaptation was able to protect only SE86. At 56 ºC and 60 ºC, non-adapted and acid-adapted SE86 strains were more thermally resistant than other serovars tested. SDS-PAGE analysis demonstrated differences in the protein profiles of non-adapted and acid-adapted cells of all serovars [15].

Using simulated gastric fluid (FGS) and germ-free mices, Perez et al. [16] evaluated the survival in the ability of intestinal invasion of SE86 and *S.* Typhimurium (ST99), whether submitted or not to acid adaptation. The microorganisms were grown in culture media supplemented with glucose in order to promote acid adaptation due to pH reduction. After the growth, approximately 8 log of SE86 and ST99 (either acid-adapted or non-adapted) were exposed to FGS with pH 1.5, and then inoculated in germ-free adult male Wistar rats. Germ-free mice were also inoculated with approximately 2 log, and the animals were observed at aseptic conditions for twelve days. Animal feces, as well as portions of the gastrointestinal tract, were examined by means of microbiological analysis, and the rats were also investigated for intestinal morphological abnormalities. The mice were analyzed by means of histopathology and then submitted to the mortality curve. The results indicated that acid-adapted SE86 had a significant higher survival rate ($p < 0.05$) than non-adapted SE86, non-adapted ST99 and also than acid-adapted ST99 in the FGS. The *in vivo* experiments demonstrated that acid-adapted SE86 and acid-adapted ST99 were capable of causing intestinal morphological abnormalities, and were then recovered from feces, jejunum and ileum-cecal junctions of rats. Acid-adapted SE86 showed higher counts in the ileum-cecal junction than the other strains, suggesting that acid adaptation influenced the virulence of this microorganism. All strains were able to rapidly multiply in germ-free animals, but mortality caused by acid-adapted SE86 was more intense. Histopathological analyses revealed greater severity of the infection caused by SE86, a fact which was confirmed by the death of animals starting at the fourth day of infection - unlike the ST99 which did not cause the death of animals until twelve days after inoculation.

The SE86 Biocide Resistance

The resistance to biocides of SE86, S. Typhimurium and S. Bredeney was evaluated using the suspension test as recommended by the Brazilian Ministry of Agriculture. Peracetic acid, quaternary ammonium and sodium hypochlorite were chosen to be tested because they are sanitizers commonly used in the Brazilian food industries. Based on the results, it was possible to observe that, when the concentrations indicated by the manufacturers were used, biocides were able to inactivate all of the microorganisms tested. However, SE86 was resistant to 400 ppm sodium hypochlorite and survived for up to 15 minutes of exposure to 200 ppm of this biocide, a fact which was not demonstrated by the other strains [17]. The same microorganisms were used in order to test biofilm formation capability on surfaces of material commonly used in food industries and food services. Coupons of stainless steel and polyethylene were immersed in bacterial suspensions of SE86, S. Typhimurium, and S. Bredeney during 15, 30 and 60 minutes, and then were submitted to different concentrations of peracetic acid, sodium hypochlorite, and quaternary ammonium. Hydrophobicity of the surfaces was evaluated by means of measurements of contact angle using the sessile drop method, and bacterial adhesion was accompanied by means of bacterial counts and scanning electron microscopy (SEM). When evaluating the results, it was possible to observe that the three serovars indicated similar counts of adhered cell to both materials (5.0 to 6.5 log cfu cm^{-2}). The time of exposure did not influence the counts of adhered cells on both surfaces; however, SEM revealed larger clusters of SE86 on both materials, which were not found in the other serovars. SE86 demonstrated a lower sessile drop angle when on polyethylene, indicating hydrophilic properties of this material. The biocides were not able to inactivate all the microorganisms adhered on both surface materials. At least 1 log cfu cm^{-2} of all serovars tested remained viable after the exposure to different sanitizer concentrations. In general, higher counts of survivors were observed on polyethylene disinfected with different concentrations of biocides. *S.* Bredeney and *S.* Typhimurium were more resistant than SE86 to peracetic acid, whilst SE86 demonstrated smaller reduction rates after sodium hypochlorite exposure. When adhered to polyethylene, the serovars *S.* Typhimurium and SE86 were more resistant to quaternary ammonium than *S.* Bredeney in all concentrations tested, and the numbers of SE86 remained almost unaltered. On stainless steel disinfected by quaternary ammonium, *S.* Bredeney presented higher numbers of survivors [18].

Since SE86 demonstrated to be resistant to high concentrations of sodium hypochlorite [17,18], the resistance of this Brazilian strain was compared to other strains of *S.* Enteritidis isolated worldwide, i. e. from Albania, Zimbabwe, Morocco and Pakistan. All the strains were chosen because they were responsible for salmonellosis and were submitted to 200 ppm sodium hypochlorite in suspension tests for 5, 10, 15, and 20 minutes, according recommended by the Brazilian Ministry of Agriculture. The results showed that none of the *S.* Enteritidis were totally inactivated after 20 minutes of exposure and the reduction rates were similar. Only the strain isolated in Albania demonstrated to be significantly more sensitive [19].

The involvement of the *rpo*S and *dps* genes in the resistance to 200 ppm sodium hypochlorite was also investigated in SE86. Mutants of SE86 were constructed by means of the Knockout method (Datsenko and Wanner, 2000) and tagged by using the 3X FLAG method (Uzzau, et al. 2001). The survival of the Wild Type (WT) strain, as well as of the attenuated strains, was determined by bacterial counts. Tagged proteins (Dps and RpoS) were detected by means of SDS-PAGE and also immunoblotting with anti-FLAG antibodies. The SE86 strain which lacked *dps* demonstrated greater sensitivity compared to the WT SE86 exposed to sodium hypochlorite, with a 2-log reduction after one minute, whilst WT demonstrated a reduction of only one log. The RpoS and Dps proteins were actively expressed under the conditions tested, strongly suggesting that these SE86 genes are related to oxidative stress resistance, since both were expressed during the exposure of the microorganism to 200 ppm sodium hypochlorite [19].

Antimicrobial Resistance of *Salmonella*

Salmonella is not only a public health concern due to the number of salmonellosis cases that it causes, but also because many strains are resistant to a number of antimicrobial agents. The concern is that if such strains cause food poisoning in humans they can be difficult to treat, making the probability of human death more likely. The resistance of *Salmonella* sp. to antibiotics is increasing rapidly throughout the world, and the indiscriminate and incorrect use of antibiotics has facilitated the emergence of resistance in many serovars. For example, we can mention the recent food-borne outbreaks in the USA and Europe caused by both multi-antibiotic-resistant *S.* Heidelberg and *S.* Kentucky, respectively. Other examples are related to several cases involving the clone of the *S.* Typhimurium DT104, which is characterized by chromosomal resistance to ampicillin, tetracycline, streptomycin, chloramphenicol, and sulphonamides. Infections with *S.* Typhimurium DT104 are associated with more severe illness, higher rates of admission to hospitals and increased mortality. Although the antimicrobial resistance in *S.* Enteritidis has been considered low when compared to the dramatic increase of resistance demonstrated by some *S.* Typhimurium isolates (Yang et al. 2002), attention should be given to the frequent isolation of multi-resistant *S.* Enteritidis [20]. The surveillance of the rising antimicrobial resistance of *S.* Enteritidis is especially important, since this serotype has become the prevalent agent of human salmonellosis in many countries in the last years, including Brazil. Over the last decade in the RS State, the resistance of *S.* Enteritidis isolated from food-borne illnesses, pork and poultry has been the subject of several studies and are presented below.

Antimicrobial Resistance of *S.* Enteritidis Isolated in Food-Borne Outbreaks in the RS State

S. Enteritidis strains isolated from foods involved in salmonellosis in 1999 - 2000 (n=73) demonstrated to be predominantly resistant to streptomycin (37 %), gentamicin (14 %), and nalidixic acid (14 %), while intermediate resistance was observed most often for tetracycline (53 %), neomycin (30 %), and gentamicin (15 %). Multiple resistance was demonstrated in 17 of the strains (23 %), and one isolate exhibited resistance to four drugs (neomycin, kanamycin, streptomycin, and nalidixic acid). Most strains demonstrated to be fully susceptible to the ten drugs tested [21]. *S.* Enteritidis strains (n=79) isolated in 2001 to 2002 showed the highest percentages of resistance for gentamicin (13 %), streptomycin (11 %), and nalidixic acid (21 %), while the most expressive intermediate resistances were demonstrated for kanamycin (29 %), neomycin (18. 7%) and streptomycin (14 %). Full susceptibility for all ten drugs tested was found in 62 % of the strains. The highest rates of sensitivity were demonstrated for ampicillin (95 %), tetracycline (91 %), and chloramphenicol (99 %). No resistance was observed regarding sulfamethoxazole/trimetoprim and sulfazotrim. Comparing the antibiotic resistance of the bacteria isolated in 2001 to those isolated in 2002, an increase in the resistance percentage of the isolates was observed concerning tetracycline (0 % in 2001 to 5 % in 2002), kanamycin (2 % in 2001 to 3 % in 2002), nalidixic acid (19 % in 2001 to 24 % in 20002), and chloramphenicol (0 % in 2001 to 3 % in 2002). Results of the intermediate resistance for neomycin, kanamycin, gentamycin, and streptomycin also increased from 2001 to 2002. Overall, resistance was verified in 30 strains (38 %) [22]. Among the 80 *S.* Enteritidis isolated from salmonellosis in RS from 1999 to 2006, only three isolates (4 %) were fully susceptible to all the antibiotics tested. The major resistances were observed for ampicillin (81 %), streptomycin (19 %), and nalidixic acid (25%) [13]. Paula et al. [23] have studied 130 *S.* Enteritidis responsible for food-borne salmonellosis occurred in RS from 2003 to 2006, and have reported that the higher percentages of resistance were demonstrated for ampicillin (100 %) and nalidixic acid (48 %). Intermediate resistance was found for neomycin (49 %) and tetracycline (25 %). Multiple drug resistance was observed in 63 % of isolates. Analysing the results published by Geimba et al. [21], Oliveira et al. [22], Oliveira et al. [11], and Paula et al. [23], it is possible to observe increasing resistance rates for nalidixic acid and ampicillin regarding *S*. Enteritidis associated with salmonellosis in RS (Figure 1).

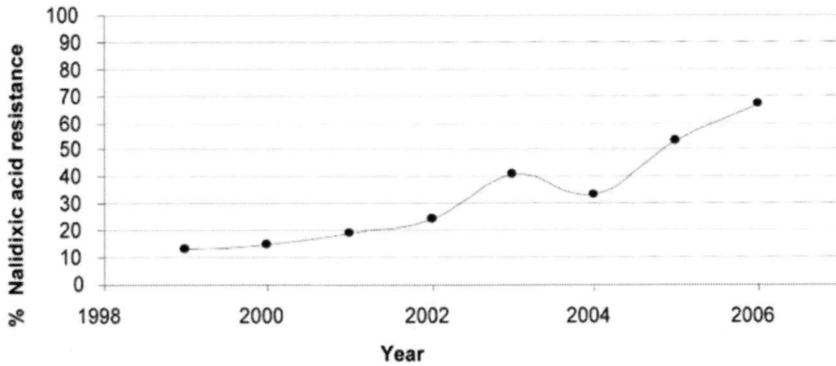

Figure 1. Resistance to nalidixic acid in the *S*. Enteritidis responsible for food-borne salmonellosis outbreaks occurred in the Rio Grande do Sul State, southern Brazil, from 1999 to 2006.

The raising resistance for nalidixic acid and the resistance for ciprofloxacin are issues of concern, because several studies have reported increasing numbers of *Salmonella* sp. strains resistant to quinolones in Germany [24], England and Wales [25] and Spain [26]. Emphasizing this concern, the CLSI added a guideline recommending clinical laboratories to routinely test for nalidixic acid resistance in extraintestinal *Salmonella* isolates in order to alert physicians about the emerging resistance (Clinical and Laboratory Standards Institute [27]. Quinolones are widely used in food animal production and are known to select for quinolone-resistant *Salmonella* sp. in animals. At the same time, quinolones are one of the few available therapies for serious *Salmonella* infections, particularly in adults.

The prevalence of resistant samples to tetracycline and streptomycin could be explained by the dissemination of resistance genes, *strA* and *strB* tet (A), as observed by Pezzella, Ricci, and Digiannatale [28] in a study about *Salmonella* strains isolated from animals in Italy. Hyeon et al. [29] also demonstrated resistance to streptomycin (22.2 %) and tetracycline (16.7 %) among *S*. Enteritidis isolated from retail meats products in South Korea in 2009. Tetracycline and streptomycin are common antimicrobials administered in veterinary medicine and their frequent use may have contributed to the resistance rates found in the RS State and South Korea. On the other hand, chloramphenicol resistance observed among *S*. Enteritidis isolated in southern Brazil could not be explained by the use of this drug in animal feed, because chloramphenicol was banned from animal feed production in Brazil more than a decade ago.

Salmonella in Pork Production and Pork Products in the RS State

The southern region of Brazil is the most important area for pork production in the country. Its pork output accounted for two thirds of the Brazilian total production, which consisted of 2.8 million tons in 2006. Approximately 70 % of the pork produced in Brazil is consumed in the form of processed meat products, such as sausages, bacon and ham. Pork contamination by *Salmonella* can occur at multiple stages along the production chain.

Moreover, the level of *Salmonella* infection of pigs on farms can be increased during transport, lairage and slaughtering-plant operations [30].

The slaughter of *Salmonella* carrier pigs is considered the first critical point for the contamination of pork products. The risk represented by positive animals tends to increase when this pathogen is found in carcass portions consumed by the population [31].

Castagna et al. [31] assessed the implication of the prevalence of *Salmonella*-positive pigs at slaughter on the contamination of ground meat used for fresh sausage production in the RS State. Mandibular lymph node/tonsil pools (LT) and intestinal contents (CI) of 16 animals were collected in each one of the three samplings conducted at an abattoir. On the day after, 99 samples of the ground meat, produced with carcass parts of pigs slaughtered in the previous day, were collected immediately before the casing. The mean prevalence of *Salmonella* carrier pigs at slaughter was 83.33 %, while 93.94 % of the ground meat samples were positive. The most prevalent serovars were Panama, Bredeney, and Typhimurium. Results demonstrated that the slaughter of *Salmonella*-positive pigs implicated on the contamination of fresh pork sausage.

Mariot et al. [*32*] studied the incidence of *Salmonella* sp. in four surface points (ham, belly, loin and neck) of 239 pork carcasses processed in a big exporter pig-slaughtering plant (3200 animals per day) in RS. *Salmonella* spp. was isolated in 30 % of the carcasses after bleeding. Other steps also demonstrated *Salmonella* contamination on the pork carcasses. As examples, *Salmonella* sp. isolation was verified after washing (17.95 %), after dehairing (16.65 %), and also after the first polishing (20 %). *Salmonella* sp. was not detected after the scalding and singeing steps, suggesting that these steps are important to control *Salmonella* in pork production.

Bessa et al. [33] evaluated the prevalence of *Salmonella*-positive pigs at slaughterhouses under federal inspection in RS. Samples of feces and lymph nodes of 300 animals were collected in three different slaughterhouses and submitted to bacteriological analysis. The prevalence of *Salmonella* carrier animals was 55.66 %, being 17.6 % of the animals *Salmonella*-positive in lymph nodes, 18.3 % in feces, and 19.6 % in both materials. Twenty-six different serovars were identified among 226 *Salmonella* isolates. The most prevalent serovars were Typhimurium (24.3 %), Agona (19.9 %), Derby (13.2 %) e Bredeney (12 %).

Schwartz et al. [34] analyzed the prevalence of *Salmonella* in slaughtered swine and the results of serology and *Salmonella* isolation were compared in order to determine the most important stage of the infection (on-farm or transport, and pre-slaughter) in relation to the number of carrier animals found at slaughter. Forty herds from three different swine raisers in the southern region of Brazil were sampled at slaughter. Blood and mesenteric lymph nodes were collected from 20 swine in each herd. *Salmonella* was isolated from 62.5 % to 85.0 % of the animals, while seroprevalence varied from 73.8 % to 83.2 % in the three swine raisers. Serovars Agona, Typhimurium and Panama were the most prevalent among the *Salmonella* isolates. Isolation and serological results demonstrated that *Salmonella* infection occurred during the on-farm stage, since a high seroprevalence was detected at slaughter.

Muller et al. [35] compared the prevalence of *Salmonella* positive pigs at the beginning of the finishing phase and at slaughter in order to identify the possible sources of contamination in the farms. In three finishing farms, environmental swabs from the barns and from the feed silos were collected during the sanitary emptiness. Feces samples from all pigs were *Salmonella*-negative at the beginning of the finishing phase; in two farms seropositive animals were found. In two farms, residual environmental contamination was detected, and in the third farm one of the feed batches was *Salmonella*-positive. At slaughter, over 90 % of the animals were positive and, in all cohorts, a variable number (12 % - 92 %) of carriers was detected. From this on, it was concluded that the finishing phase was critical for the amplification of *Salmonella* infection, and the residual environmental contamination in the farms, as well as *Salmonella*-positive feed batches, were the probable sources of infection.

A total of 336 samples of fresh pork sausage randomly obtained from supermarkets and butcher shops in Porto Alegre city, the capital of the RS State, were examined for the presence of *Salmonella* sp. *Salmonella enterica* was detected in 24.4 % of the samples, with a most probable number count ranging from 0.03 MPN g^{-1} to 460 MPN g^{-1}. Strains belonging to the most isolated *S. enterica* serovars (Brandenburg, Panama, Derby, and Typhimurium) were further analysed for antimicrobial resistance, and the results demonstrated that the resistance for tetracycline was the most prevalent among the *Salmonella* isolates. *S.* Panama and *S.* Typhimurium presented the greatest number of resistance phenotypes [30].

The survival of *Salmonella* sp. in pig slurry submitted to treatment in successive stabilization ponds on a pig-breeding farm was investigated. The isolated *Salmonella* strains were tested for their resistance against 14 antibiotics, using the agar diffusion method. Of a total of 20 samples taken from different points in the stabilization ponds system, 13 were positive for *Salmonella* sp. in the beginning, and only one at the end of the system. Most of the isolated *Salmonella* (161/163) belonged to sorovar Typhimurium. These strains were resistant to sulfonamide (100 %), tetracycline (9.4 %), sulfamethoxazole/trimethoprin (84.5 %), ampicillin (76.4 %), cloramphenicol (29.2 %), streptomycin (90.1 %), nalidixic acid (77.6 %), tobramycin (13.7 %), neomycin (5 %), amikacin (3.7 %), cefaclor (25.5 %), gentamicin (6.2 %) and amoxacilin/clavulanic acid (5 %). Most *S.* Typhimurium strains (94.5 %) were resistant to four or more antibiotics. The multi-resistance level and the pattern variability of these strains were similar in the beginning and at the end of the stabilization ponds system [36].

Salmonella Isolated from Pork and Resistance to Biocides

The effectiveness of six biocides (quaternary ammonium, glutaraldehyde, iodophor, sodium hypochlorite, phenol and peracetic acid) in strains of *Salmonella* sp. isolated from pigs was evaluated. The disinfectants were evaluated against 8 porcine *S.* Typhimurium strains presenting different antibiotic resistance profiles, with a contact time of five minutes, with and without organic matter. All disinfectants were effective in the absence of organic matter. However, when organic matter was included on the assay, only sodium hypochlorite, phenol and peracetic acid were effective. Furthermore, sodium hypochorite, phenol and peracetic acid were also the most effective against porcine *S.* Typhimurium strains after five minutes of contact. These results indicate that the effectiveness of the tested disinfectants was more related to the presence of organic matter and exposure time than to the resistance profile presented by the tested strains [37].

The sensitivity of 96 *S.* Typhimurium strains isolated from slaughter pigs in the RS State was evaluated. The isolates were tested against quaternary ammonium and iodophor, which represent two commercial disinfectants commonly used in animal production. The tested disinfectants were used in the concentration recommended by the fabricant and in a sub-concentration in order to simulate a possible field situation. Dilution suspension tests were conducted observing the inactivation of each *S*. Typhimurium isolate after 5, 15, 30 and 60 minutes of contact with each compound. All tested isolates were inactivated by the quaternary ammonium compound in both concentrations. Four isolates revealed resistance to iodophor in the recommended concentration, and 59 isolates were resistant when a sub-concentration was used [38].

Salmonella in Brazilian Poultry

Brazil is the third biggest poultry producer in the world, staying behind only China and the USA. However, concerning the exportations, Brazil is the biggest exporter in the world since 2006, when this country exported 2,900 thousand tons of poultry meat. Approximately 40 % of the poultry meat in the world comes from Brazil [39]. Even though poultry meat produced in Brazil presents high quality standards, the growth of the Brazilian poultry industry in the 1990s, as well as the increasing number of birds reared in high density environments, have created favorable conditions for the presence of *Salmonella* in some flocks [40].

The control of *Salmonellae* in Brazil is regulated by the Poultry National Health Plan developed by the Ministry of Agriculture, Livestock and Food Supply. In 2003, a vaccination for broiler breeders using killed vaccine against *S.* Enteritidis was approved. It has been suggested that the presence of one serovar in a flock will reduce the accumulation of others. For example, it is believed that either the reduction of *S.* Gallinarum resulted in the increase of *S.* Enteritidis in flocks or the increased presence of *S.* Enteritidis displaced other serovars. In broiler production, when cecal tonsil colonization is established by *Salmonella*, such bacteria are consistently excreted in the feces [40].

Santos et al. [41] evaluated samples of broiler carcasses produced in poultry companies located at the highlands region of RS, which were all submitted to a microbiological monitoring program carried out during the years 1995 and 1996. During this period, 1,344 carcasses were analysed, from which 15.10 % were positive for *Salmonella* sp. (111 of the later identified as *S.* Enteritidis). The 111 isolates of *S.* Enteritidis were phage-typed and the results indicated that 93.3 % of them belonged to the PT4. The same isolates were evaluated for RAPD, and it was verified that 91.8 % were classified as pattern A [40]. However, lesser percentages of *Salmonella*-positive samples were verified by the Brazilian Sanitary Agency (ANVISA), who analyzed 180 poultry carcasses produced in RS, demonstrating that 95.56 % of them were negative for *Salmonella* sp [42].

Salmonella strains were isolated from ill and shedding birds in several regions of Brazil between 1962 and 1991. Serotyping of 2123 isolates showed 90 serovars pertaining to 14 serogroups. There was a predominance of groups O:9 (40.0%), O:4 (33.3%), O:7 (10.6%) and O:3,10 (6.7%). Major serovar diversity was found in the serogroup O:7, which accounted for 22 different types, followed by the serogroups O:4, O:3,10 and O:9, with 19, 15 and 10 serotypes respectively.

An average of 10.8 serovars was isolated per year. S. Gallinarum, S. Pullorum, S.Typhimurium, S. Heidelberg, S. Enteritidis and S. Infantis were the most frequent serovars found over 30 years, representing 65 % to 67 % of the total of isolates [43].

Antimicrobial Resistance of *Salmonella* sp. Isolated from Poultry

The antimicrobial resistance of 96 *S.* Enteritidis isolated from salmonellosis outbreaks (n=43) and poultry-related products not involved with food-borne outbreaks (n=53), in the period from 1995 up to 2003, was investigated. Although 43.75 % of the samples were sensitive to all drugs tested, and resistance to sulfonamide (34.37 %), trimethoprim-sulfamethoxazole (25.00 %), nalidixic acid (14.58 %), streptomycin (2.08 %), gentamicin and tetracycline (1.04 %) was identified. *S.* Enteritidis resistance to nalidixic acid (14.58 %) was identified only in strains isolated from poultry, and this result could be explained because nalidixic acid is commonly used in poultry therapy in Brazil [44]. Ribeiro et al. [45] evaluated the occurrence of *Salmonella* sp. in raw broiler parts and analysed the antimicrobial resistance profile of the microorganisms isolated. The study was carried out using 61 broiler chicken parts (wings, whole legs, boneless breasts and backs) collected in the period from September to December of 1996 in a processing plant located in southern Brazil. Regarding the antimicrobial resistance, the results indicated that 88 % of the *Salmonella* isolates were resistant to one or more antimicrobial agents, presenting eight different patterns of resistance. Multiple resistance was not observed in five of the 21 *S.* Enteritidis isolates, while 3 were susceptible to all antimicrobials tested, and two were resistant only to tetracycline. Multiple resistance was also found in the *S.* Typhimurium, and in all three *S.* Hadar isolates. Three *S.* Enteritidis isolates were susceptible to all antimicrobials tested, and two were resistant only to tetracycline. The results emphasized the need for the responsible use of antimicrobials in animal production.

During the years of 1999, 2000 and 2001, the antimicrobial resistance of *S.* Enteritidis isolated from clinical and environmental poultry samples was evaluated in southern Brazil. Among the 79 isolated samples, 81 % were resistant to at least one of the antimicrobial agents tested, showing 22 different resistance patterns. Tetracycline showed the highest percentage of resistance (64.5 %) among the antimicrobial agents used. Resistance to drugs at different levels was found as the following: ampicillin (1.2 %), kanamycin (1.2 %), ciprofloxacin (2.5 %), enrofloxacin (8.8 %), gentamicin (21.5 %), streptomycin (20.2 %), nitrofurantoin (26.6 %), and nalidixic acid (30.4 %). None of the *S.* Enteritidis strains were resistant to chloramphenicol, norfloxacin, and polimycin B. Among the 64 *S.* Enteritidis strains that showed resistance, 67.2 % were resistant to two or more antimicrobial drugs. Twenty-one isolates (32.8 %) were resistant to only one of the antimicrobial agents, 14 to tetracycline, three to nalidixic acid, three to nitrofurantoin, and one to gentamycin. These levels of antimicrobial resistance suggest a high occurrence of tetracycline-resistant *S.* Enteritidis strains, as well as resistance to two or more antimicrobial drugs [46].

CONCLUSION

Salmonella sp. was recognized as the first cause of food-borne illnesses in Brazil in the last decade, being that, in the southern region, this microorganism has been identified as the first cause for food-borne outbreaks for almost two decades. A specific strain of *S.* Enteritidis (SE86) was identified as the microorganism responsible for more than 95 % of salmonellosis in RS. When compared to other *Salmonella* serovars, SE86 demonstrated higher acid-and-thermal adaptation capability and also has demonstrated to be able to grow faster in home-made mayonnaise, the food vehicle most involved with salmonellosis in RS. When exposed to sub-letal pHs, SE86 increased its virulance in germ-free mices, which was not verified for *S.* Typhimurium and *S.* Bredeney. The antibiotic surveillance of the *S.* Enteritidis isolated in RS demonstrated an increasing resistance for nalidixic acid and ampicilim, even though high levels of suceptibility were reported for many antibiotics. SE86 was tested against different sanitizers and demonstrated to be more resistant than other *Salmonella* serovars, mainly to sodium hypochlorite, the most used biocide in RS. The involvement of *rpo*S and *dps* genes with this resistance was studied and it was demonstrated that both genes are expressed during sodium hypochlorite exposure. However, the mutant *dps* demonstrated lesser survival rates than the wildtype SE86. All those characteristics of SE86 could be related to the frequent involvement of this strain with salmonellosis outbreaks in RS. Also corroborating this possibility is the fact of the presence of some other *Salmonella* serovars in pork and poultry meat produced in RS, which were not responsible for salmonellosis outbreaks.

References

[1] Brasil. Ministério da Saúde. Secretaria de Vigilância em Saúde- SVS. Dados Epidemiológicos- DTA- Período de 2001 a 2011. Disponível em www.saude.gov.br/svs.

[2] Rio Grande do Sul. Secretaria Estadual da Saúde. (2001) Divisão de Vigilância Sanitária. Relatórios anuais de DTA. Porto Alegre.

[3] Costalunga, S,. and Tondo, E. C. (2002) Salmonellosis in Rio Grande do Sul, 1997 to 1999. *Brazilian Journal of Microbiology*, 33, 342-346.

[4] Silveira, J. B. and Tondo, E. C. (2006) Salmonellosis outbreaks occurring in Rio Grande do Sul, Southern Brazil, during 2000 to 2001. In: *International Symposium Salmonella and Salmonellosis* (I3S), Saint-Malo. Proceedings. v. 1. p. 521-522.

[5] Wagner, V. R., Silveira, J. B., Tondo, E. C. Salmonellosis in Rio Grande do Sul State, Southern Brazil, 2002 to 2004 *Brazilian Journal of Microbiology submitted.*

[6] Geimba, M. P., Tondo, E. C., Oliveira, F. A., Cardoso, M. I. (2004) Serological characterization and prevalence of spvR genes in *Salmonella* isolated from foods involved in outbreaks in *Brazil. Journal of Food Protection*, 67, 1229-1233.

[7] Oliveira, F. A., Frazzon, A. P., Brandelli, A., Tondo, E. C. (2007) Use of PCR-ribotyping, RAPD, and antimicrobial resistance for typing of *Salmonella* Enteritidis involved in food-borne outbreaks in Southern *Brazil. J. Infect. Dev. Countries*, 1, 170-176.

[8] Usera, M. A., Popovic, T., Bopp, C., Strockbine, N. A. (1994) Molecular subtyping of *Salmonella enteritidis* phage type 8 strains from United States. *J. Clin. Microbiol.*, 32, 194-198.

[9] Agron, P. G., Walker, R. I., Kinde, H., Sawier, S. J., Hayes, D. C., Wollard, J., Andersen, G. I. (2001) Identification by subtractive hibridization of sequences specific for *Salmonella enterica* serovar Enteritidis. *Appl. Environ. Microbiol.*, 67, 4984-4991.

[10] Bäumler, A. J., Hargis, B. M., Tsolis, R. M. (2000) Tracing the origins of *Salmonella* outbreaks. *Science*, 287, 50-52.

[11] Oliveira, F. A., Geimba, M. P., Pasqualotto, A. P. and Tondo, E. C. (2009) Clonal relationship among *Salmonella* enterica serovar Enteritidis involved. *Food Control*, 20, 606-610.

[12] Murmann, L., Santos, M. C. M., Longaray, S., Both, J., Cardoso, M. R. I. (2008) Quantification and molecular characterization of *Salmonella* isolated from food samples involved in salmonellosis outbreaks in Rio Grande do Sul, Brazil. *Brazilian Journal of Microbiology*, 39, 529-534.

[13] Oliveira, F. A., Pasqualotto, A. P., Padilha, W., Tondo, E. C. (2010) Characterization of *Salmonella* Enteritidis isolated from human samples. *Food Research International*, 1, 2-5.

[14] Malheiros, P. S., Paula, C. D. M. and Tondo, E. C. (2007) Avaliação da cinética de crescimento de *Salmonella* Enteritidis envolvida em surtos alimentares no RS: uma comparação com outros sorovares. *Ciência e Tecnologia de Alimentos*, 27, 751-755.

[15] Malheiros, P. S., Brandelli, A., Tondo, E. C. (2008) Acid and thermal resistance of a *Salmonella* Enteritidis strain involved in several foodborne outbreaks. *Journal of Food Safety*, 29, 302-317.

[16] Perez, K. J., Martins, F. S., Cara, D. C., Nicoli, J. R., Tondo, E. C. (2011) Evaluation of intestinal invasion in germ free mice challenge with acid-adapted and non acid-adapted *Salmonella* Enteritidis SE86 and *Salmonella* Typhimurium ST99. *Journal of Food Safety*, "in press".

[17] Machado, T. R. M., Malheiros, P. S., Brandelli, A., Tondo, E. C. (2010) Avaliação da Resistência de *Salmonella* à ação de desinfetantes ácido peracético, quaternário de amônio e hipoclorito de sódio. *Revista do Instituto Adolfo Lutz*, 69, 475-481.

[18] Tondo, E. C., Machado, T. R. M., Malheiros, P. S., Padrão, D. K., Carvalho, A. L. and Brandelli, A. (2010) Adhesion and biocides inactivation of *Salmonella* on stainless steel and polyethylene. *Brazilian Journal of Microbiology*, 4, 10-20.

[19] Ritter, A. C., Bacciu, D., Santi, L. Silva, W. O. B., Vainstein, M. H., Rubino, S., Uzzau, S. Tondo, E. C. (2011) Investigation of *rpoS* and *dps* genes in sodium hypochlorite resistance of *Salmonella* Enteritidis SE86 isolated from foodborne illness outbreaks in Southern Brazil. *Journal of Food Protection*, "in press".

[20] Breuil, J., Brisabois, A., Casin, I., Armand-lefèvre, L., Frémy, S., Collatz, E. (2000) Antibiotic resistance in salmonellae isolated from humans and animals in France: comparative data from 1994 and 1997. *Journal of Antimicrobial Chemotherapy*, 46, 965-971.

[21] Geimba, M. P., Tondo, E. C., Brandelli, A. (2005) Antimicrobial Resistance in *Salmonella* Enteritidis Isolated from Foods Involved in Human Foodborne Outbreaks Occurred in the South of Brazil, 1999 to 2000. *Journal of Food Safety*, 25, 3, 173-182.

[22] Oliveira, F. A., Brandelli, A., Tondo, E. C. (2006). Antimicrobial resistance in *Salmonell*a Enteritidis from foods involved in human salmonellosis occurred in southern Brazil. *The New Microbiologica*, 29, 49-54.

[23] Paula, C. M. D., Ritter, A. C., Pieta, L., Amaral, P. H., Tondo, E. C. (2011) Antimicrobial resistance in *Salmonella* Enteritidis from foods involved in human salmonellosis outbreaks in Southern Brazil from 2003 to 2006. *Journal of Microbiology and Antimicrobials*, 3, 233-240.

[24] Malorny, B., Schroeter, A. and Helmuth, R. (1999) Incidence of quinolone resistance over the period 1986 to 1998 in veterinary Salmonella isolates from Germany. *Antimicrobial agents and Chemotherapy*, 43, 2278–2282.

[25] Threlfall E. J., Day, M., de Pinna, E. (2006) Drug-resistant enteric fever in the UK. *Lancet*, 367:1576.

[26] Marimon, J. M., Goariz, M., Zigorraga, C., Cilla, G. and Perez-Trallero, E. (2004) Increasing prevalence of quinolone resistance in human nontyphoid Salmonella enterica isolates obtained in Spain from 1981 to 2003. *Antimicrob Agents Chemother,* 3, 576–577.

[27] NCCLS (2005). Clinical and Laboratory Standards Institute/NCCLS. Performance Standards for Antimicrobial Susceptibility Testing, Fifteenth Informational Supplement. CLSI/NCCLS document M100- S15. Clinical and Laboratory Standards Institute, 940 West Valley Road, Suite 1400, Wayne, *Pennsylvania*, 19087-1898 USA.

[28] Pezzella, C., Ricci, A., DiGiannatale, E., Luzzi, I., Carattoli, A. (2004) Tetracycline and Streptomycin Resistance Genes, Transposons, and Plasmids in *Salmonella* enterica Isolated from Animals in Italy. Antimicrob. *Agents Chemother*., 48, 903–908.

[29] Hyeon, J. H. Chon, J. W. Hwang, I. G., Kwak, Moo-Sang, H. S., Kim, S. (2011) Prevalence, Antibiotic Resistance, and Molecular Characterization of *Salmonella* Serovars in Retail Meat Products. *Journal of Food Protection*, 74, 161–166.

[30] Muzmann, L., Santos, M. C. M., Cardoso, M. R. I. (2009) Prevalence, genetic characterization and antimicrobial resistance of *Salmonella* isolated from fresh pork sausages in Porto Alegre, Brazil. *Food Control*, 20, 191-195.

[31] Castagna, S., Schwarz, P., Canal, C., Cardoso, M. R. I. (2004) Presença de *Salmonella* sp no trato intestinal e em tonsilas/linfonodos submadibulares de suínos ao abate. *Arquivo Brasileiro de Medicina Veterinária e Zootecnia*, 56, 300-306.

[32] Mariot, R. F., De Paula, C. M., Do Amaral, P. H., Tondo, E. C. Evaluation of microbial contamination and the incidence of *Salmonella* spp. at various stages of pork slaughter lines. *Food Control*, submitted.

[33] Bessa, M. C., Costa, M., Cardoso, M. R. I. (2004) Prevalência de *Salmonella* sp. em suínos abatidos em frigoríficos do Rio Grande do Sul. *Pesquisa Veterinária Brasileira*, 24, 80-84.

[34] Schawarz, P., Calveira, J., Sella, A, Bessa, M. C., Barcellos, D., Cardoso, M. (2009) *Salmonella* enterica: isolamento e soroprevalência em suínos abatidos no Rio Grande do Sul. *Arquivo Brasileiro de Medicina Veterinária e Zootecnia*, 61, 1028-1034.

[35] Muller, M., Schwarz, P., Silva, L. E., Cardoso, M. R. I. (2009) Perfil sorológico e de isolamento de *Salmonella* sp. em suínos no início da terminação e ao abate. *Ciência Animal Brasileira*, (UFG), 10, 931-937.

[36] Schmidt, V. and Cardoso, M. R. I. (2003) Sobrevivência e perfil de resistência a antimicrobianos de amostras de *Salmonella* sp. isoladas em um sistema de tratamento de dejetos de suínos. *Ciência Rural*, Santa Maria, 33, 881-888.

[37] Kich, J. D., Mores, N., Piffer, I., Barioni Junior, W., Amaral, A., Ramminger, L., Cardoso, M. R. I. (2005) Fatores de risco associados com a prevalência sorológica de *Salmonella* em granjas comerciais de suínos do sul do Brasil. *Ciência Rural*, Santa Maria, 35, 398-405.

[38] Borowsky, L. M., Bessa, M. C., Cardoso, M. R. I., Avancini, C. A. (2006) Sensibilidade e resistência de amostras de *Salmonella* Typhimurium isoladas de suínos

abatidos no Rio Grande do Sul frente aos desinfetantes quaternário de amônio e iodofor. *Ciência Rural*, 36, 1474-1479.

[39] PREBAF (2008) National Programme for Monitoring of Prevalence and Bacterial Resistance in Chicken (Programa Nacional de Monitoramento da Prevalência e da Resistência Bacteriana em Frango).

[40] Borsoi, A., Santos, L. R., Rodrigues, L. B., Moraes, H. L., Salle, C. T. P., Nascimento, V. P. (2011) Behavior of *Salmonella heidelberg* and *Salmonella enteritidis* strains following broiler chick inoculation: evaluation of cecal morphometry, liver and cecum bacterial counts and fecal excretion patterns. *Brazilian Journal of Microbiology*, 42, 266-273.

[41] Santos, L. R., Oliveira, S. D., Rodrigues, D. P., Ribeiro, A. R., Lopes, R. F. F., do Nascimento, V. P. (2003) Phage types of *Salmonella* Enteritidis isolated from clinical and food samples, and from broiler carcasses in southern Brazil. Revista do Instituto de Medicina Tropical de São Paulo, 45, 1, 001-004.

[42] Santos, L. R., Oliveira, S. D., Rodrigues, L. B., Ribeiro, A. R., Flores, M. L., Lopes, R. F. F., Nascimento, V. P. (2008) RAPD/PCR and phage typing of *Salmonella* Enteritidis isolated from poultry and food poisoning outbreaks. Arquivos do Instituto Biológico, São Paulo (SP), 75, 91-95.

[43] Hofer, E., Filho, S. J. S., Reis, E. M. (1997) Prevalência de sorovares de *Salmonella* isolados de aves no Brasil, *Pesq. Vet. Bras*. 17, 2, 55-62.

[44] Vaz, C., Streack, A. F., Michael, G. B., Marks, F., Rodrigues, D. P., Reis, E., Cardoso, M. R. I., Canal, C. W. (2010) Antimicrobial resistance and subtyping of *Salmonella* enterica subsp. enterica serovar Enteritidis isolated from human outbreaks and poultry. *Poultry Science*, 89, 1530-1536.

[45] Ribeiro, A. R., Kellermann, A., Santos, L. R., Fittel, A. P., Nascimento, V. P. (2006) Resistência antimicrobiana em *Salmonella* Enterica subsp. Enterica sorovar Hadar isoladas de carcaças de frango. Arquivos do Instituto Biológico, São Paulo (SP), 73, 357-360.

[46] Ribeiro, A. R., Kellermann, A., Santos, L. R., Nascimento, V. P. (2008) Resistência antimicrobiana em *Salmonella* Enteritidis isoladas de amostras clínicas e ambientais de frangos de corte e matrizes pesadas. *Arquivo Brasileiro de Medicina Veterinária e Zootecnia*, 60, 1259-1263.

In: Salmonella: Classification, Genetics and Disease Outbreaks ISBN: 978-1-61942-928-4
Editors: Adelaide S. Monte, Paulo Eduardo De Santos

Chapter 8

SALMONELLA ENTERICA ISOLATED FROM FOOD, ENVIRONMENT, ANIMAL, AND HUMAN: TRENDS AND CONSEQUENCES FOR PUBLIC HEALTH

***Ben Salem Imen*[1,*]*, Hassine Fraj*[2]*, Mzoughi Ridha*[3]**
***and Aouni Mahjoub*[1]**
Monastir University
[1]Laboratory of Infectious Diseases and Biological Agents,
Faculty of Pharmacy, Monastir, Tunisia
[2]Polyclinique CNSS Sousse - Khzema Sousse, Tunisia
[3]Laboratory of Hygiene, 5 Rue de Kairouan, Tunisia

ABSTRACT

Salmonella spp. are ubiquitous enteric bacteria. These gram-negative rods are the etiologic agents of food-borne salmonellosis and other food borne diseases (1, 2). It is also the agents that cause typhoid and paratyphoid fevers. An estimated 2 to 4 million cases of salmonellosis occur annually in the United States (3). In Tunisia, bacteriological results showed that the rate of *salmonella* contamination remains quite high. In fact, the infection progresses, mostly under sporadic and rarely in an epidemic mode.

Salmonella spp. can survive for long periods in natural waters, and the persistence of specific and epidemic strains is of great concern in public health. However, information on the diversity and occurrence of *Salmonella* strains is very scarce (4, 5), and as a consequence, the ecology of these species remains unknown. *Salmonella* bacteria cause, also, much of the food poisoning in the world, including an estimated 1,400,000 cases of salmonellosis in the United States each year. Although foods of animal origin (eggs, poultry, beef, dairy products…) are the vehicles of transmission in most *Salmonella* outbreaks, contaminated fresh fruits and vegetables are now recognized as the main cause of salmonellosis (1, 2).

The purpose of the present review was to provide information on the diversity of *Salmonella* strains isolated from environmental, animal, food and human samples which

[*] Corresponding authors: Ben Salem Imen; E-mail: imen.ben-salem@laposte.net.

allows to follow trends in *salmonella enterica* seotypes that provide information about source of infection and the efficacy of prevention and control measures.

Salmonella is an important source of food-borne disease in humans throughout the world. An important change in the epidemiology of *Salmonella* occurred since the mid 1980s, when *Salmonella Enteritidis* (*S. Enteritidis*) became a major contaminant of eggs and egg products, hereby causing a worldwide pandemic. In France, salmonellosis is also the largest documented cause of foodborne infections (6). A total of 21 *S. Muenster* isolates had been received by the the French Food Safety Agency (Afssa) between January 2006 and February 2008. Among them, four were food isolates (poultry); the other 17 strains were from different origins (meat and bone meal, environmental isolates).

In Canada, in 1982, a documented food poisoning outbreak caused by *S. Muenster* occurred and implicated cheddar cheese made from unpasteurised milk as the source of infection (7). On March 2008, the National Reference Centre (NRC) for *Salmonella* reported three laboratory-confirmed cases of *S. Muenster* to the (Institut de veille sanitaire, InVS).

In Tunisia, during the study period (1994-2004), Nazek and coll showed that the top three *Salmonella* serotypes frequentely isolated with interchangeable ranking were: *Anatum, Enteritidis* and *Corvallis* (8). Aknown food origine was reported for all *Salmonella* isolates: red meat for *S.enterica* and *S.Anatum*. Whereas, *S.Enteritidis*, *Corvallis* and *Anatum* were most commonly isolated from poultry. The highest serotype commonly isolated from vegetables and fruits were *S.enterica* serotypes: *Anatum, Enteritidis* and *Corvallis*. Serotypes most frequentely isolated from milk and dairy products was *S.enterica* serotype *Anatum*.

Finally, on November 2007, the Singapore Ministry of Health was notified of an outbreak of food poisoning. This outbreak was the largest common source outbreak of gastroenteritis caused by *Salmonella enterica* subspecies *enterica* serotype *Enteritidis* in Singapore. The epidemiological evidence implicates cream cake as the vehicle of transmission (9).

In addition to food contamination, *Salmonella* species are pathogenic bacteria often detected in wastewater, freshwater, marine coastal water, and groundwater. Municipal sewage and storm water runoff become the conduits for the passage of pathogens into surface waters (10, 11). Serotype *Typhimurium* was dominant in all river samples and in marine and freshwater sediments. A high occurrence of this serotype has already been reported for polluted freshwaters (12, 13). In contrast, serotype *Newport* was the dominant serotype in wastewater, and consequently, it was also found in river samples.

In Tunisia, Nazek and coll. reported that *S.enterica* serotype *Corvallis* was the most frequentely reported *Salmonella* serotype, accounting for 17.3% of all environmental isolates. Whereas, *S.enterica* serotype *Enteritidis* and *S.enterica* serotype *Anatum* came in second and third position, respectively, with non consistent trends during the study period (8). The most frequent source of isolation was tap water samples (8). Another study analyzing 60 wastewater samples showed that in entrance point 66.6% of samples were contaminated with *Salmonella* whereas, in exit points, a percentage of 20% were found. In entrance points, three serotypes of *Salmonella spp*. were detected: *Typhimurium, Enteritidis* and *Montevideo*; however, in exit points only the *Typhimurim* serotype was isolated (14). In 1999 and 2000, in Spain, the most frequent serotypes isolated from wastewater were *S. Enteritidis* and *S. Anatum* (15).

Regarding *Salmonella* strains isolated from animal, the most frequently isolated *Salmonella* serotype during the study period was *S.enterica* serotype *Enteritidis* followed by *S.enterica* serotype *Corvallis*. For *Enteritidis* serotypes, the source of isolation was poultry (70%), cattle (69%) and fish and shellfish (22%). While, *S.enterica* serotype *Amesterdam* and *S. enterica* serotype *Corvallis* were in a lead for cattles (8).

Salmonella strains present a great impact on human health. In Tunisia, during 11 year surveillance periode (1994-2004), the top three reported *Salmonella* serotypes

(*Enteritidis, Corvallis and Linvingstone*) accounted for 48.4% of all human isolates (8). *S.enterica* serotype *Enteritidis* came in first position during the study period, except for the years 2001, 2002, and 2003 where it came in the second position, prececed by *S.enterica* serotype *Livingstone* (8). The next not frequently reported serotype was *Corvallis*. Data from 2000 to 2004 suggest that *Salmonella Corvallis* infections are decreasing. *S. enterica* serotype *Linvingstone* was the third most common serotype (8). The most frequent source of isolation was stool samples (95% of *Salmonella* serotypes that were most commonly isolated) (8).

Human infection due to *Salmonella enterica* serovar *Senftenberg* is infrequent in the United States. This bacterium colonizes the gastrointestinal tract of birds and mammals, and has been isolated from sewage systems, poultry processing plants, and different animal feeds (16, 17). *S. Senftenberg* infections in humans have been documented, mainly in Africa (18, 19) and India (20, 21), as well as in 1 US outbreak of gastroenteritis (22). Nonintestinal infectious syndromes due to *S. Senftenberg* were also reported in the Indian study (23, 24).

At the end of February 2005, the National Institute for Health Surveillance was informed by the National Reference Centre for *Salmonella* of an increase of *Salmonella enterica* serotype *Agona* isolated in infants in January-February 2005. This is the first documented outbreak of *Salmonella Agona* in France. This investigation shows that regular microbiological examinations of formula were insufficient to detect low-grade or inhomogeneous contamination (http://www.invs.sante.fr).

Our study highlighted the role of *Salmonella* as a pathogen widely dispersed in nature. These organisms can cause disease states that range from self-limited diarrhea to bacteremia considered as a public health problem. Thus, routine controls of all food, animal and human samples must be done in order to prevent community wide outbreaks of *salmonellosis*. The availability of routine molecular typing techniques in outbreak settings would facilitate tracing the source of infection and confirming epidemiological linkages of the *Salmonella* strains isolated from humans, food, animals and the environment.

Keywords: *Salmonella:* serotypes, surveillance, outbreak reports

Introduction

Salmonella spp. have been recognized as human and animal pathogens for over a century. The genus Salmonella includes more than 2400 different known serotypes (1, 2). According to recent data from FoodNet, the incidence of salmonellosis has not diminished significantly over the past ten years but some serotypes have increased or decreased in importance (3). Most serotypes are not hostspecific, but a few species are restricted to one kind of animal such as *S. Pullorum* in chickens and *S. Typhi* in humans.

Several large outbreaks of salmonellosis have occurred during the past year. *S. Typhimurium,* believed to be carried in pork, has made more than 1000 people ill in Denmark (4) and *S. Typhimurium* present in municipal tap water affected over 400 people in Colorado (5). Perhaps the most noteworthy outbreak in 2008 was the nationwide illness caused by *S. Saintpaul* that extended for several months while investigators sought to pinpoint the fresh produce vehicles of infection (6). *Salmonella spp.* are estimated to cause about 1.4 million non-typhoidal infections in humans per year in the U.S., and it has been estimated that 95% of these cases were due to consumption of contaminated food (7). According to the world Health

Organisation, annually there are about 17 million cases of acute gastroenteritis or diarrhea due to non-typhoidal salmonellosis with 3 million deaths (8, 9). Additionally, 300–400 cases of typhoid fever are reported yearly in the U.S. (10). The large number of cases that occur annually does have a significant economic impact on individuals, the health care system, and businesses associated with outbreaks.

Phenotypic and molecular methods play an important role in the identification to the genus level (11-12). Serotyping, according to the Kauffmann-White schema, was the standard for classification of Salmonella isolates in outbreak investigation. It is a useful classification schema that allows for trends in salmonella surveillance data to be followed over time. Such surveillance is needed to help in preventing foodborne disease outbreak and also to detect, respond, and prevent foodborne diseases.

In Tunisia, the surveillance for Salmonella species is carried out by the national Centre of Enteropathogenic Bacteria in Pasteur Institute- Tunis- Tunisia. Annually, approximately 2000 Salmonella strains are reported from all over Tunisia to the National Centre of Enteropathogenic Bacteria at Pasteur Institute (13).

The objectives of this bibliographical minireview were: to report trends of Salmonella in environment, food products, animal and human in Tunisia and all over the world. This information would facilitate tracing the source of infection and helps to improve the prevention of Salmonella infections.

1. Food-Associated Serotypes in Tunisia and Abroad

1.1. Tunisian Case Finding

To find Tunisian cases, we reviewed the control study conducted in "laboratoire de controle des Eaux et Denrées Alimentaire de l'institut Pasteur de Tunis", Tunis, Tunisia. This Salmonella study was elaborated by Nazek and coll (13) during the 11-year period (1994-2004). It reported that, the annual isolation percentage considerably increased during the years from 1999 to 2002, and then decreased in the years 2003, 2004. A confirmed case reported that Salmonella serotypes did not have a consistent trend during the years from 1994 to 2004. But, the three serotypes *Anatum*, *Enteritidis*, and *Corvallis* were frequently isolated. *S.enterica* serotype *Anatum* was the most common serotype reported from food isolates and was strongly in the first position from 1997 to 2004. During the 11-year period, this serotype was frequently isolated from red meat. *S.enterica* serotype *Enteritidis* was the second most common serotype followed by *S.enterica* serotype *Corvallis* that occupied the third position during the study period (13). Also, Nazek and coll. reported that, from 2002 to 2004, a new serotypes (*Amesterdam, Cerro,* and *Infantis*) came forward and occupied a position among the top three frequently isolated serotypes.

The most commonly Salmonella serotypes isolated from poultry from 1994 to 2004 were *S. enterica* serotypes: *Enteritidis*, *Corvallis* and *Anatum*. Serotype most commonly isolated from milk and dairy products was *S.enterica* serotype *Anatum*. Whereas, the highest serotype commonly isolated from vegetables and fruits were *S.enterica* serotypes: *Anatum*, *Enteritidis* and *Corvallis*. Finally, *S.enterica* serotype Anatum was in a lead in fish and seafoods, and cereals. Whereas, pastries were frequently contaminated by *S.enterica* serotypes *Enteritidis* (13).

1.2. Food *Salmonella Enterica* Status: Outbreaks and Cases

A majority of Salmonella cases are never linked to outbreaks. In fact, at FoodNet sites in 2007, Salmonella isolates from outbreaks comprised only 5.4% of the total Salmonella cases identified; the remaining 94.6% of cases were sporadic with no known connection to other cases (3). Data from the European Union, Australia, Canada, and the CDC in the U.S. from 1996 to 2007 demonstrate a marked decrease in salmonellosis in Europe, an increase in Australia, and slight decreases in Canada and the U.S. (10, 14). Large outbreaks (greater than 200 cases) of salmonellosis were occurred during the past ten years. Of the next ten outbreaks, vehicles included chicken, pork, eggs, fresh produce, dried squid, cheese, and cake. Three outbreaks in Japan, associated with "boxed lunch" or "school lunch," were caused by *S. Enteritidis*. One or more of these outbreaks may have been due to contaminated eggs or chicken but the exact food vehicle is unknown. The Canadian cheese outbreak was caused by contaminated cheese in a commercial lunch pack product. In 2010, Egypt was the country most frequently reported and was associated with 36 (33%) outbreaks. This was higher than 2009 when Egypt was associated with 15 (21%) (15). In 2009 Turkey had been the most frequently reported country with 19 (27%) outbreaks but in 2010 it was the second most frequently reported country, associated with 22 (20%) outbreaks (15). Spain, including the Balearic Islands, was associated with 12 outbreaks compared to 15 the previous year. Eleven outbreaks were associated with Tunisia (15). Five outbreaks were associated with Morocco (15). The USA, Cuba and cruises were each associated with three outbreaks (15). India and Kenya were each associated with two outbreaks (15). Thus, Salmonella was the most frequently identified pathogen associated with overseas outbreaks in 2010 and was reported from 62 (57%) outbreaks. Within the 62 outbreaks of Salmonella, *S. Enteritidis* was the most frequently identified serotype, associated with 14 outbreaks. Of the total, 19 (31%) of the outbreaks were associated with travel to Egypt, 13 with travel to Turkey, and nine with travel to Tunisia (15).

Meat represent the most important food considerated as vehicles for human salmonellosis. Poultry and pork together were responsible for 63% of the outbreaks and 79% of the cases included here. An estimation of the percentage distribution of salmonellosis cases in 1998–2003 due to different types of meat stated that poultry accounted for 26%, ground beef for 19%, and pork for 2%. Cases attributed to ground beef and pork decreased by about one-half from 1998 to 2003; while cases related to consumption of chicken increased by 1.6-fold (16). Several large outbreaks in Europe and Australia due to contaminated pork increased the importance of this vehicle from an international perspective. Processed meats, such as ham, salami and sausage accounted for about 6% of the meat outbreaks. In addition, a small number of cases and outbreaks were traced to other meats, including lamb, pigeon, rabbit, horse, and turtle. Eggs are also an important vehicle for salmonellosis, particularly for *S. Enteritidis*. Despite antimicrobial compounds in egg albumen, *S. Enteritidis* can grow well in eggs stored at 21°C (17). Seafood is not usually considered an important vehicle for salmonellosis. However, shellfish harvested from inshore areas may be exposed to runoff from human sewage or animal manure or droppings from seagulls that contain salmonella

(18). A survey of oysters from the Atlantic, Pacific, and Gulf coasts of the U.S. found that an average of 7.4% contained salmonella, with *S. Newport* most frequently isolated (19). Other seafood salmonellosis outbreaks have been associated with contaminated egg used in preparation (20) and fish dried in the open under the sun, presumably contaminated by bird and/or rodent droppings (21). Fresh produce has become an important vehicle for foodborne infections in recent years. Tomatoes caused the largest number of outbreaks whereas sprouts caused the greatest number of cases. Trace back of tomatoes from outbreaks in 2002 and 2005, caused by *S. Newport,* to a farm in Virginia identified a contaminated pond used for irrigation as the source of the bacteria (22). A survey of 170 sources of irrigation water in Texas found that 16 contained salmonella (23). A 1993 outbreak in Germany caused by a contaminated spice, paprika, demonstrated the potential impact of such a vehicle. A total of 94 different serotypes were isolated from the paprika and about 1000 case patients, although three serotypes, *Saintpaul, Rubislaw, and Javiana*, accounted for about 42% of isolates. Dairy products are occasionally identified as vehicles for salmonellosis. The most notorious dairy-related outbreak occurred in 1994 caused illness with *S. Enteritidis* in an estimated 224,000 persons (24). In the 2006–2007 outbreak of Salmonella Tennessee associated with peanut butter, at least 628 persons in 47 states became ill with about 20% requiring hospitalization (25).

2. Environmental-Associated Serotypes in Tunisia and Abroad

2.1. Tunisian Case Finding

Our research study made in laboratory "Laboratoire des Maladies Transmissibles et Substances Biologiquement Actives – Monastir", Tunisia reported that in entrance points of fifteen wastewater treatment stations located in the Sahel and the central of Tunisia, twenty from thirty samples were contaminated with Salmonella (66.6%). Whereas, in exit points a percentage of 20% was found (26). Molecular serotyping results showed that, in entrance points, three serotypes of *Salmonella spp.* were found: *Typhimurium, Enteritidis* and *Montevideo*; whereas, in exit points only the *Typhimurim* serotype was detected (personal data). In 1999 and 2000, in Spain, the most frequent serotypes isolated from wastewater were *S.Enteritidis* and *S. Anatum* (27).

Another study elaborated by Nazek and coll., during the year of study (from 1994 to 2004), reported that the rate of Salmonella species in Tunisia increased gradually reaching to highest levels from 2000 to 2002 (13). *S. enterica* serotypes *Corvallis* (17,3%) was the most frequently reported Salmonella serotypes. The annual incidence rate rose from 9,5 in 1994 to 34% in 1998. Then decreased to 2,3% in 2004 (13). *S.enterica* serotype *Enteritidis* and *S.enterica* serotype *Anatum* came in second and third position, respectively, with no consistent trends during the study period (13). The top three serotypes during the 11 year study period were *Typhimurium, Braenderup,* and *Infantis.* S.enterica serotype *Typhimurium* increased suddenly in the year 1996 and 2003 (13). *S.enterica* serotype *Braenderup* came in second position in 1994 and in third position in the year 2000. Finally, *S.enterica* serotype *Infantis* occupied the third position in the years 1997 and 1998 (13). These salmonella strains were mostly isolated from tap water (73,2%) (13). *Corvallis, Enteritidis,* and *Anatum* serotypes were frequently founded (16-17%). Whereas, other salmonella serovars were also isolated: *Haddar, Wien,* and *Montevideo* (<2%) (13).

2.2. Environmental *Salmonella Enterica* Status: Outbreaks and Cases

S. Typhi is the most virulent salmonella and still causes large, often waterborne, outbreaks in developing countries, including one in Nepal in 2002 affecting nearly 6000 people (28). Thus, water used for drinking has been reported as the vehicle of infection for nine outbreaks, including one in Spain attributed to bottled water (29). For the other outbreaks, wells or water storage containers were probably contaminated with fecal material from infected domestic and/or wild animals. Examination of the 2008 Colorado outbreak identified an underground cement-lined water storage tank as the site of contamination (30). Such large outbreaks do not occur in more developed countries with chlorinated drinking water, and adequate sewage treatment facilities. The most recent large outbreak (over 200 cases) in the U.S. occurred in a migrant labor camp in Florida in 1973 (31). Nevertheless, 321 to 377 cases of typhoid fever have been reported annually in the U.S. during the past 10 years (10).

3. Animal-Associated Serotypes in Tunisia and Abroad

3.1. Tunisian Case Finding

Nazek and coll examined trends in Salmonella serotypes known to be associated with animals. The study revealed that, the percentage of the isolates were not steady. However, a general increase was noted in the years 2000 to 2004 (13). The most frequently isolated Salmonella serotype from animal origin during the 11 year study period was *S.enterica* serotypes *Enteritidis* (69%). This serotype decreased from 94,5% in 1994 to 63% in 2004 (13). Then *S.enterica* serotype *Corvallis* except in the years 2002, 2003, and 2004 were *S.enterica* serotypes: *Hadar, Anatum,* and *Livingstone* came in second position, respectively (13). Also, this research study showed that *S.enterica* serotype *Typhimurium* revealed a sudden peak in the year 2001. The same study demonstrated that the *Enteritidis* serotype was the most frequently isolated from the three different categories of the animal included in the study (13). It was followed by *S.enterica* serotype *Corvallis* for poultry and fish and shellfish. While *S.enterica* serotype *Amesterdam* and *S.enterica* serotype *Corvallis* were in a lead for cattles (13).

3.2. Animal *Salmonella Enterica* Status: Outbreaks and Cases

Farm Animals

Farm animals are considered to be a primary reservoir for important Salmonella serotypes associated with human infections. *S. Typhimurium* and *S. Enteritidis*, the most common serotypes causing human infection, are frequently detected in farm animals as are other serotypes known to be human pathogens (32).

Pets

Turtles are the most commonly identified pets that are vehicles for human salmonellosis. However, in recent years a variety of other reptilian pets as well as some mammals have been found to carry salmonella and pass them on to their human caretakers. It has been estimated that 6–7% of all sporadic Salmonella infections in the U.S. can be attributed to contact with reptiles and amphibians (33). Although pet snakes at a breeding facility were found to be frequent carriers of *S. diarizonae* (34). Aquaria housing tropical fish have also been vehicles for human salmonellosis. Salmonella were found in more than 50% of aquaria from homes, wholesale facilities, and pet shops that were tested during a survey to determine incidence of *S. Paratyphi B* (26, 35). Pet rodents (hamsters, mice, and rats) purchased at retail stores have been found to carry multidrugresistant *S. Typhimurium* (37). Cats and dogs may also carry salmonella and have been implicated in some cases and outbreaks (38, 39).

Wild Animals

Mammals and birds serve as reservoirs for salmonella and may also be vehicles of infection for humans. Salmonellosis is known to be a significant cause of mortality in some species of wild birds, and humans have acquired salmonellosis from infected birds (40). In New Zealand during the winter of 2000, hundreds of small birds died from infection with a virulent *S. Typhimurium* strain. Human cases also occurred in the same areas, and *S. Typhimurium* isolates from birds and humans were indistinguishable (41). Other studies of serotypes of salmonella isolated from birds captured on a dairy farm in California (42) and in Norway and the UK indicated that many strains commonly detected in birds are seldom isolated from farm animals or humans, suggesting that some avian strains are host adapted and may not pose a health threat to humans (43, 44). Investigation of outbreaks of *S. Typhimurium* 4,5,12:i:1,2 in humans in Norway in 2000 revealed that the identical serotype was present in a high percentage of hedgehogs that came to feeding stations (45). Identical or very similar strains of *S. Enteritidis* were detected in mice and rats associated with layer houses and in eggs from these houses, indicating that these rodents may be reservoirs that maintain infections in these houses (46, 47). Numerous other wild animals harbor salmonella and in some cases appear to be the source of human infections (48). *S. Newport*, one of the most common human isolates in the U.S., accounted for 22% of the raccoon isolates (49). In recent studies, approximately 50% of 132 individuals of several species of turtles in Texas were found to carry salmonella in cloacae/feces or in biofilms growing on their shells. Isolates of known human pathogens included *S. Newport, S. Rubislaw, S. Thompson,* and *S. Gaminara* (50) were also found.

4. Human-Associated Serotypes in Tunisia and Abroad

4.1. Case Finding

In our prospective study that aimed to investigate the etiology of infantile diarrhea in Sousse, Tunisia from December 2008 to November 2009; we have isolated 12 strains of *Salmonella Spp.* (9.7%) among the 124 children patients, who suffered from diarrhea. Molecular serotyping of these strain revealed the following serotypes: *Enteritidis* (n=7), *Braenderup* (n=3), *Cerro* (n=1) and *Kottbus* (n=1) (personal data).

Nazek and coll reported that, during the 11-year surveillance period (1994-2004), the top three reported Salmonella serotypes were *Enteritidis, Corvallis,* and *Livingstone.* These three serotypes accounted for 48,4% of all human isolates. During the study period, the most frequentely isolated serotype was *S.enterica* serotype *Enteritidis* except for the years 2001, 2002, and 2003 where it came in the second position, preceded by *S.enterica* serotype *Livingstone* (13). From 1994 to 1999, serotype *Corvallis* was the second most frequentely reported serotype in Tunisia accounting for 12,5% of all human isolates (13). The third common serotype was *S.enterica* serotype *Livingstone.* In 1999, isolation of this serotype from human salmonellosis occurred in patients hospitalized in a pediatric wards in Sfax Hospital (13). No death cases were reported (51). Whereas in 2002, an outbreak of human salmonellosis infection was occurred in the neonatal ward of maternity department Farhat Hached Hospital in Sousse City. This outbreak was associated with death cases (52).

Also Nazek and coll reported that the three serotypes *Mbandaka*, *Typhi Vi+*, and *Typhimurium* showed obvious peaks throughout the 11-year study period (13).

Concerning source of isolation, among the detected Salmonella serotypes, Nazek and coll reported that the most frequent source of isolation was stool samples ranging from high of 24% for serotype *S.enterica* serotype *Enteritidis* to a law of 1% for *S.enterica* serotypes: *Typhi Vi+*, *Amesterdam*, *Hadar*, and *Montevideo* (13). From blood samples, the most commonly isolated Salmonella serotypes were: *S. enterica* serotype *Typhi Vi+* (38,6%), and *S.enterica* serotype *Enteritidis* (20%) (13). Finally, Nazek and coll showed that Salmonella serotypes most commonly isolated from urine were *S.enterica* serotypes *Typhimurium* (20%), *Wien* (20%), *Enteritidis* (14,4%) and *Mbandaka* (14,4%) (13).

4.2. Human *Salmonella Enterica* Status: Outbreaks and Cases

In many countries, the incidence of salmonellosis has markedly increased; however, a paucity of good surveillance data exists. In 2000, approximately 21.6 million worldwide cases of typhoid fever caused 216,500 deaths **(53)**. The incidence of typhoid fever in south-central Asia, and Southeast Asia, was high (>100 cases per 100,000 population per year). The rest of Asia, Latin America, Africa (except for southern Africa), and Oceania (except for Australia and New Zealand) typically see intermediate rates of typhoid fever (10-100 cases per 100,000 population), while the incidence is low in the other parts of the world (< 10 cases per 100,000 population). In countries where typhoid fever is endemic, most cases of the disease occur in children aged 5-19 years and young adults (54).

In the United States, the incidence of Salmonella infections has been stable since 2004 but has decreased approximately 8% from 1996-1998 levels (55). In 2007, the reported annual incidence of salmonellosis was 14.9 cases per 100,000 population (55). The true annual burden of nontyphoidal *Salmonella* infection in the United States was estimated to approximately 38.6 cases of nontyphoidal *Salmonella* infection for each culture-confirmed case (56). In 2007, four large multistate outbreaks of *Salmonella* infections that included FoodNet sites were investigated: an outbreak of *S enterica* serotype Tennessee infections caused by contaminated peanut butter, an outbreak of *S enterica* serotype I 4,5,12:i:- caused by contaminated frozen pot pies, an outbreak of *S enterica* serotype Wandsworth and *Styphimurium* infections attributed to a puffed vegetable snack, and an outbreak of *S paratyphi* B variant Java associated with exposure to turtles (55). In 2008-2009, a nationwide outbreak of *S typhimurium* was traced to peanut products and frozen chicken products (57). Although the prevalence of *Salmonella* infections is highest in children, in fact salmonellosis outbreaks are common among individuals who are institutionalized and residents of nursing homes. Finally, typhoid fever is increasingly associated with travel to developing countries (currently 72% of approximately 400 cases per year). Common sources of infection include Haiti (5%), Philippines (8%), Bangladesh (8%), Mexico (12%), Pakistan (13%), and India (30%) (58).

Regarding mortality and morbidity, infection with nontyphoidal salmonella typically produces a self-limiting gastroenteritis, and dehydrated patients occasionally require hospitalization. Death is rare. The mortality rate associated with *S. Enteritidis* infection outbreaks in the United States from 1985-1991 was 0.4%. Case-fatality rates were 70 times higher in nursing homes and hospitals. Between 1996 and 1999, an estimated 1.4 million nontyphoidal Salmonella infections occurred in the United States, with an estimated 15,000 hospitalizations and 400 deaths annually. A related study during the same period found that 22% of people infected with nontyphoidal Salmonella required hospitalization, with an annual incidence of 0.08 deaths per 100,000 population. In the 1990s, at Massachusetts General Hospital, 18% of 45 patients with Salmonella bacteremia died (59).

5. Impact of *Salmonella Enterica* Infection in Human Health

Most people infected with Salmonella develop diarrhea, fever and abdominal cramps 6 to 72 hours after being infected. The illness usually lasts four to seven days and most people recover without treatment. As with any disease causing diarrhea or vomiting, those infected should drink plenty of liquids to replace lost body fluids. This is particularly important with very young children and seniors. In severe cases, patients may need to be given fluids intravenously, which is usually done in hospital. In a small number of cases, Salmonella may spread from the intestines to the blood stream and other body sites, causing severe illness and, in vulnerable people, death. In cases of severe illness, patients may be treated with antibiotics. However, some Salmonella bacteria have become resistant to many commonly used antibiotics. A small number of infected people go on to develop pains in their joints, irritation of the eyes and painful urination, a condition called Reiter's Syndrome. It can last for months or years, sometimes leading to chronic arthritis, which is difficult to treat.

To minimize risk to contact pathogenic Salmonella strains, there is no vaccine to prevent, but we can minimize our chances of contracting it by following the steps that was mentioned mainly: thoroughly cook foods to destroy the bacteria, do not eat raw or undercooked eggs, poultry or meat, poultry and meat, including hamburgers, should be well-cooked, avoid raw or unpasteurized milk, thoroughly wash fruits and vegetables before eating them, always defrost food in the refrigerator, in cold water or in the microwave, never at room temperature.

In bref, following recognition of the importance of Salmonella organisms as the cause of potentially preventable infectious disease, surveillance systems for salmonella infections was established in different part of the world. Surveillance system accurate assessment of the number of infections which is important for determining complication rates and for evaluating the efficacy of control programs.

REFERENCES

[1] Nair S, Lin TK, Pang T, Altwegg M. Characterization of Salmonella serovars by PCR-single-strand conformation polymorphism analysis. *J Clin Microbiol* 2002; 40:2346-51.

[2] Martinez-Urtaza J, Liebana E, Garcia-Migura L, Perez-Pineiro P, Saco M. Characterization of *Salmonella enterica* serovar *Typhimurium* from marine environments in coastal waters of Galicia (Spain). *Appl environ Microbiol* 2004; 70:4030-4.

[3] Centers for Disease Control. 2008. Preliminary FoodNet data on the incidence of infection with pathogens transmitted commonly through food—10 states, United States, 2007. *Morbid Mortal Wkly Rep* 57:366–370.

[4] Ethelberg S, Wingstrand A, Jensen T, Sørensen G, Müller L, Lisby M, Nielsen EM, Mølbak K. 2008. Large outbreaks of Salmonella typhimurium infection in Denmark in 2008. *Euro Surveill* 13(44):pii=19023.

[5] Berg R. 2008. The Alamosa Salmonella outbreak; a gumshoe investigation. *J. Environ Health* 71:54–55.

[6] Centers for Disease Control. 2008. Outbreak of Salmonella serotype Saintpaul infections associated with multiple raw produce items—United States, 2008. *Morbid Mortal Weekly Rep* 57:929–934.

[7] Mead PS, Slutsker L, Dietz V, McCaig LF, Bresee JS, Shapiro C, Griffin PM Tauxe RV. 1999. Food-related illness and death in the United States. *Emerg Infect Dis* 5:607–25.

[8] Rabsch W, Tschape H, Baumler AJ. Non-typhoidal salmonellosis: emerging problems. *Microbes Infect* 2001; 3:237-47.

[9] Ling ML, Wang BCY. Epidemiological analysis of Salmonella enteritidis isolates in Singapore. *J Infect* 2001; 43:169-72.

[10] Centers for Disease Control. 2008. Summary of notifiable diseases—United States, 2006. *Morbid Mortal Weekly Rep* 55:77–81.

[11] Botteldoor N, Herman L, Rijpens N, Heyndrickx M. Phenotypic and molecular typing of Salmonella strains reveal different contamination source in two commercial pig slaughterhouses. *Appl Environ Microbiol* 2004; 70: 5305-14.

[12] Burr MD, Josephson KL, Pepper IL. An evaluation of ERIC and AP PCR for discriminating Salmonella serotypes. *Lett Appl Microbiol* 1998; 27: 24-30.

[13] Ridha ben Aissa, Nazek Al-Gallas, Hinda Troudi, Nabiha Belhadj, Abderazzaque Belhadj. Trends in *Salmonella enterica* serotypes isolated from human, food, animal, and environment in Tunisia, 1994-2004. *Journal of infection.* 2007; 55, 324- 339.

[14] Amato-Gauci A, Ammon A, eds. 2007. Annual epidemiological report on communicable diseases in Europe. European Centre for Disease Prevention and Control. ecdc.europa.eu/documents/pdf/Epi_report_2007.

[15] Alison Smith-Palmer and Mary Locking. Gastro-intestinal and foodborne infections: overseas outbreaks of infectious intestinal disease. *HPS weekly report*, Volume 45 No.2011/25

[16] Guo C. A statistical model for attributing human salmonellosis to meat poultry and eggs. 2007.

[17] Chen J, Thesmar HS, Kerr WL. 2005. Outgrowth of salmonellae and the physical property of albumen and vitelline membrane as influenced by egg storage conditions. *J Food Prot* 68:2553–2558.

[18] Albarnaz JD, Toso J, Correa AA, Simoes CM, Barardi CR. 2007. Relationship between the contamination of gulls (Larus dominicanus) and oysters (Crassostrea gigas) with Salmonella serovar Typhimurium by PCR-RFLP. *Int J Environ Health Res* 17:133–140.

[19] Brands DA, Inman AE, Gerba CP, Mare CJ, Billington SJ, Saif LA, Levine JF, Joens LA. 2005. Prevalence of Salmonella spp. in oysters in the United States. *Appl Environ Microbiol* 71:893–897.

[20] Guerin PJ, De Jong B, Heir E, Hasseltvedt V, Kapperud G, Styrmo K, Gondrosen B, Lassen J, Andersson Y, Aavitsland P. 2004. Outbreak of Salmonella Livingstone infection in Norway and Sweden due to contaminated processed fish products. *Epidemiol Infect* 132:889–895.

[21] Ling ML, Goh KT, Wang GC, Neo KS, Chua T. 2002. An outbreak of multidrug-resistant Salmonella enterica subsp. enterica serotype Typhimurium, DT104L linked to dried anchovy in Singapore. *Epidemiol Infect* 128:1–5.

[22] Greene SK, Daly ER, Talbot EA, Demma LJ, Holzbauer S, Patel NJ, Hill TA, Walderhaug MO, Hoekstra RM, Lynch MF, Painter JA. 2008. Recurrent multistate outbreak of Salmonella Newport associated with tomatoes from contaminated fields, 2005. *Epidemiol Infect* 136:157–165.

[23] Duffy EA, Lucia LM, Kells JM, Castillo A, Pillai SD, Acuff GR. 2005. Concentrations of Escherichia coli and genetic diversity and antibiotic resistance profiling of Salmonella isolated from irrigation water, packing shed equipment, and fresh produce in Texas. *J Food Prot* 68:70– 79.

[24] Hennessy TW, Hedberg CW, Slutsker L, White KW, Besser-Wiek JM, Moen ME, Feldman J, Coleman WW, Edmonson LM, MacDonald KL, Osterholm MT. 1996. A national outbreak of Salmonella enteritidis infections from ice cream. *N Engl J Med* 334:1281–1286.

[25] Centers for Disease Control. 2007. Multistate outbreak of Salmonella serotype Tennessee infections associated with peanut butter—United States, 2006–2007. *Morbid Mortal Wkly Rep* 56:521–524.

[26] Imen Ben Salem, Imen Ouardani, Mouna Hassine and Mahjoub Aouni. Bacteriological and physico-chemical assessment of wastewater in different region of Tunisia: impact on human health. 2011; *BMC Research Notes*, 4:144.
[27] Usera MA, Aladuen˜ a A, Diez R, De La Fuente M, Gutie'rrez R, Cerda' n P, Arroyo M, Gonza' lez R, Echeita A: Ana' lisis de las cepas de Salmonella spp aisladas de muestras clı'nicas de origen humano en Espan˜ a del 2000 (I). *Bol Epidemiol Semanal* 2001, 9:221-228.
[28] Lewis MD, Serichantalergs O, Pitarangsi C, Chuanak N, Mason CJ, Regmi LR, Pandey P, Laskar R, Shrestha CD, Malla S. 2005. Typhoid fever: a massive, single-point source, multidrug-resistant outbreak in Nepal. *Clin Infect Dis* 40:554–561.
[29] Palmera-Suárez R, García P, García A, Barrasa A, and Herrera D. 2007. Salmonella Kottbus outbreak in infants in Gran Canaria (Spain), caused by bottled water, August–November 2006. *Euro Surveill* 12(28):pii=3235.
[30] Berg R. 2008. The Alamosa Salmonella outbreak; a gumshoe investigation. *J. Environ Health* 71:54–55.
[31] Olsen SJ, Bleasdale SC, Magnano AR, Landrigan C, Holland BH, Tauxe RV, Mintz ED, Luby S. 2003. Outbreaks of typhoid fever in the United States, 1960–99. *Epidemiol Infect* 130:13–21.
[32] Foley SL, Lynne AM. 2008. Food animal-associated Salmonella challenges: pathogenicity and antimicrobial resistance. *J Anim Sci* 86:E173–E187.
[33] Mermin J, Hutwagner L, Vugia D, Shallow S, Daily P, Bender J, Koehler J, Marcus R, Angulo FJ. 2004. Reptiles, amphibians, and human Salmonella infection: a populationbased, case-control study. *Clin Infect Dis* 38 Suppl 3:S253– S261.
[34] Schroter M, Roggentin P, Hofmann J, Speicher A, Laufs R, Mack D. 2004. Pet snakes as a reservoir for Salmonella enterica subsp. diarizonae (Serogroup IIIb): a prospective study. *Appl Environ Microbiol* 70:613–615.
[35] Gaulin C, Vincent C, Ismail J. 2005. Sporadic infections of Salmonella Paratyphi B, var. Java associated with fish tanks. *Can J Public Health* 96:471–474.
[36] Mitchell MA, Shane SM. 2000. Preliminary findings of Salmonella spp. in captive green iguanas (Iguana iguana) and their environment. *Prev Vet Med* 45:297–304.
[37] Swanson SJ, Snider C, Braden CR, Boxrud D, Wünschmann A, Rudroff JA, Lockett J, Smith KE. 2007. Multidrug-resistant Salmonella enterica serotype typhimurium associated with pet rodents. *N Engl J Med* 356:21– 28.
[38] Centers for Disease Control. 2001. Outbreaks of multidrugresistant Salmonella Typhimurium associated with veterinary facilities—Idaho, Minnesota, and Washington, 1999. *Morbid Mortal Wkly Rep* 50:701–704.
[39] Cherry B, Burns A, Johnson GS, Pfeiffer H, Dumas N, Barrett D, McDonough PL, Eidson M. 2004. Salmonella Typhimurium outbreak associated with veterinary clinic. *Emerg Infect Dis* 10:2249–2251.
[40] Hall AJ, Saito EK. 2008. Avian wildlife mortality events due to salmonellosis in the United States, 1985–2004. *J Wildlife Dis* 44:585–593.
[41] Alley MR, Connolly JH, Fenwick SG, Mackereth GF, Leyland MJ, Rogers LE, Haycock M, Nicol C, Reed CE. 2002. An epidemic of salmonellosis caused by Salmonella Typhimurium DT160 in wild birds and humans in New Zealand. *N Z Vet J* 50:170–176.

[42] Kirk JH, Holmberg CA, Jeffrey JS. 2002. Prevalence of Salmonella spp in selected birds captured on California dairies. *J Am Vet Med Assoc* 220:359–362.

[43] Hughes LA, Shopland S, Wigley P, Bradon H, Leatherbarrow AH, Williams NJ, Bennett M, de Pinna E, Lawson B, Cunningham AA, Chantrey J. 2008. Characterisation of Salmonella enterica serotype Typhimurium isolates from wild birds in northern England from 2005–2006. *BMC Vet Res* 4:4.

[44] Nesse L, Refsum T, Heir E, Nordby K, Vardund T, Holstad G. 2005. Molecular epidemiology of Salmonella spp. isolates from gulls, fish-meal factories, feed factories, animals and humans in Norway based on pulsed-field gel electrophoresis. *Epidemiol Infect* 133:53–58.

[45] Handeland K, Refsum T, Johansen BS, Holstad G, Knutsen G, Solberg I, Schulze J, Kapperud G. 2002. Prevalence of Salmonella typhimurium infection in Norwegian hedgehog populations associated with two human disease outbreaks. *Epidemiol Infect* 128:523–527.

[46] Garber L, Smeltzer M, Fedorka-Cray P, Ladely S, Ferris K. 2003. Salmonella enterica serotype enteritidis in table egg layer house environments and in mice in U.S. layer houses and associated risk factors. *Avian Dis* 47:134–142.

[47] Lapuz R, Tani H, Sasai K, Shirota K, Katoh H, Baba E. 2008. The role of roof rats (Rattus rattus) in the spread of Salmonella enteritidis and S. infantis contamination in layer farms in eastern Japan. *Epidemiol Infect* 136:1235–1243.

[48] Ashbolt R, Kirk MD. 2006. Salmonella Mississippi infections in Tasmania: the role of native Australian animals and untreated drinking water. *Epidemiol Infect* 134:1257–1265.

[49] Compton JA, Baney JA, Donaldson SC, Houser BA, Julian GJS, Yahner RH, Chmielecki W, Reynolds S, Jayarao BM. 2008. Salmonella infections in the common raccoon (Procyon lotor) in western Pennsylvania. *J Clinical Microbiol* 46:3084–3086.

[50] Gaertner JP, Hahn D, Jackson J, Forstner MRJ, Rose FL. 2008. Detection of salmonellae in captive and free-ranging turtles using enrichment culture and polymerase chain reaction. *J Herpetol* 42:223–231.

[51] Ktari S, Mahjoubi F, Jaoua S, Karray A, Marty N, Ben Redjeb S, et al. Application de marqueurs génotypiques dansl'investigation de deux épidémies d'infections nosocomiales à Salmonella linvingsones dans le CHU de sfax, Tunisie. *Pathol Biol* (Paris) 2006; 54: 331-6.

[52] Bouallègue-Godet O, Ben salem Y, Fabre L, Demartin M, Grimont P, Mzoughi R, et al. Nosocomial outbreak caused by Salmonella enterica serotype Linvingstone producing CTX-M-27 Extented-Spectrum β-lactamase in a neonal unit in Sousse, Tunisia. *J Clin Microbiol* 2005; 43:2940-5.

[53] Crump JA, Luby SP, Mintz ED. The global burden of typhoid fever. *Bull World Health Organ*. May 2004;82 (5):346-53.

[54] Bhan MK, Bahl R, Bhatnagar S. Typhoid and parattyphoid fever. *Lancet*. Aug 2005;366:749-62.

[55] Centers for Disease Control and Prevention. Preliminary FoodNet data on the incidence of infection with pathogens transmitted commonly through food--10 states, 2007. *MMWR Morb Mortal Wkly Rep*. Apr 11 2008;57(14):366-70.

[56] Voetsch AC, Van Gilder TJ, Angulo FJ, Farley MM, Shallow S, Marcus R, et al. FoodNet estimate of the burden of illness caused by nontyphoidal Salmonella infections in the United States. *Clin Infect Dis*. Apr 15 2004;38 Suppl 3:S127-34.

[57] Cavallaro E, Date K, Medus C, Meyer S, Miller B, Kim C, et al. Salmonella typhimurium infections associated with peanut products. *N Engl J Med.* Aug 18 2011;365(7):601-10.

[58] Linam WM, Gerber MA. Changing epidemiology and prevention of Salmonella infections. *Pediatr Infect Dis J*. Aug 2007;26(8):747-8.

[59] Hohmann EL. Nontyphoidal salmonellosis. *Clin Infect Dis*. Jan 15 2001; 32(2):263-9.

In: Salmonella: Classification, Genetics and Disease Outbreaks ISBN: 978-1-61942-928-4
Editors: Adelaide S. Monte, Paulo Eduardo De Santos

Chapter 9

SELECTIVE PRESSURE POTENTIAL OF ANTIMICROBIAL AGENTS TO FACILITATE SPREAD OF RESISTANCE PLASMID

Keri E. Powell, Maria C. Garcia and Aaron M. Lynne*
Department of Biological Sciences, Sam Houston State University, Huntsville, TX, US

ABSTRACT

Salmonellosis is of public health concern, accounting for about a quarter of all bacterial foodborne infections. According to the CDC, Salmonella enterica serovar Typhimurium is the most common Salmonella serotype reported. Of great concern is the possession and dissemination of antimicrobial resistance among Salmonella strains. Many antimicrobial resistance genes associated with Salmonella are found on conjugative plasmids. The misuse of antimicrobials in medical and animal-production settings may provide selective pressures that contribute to the proliferation of antimicrobial resistance, primarily by plasmid transfer. This study aims to present a selective pressure (i.e., varying antibiotic concentrations of four antibiotics) on the plasmid transfer rates of Salmonella via conjugation in-vitro. The four antimicrobials were selected for their plasmid-encoded resistance genes, activity against gram negative bacteria, and FDA approval for use in animal production. Successful conjugation pairs of S. Typhimurium isolates were mated under varying pressure conditions, plated on double antibiotic plates to select for transconjugants, and then conjugation rates were calculated. Preliminary results indicate a difference in conjugation rates across the four antimicrobials and within antimicrobials of varying concentration. Final results of the study may be useful in identifying antibiotics that may be more or less likely to initiate plasmid transfer between S. Typhimurium isolates in-vitro.

Keywords: Salmonella, antibiotic resistance, selective pressure, conjugative resistance, plasmids

---

* Corresponding Author. Correspondence Address: Department of Biological Sciences, Box 2116, Sam Houston State University, Huntsville, TX 77341. aaronlynne@shsu.edu.

INTRODUCTION

Salmonella belong to the bacterial family Enterobacteriacae. As such, they are motile, gram-negative, facultative anaerobic rods found in soil, water, and vegetation [1]. Historic taxonomic classifications of the genus characterized each of the 2,500 identified serotypes as being an individual species [1]. Recent DNA homology studies have revealed that despite the great number of serotypes, there are only two distinct species of Salmonella [1,2]. Around 99% of these serotypes belong to the species *Salmonella enterica*, and the remaining serotypes are grouped into Salmonella bongori. Furthermore, approximately 99% of the serovars that are pathogenic in humans belong to *Salmonella enterica* [2].

While *Salmonella* can colonize almost all animals, the many different strains present a variety of host-specific preferences [1]. Serotypes Typhi and Paratyphi are highly adapted to human hosts, causing devastating diseases such as Typhoid fever and bacteremia, yet are nonpathogenic in nonhuman hosts [1]. There are a number of different strains associated with human infection, of which the majority of cases result from foodborne and fecal-oral transmission [1]. The infectious dose of most serovars ranges from 30 to 10^8 bacteria [1]. Although a relatively large amount of bacteria are required for symptomatic infection to present itself, improper food handling and storage conditions (e.g., contaminated cutting boards or improper storage temperature) allow for rapid multiplication of bacteria in a short amount of time [1].

Salmonella account for about a quarter of all bacterial foodborne pathogens and is the second-most common etiological agent of domestically acquired foodborne illness [2,3]. The two most common serovars associated with foodborne illness are Typhimurium and Enteritidis [2,4]. Although *Salmonella* is only the number two leading cause of foodborne illnesses acquired domestically, it is the number one cause of foodborne illnesses resulting in death [3]. According to the CDC, *S.* Typhimurium is the most common *Salmonella* serotype of bacterial foodborne pathogens reported since 1997 [3]. The most common multidrug resistant (MDR) profile of *S.* Typhimurium is to five antimicrobial agents- ampicillin, chloramphenicol, streptomycin, sulfonamides, and tetracycline (ACSSuT; 3). The most common contaminated food products that lend to human infection include poultry, eggs, produce, beef and diary [1].

Gastroenteritis is the most common manifestation of foodborne Salmonella infection, with symptoms such as nausea, vomiting, and non-bloody diarrhea appearing anywhere from 6-48 hours after ingestion of contaminated food or water and persisting for two days to a week [1]. Thus, salmonellosis is generally self-limiting and does not require antibiotic therapy [1]. After ingestion, Salmonella must travel through the stomach. In order to survive the acidity of the stomach, Salmonella produce an acid tolerance response that enables them to proceed unharmed by the low pH [1,2]. The bacteria eventually colonize the small intestine, colon, or cecum where they are able to attach to specific host cells with the aid of many types of fimbriae or pili present on the surface of the bacteria cell [2]. After attachment, a syringe-like apparatus designed to secrete bacterial effector proteins across membranes-known as a type III secretion system (T3SS)- aids the bacteria in internalization and invasion into the host cell [2]. Once engulfed by the host cell, the microorganism is confined to a membrane-bound vesicle, called a Salmonella containing vacuole (SCV), where it is able to survive host immune responses [2].

In extreme cases, those microorganisms that invade migratory immune cells are able to hematogenously or lymphatogenously spread to other organs [2]. This risk for bacteremia is more likely to occur in pediatric, geriatric, and immunocompromised patients, as well as, patients with reduced gastric acid levels [1].

Bacteria do not sexually reproduce, as they remain haploid throughout their lives [5]. However, bacterial sex does occur in a sense. In a mechanism called conjugation, one bacteria (i.e., the donor) transfers genetic information to another bacteria (i.e., the recipient). The transfer occurs after physical contact between the bacteria, via a connective tube called the sex pilus. The process is nonreciprocal, as it is a one-way transfer of genetic information instead of a combination of two separate genomes. It is replicative, however, in that the donor retains the genetic information that is transferred to the recipient. Conjugation is a very promiscuous process, capable of occurring between bacteria from different species and even genuses.

The genetic information that is typically transferred in conjugation is called a plasmid. A plasmid is a small, extra-chromosomal piece of double-stranded DNA that can replicate independently of the host chromosome. Plasmids differ in their size, copy number, spread, and function [4]. There are several types of plasmids that encode various nonessential genes related to advantageous functions such as virulence, antimicrobial resistance, metabolism, conjugation, and colicin production [4].

In order for a plasmid to be transferable through conjugation it needs to either: 1) possess a group of genes responsible for conjugal functions, called the transfer operon (i.e., tra genes), or 2) it needs to use the proteins expressed from these tra genes by another plasmid. These latter plasmids, called mobilizable plasmids, lack the tra genes necessary for conjugation, but encode genes needed for their own DNA transfer [9]. Thus, mobilizable plasmids are able to be co-transferred with the use of proteins expressed by the co-resident conjugative plasmid.

Plasmid transfer enables rapid, widespread dissemination and persistence of genes that contribute to the pervasiveness of bacteria in many environments. Although conjugation is only one of the three mechanisms, which are collectively known as horizontal gene transfer mechanisms, by which bacteria can exchange DNA, it is the only process described here due to the nature of the current experiment.

The process by which many plasmids are replicated and transferred during conjugation is called rolling-circle replication. The first step involves one strand of the double-stranded plasmid DNA to be nicked at a site-specific sequence called the origin of transfer [2]. The free 3'-hydroxyl group is covalently extended by DNA polymerase, while the 5'-phosphate end is displaced to form an increasingly-lengthened tail of single-stranded DNA (ssDNA) that gets transferred into the recipient through the sex pili [2]. Once transferred, ssDNA can be converted to double-stranded DNA (dsDNA) by the recipients' replication machinery [2].

Technically, the term antibiotic refers to a chemical produced by a living microbe as a defense mechanism against other microbes, such that exposure to the chemical inhibits growth or kills. The term is often mistakenly used to encompass synthetic drugs that have antibiotic properties, such as the sulfa drugs. Regardless, any antibiotic is only effective against bacteria. 'Antimicrobial' is the preferred, all-inclusive term used to describe drugs that target microbes in general. The effectiveness of any given antimicrobial is dependent upon a few factors- the most obvious being that the pathogen must be susceptible to the antimicrobial [1]. Treating viral or fungal infections with antibiotics is useless, and potentially harmful as it poses risk for resistance acquisition by present bacteria (described later).

Antimicrobials target structures or metabolic processes that are different from those structures or processes of the host. While the host is generally not susceptible to the direct actions of the antimicrobial, there is still a concern over the selective toxicity of the given antimicrobial. The more different the pathogen's cellular anatomy and physiology is from the hosts', the more selective the antimicrobial is, and hence, the more effective.

The route of administration of the antimicrobial also plays a crucial role in its effectiveness, as it must reach the site of infection to exert its actions [1]. Attention to the pharmacokinetic and pharmacodynamic properties of a given antimicrobial and the nature of the infection is critical in effectively treating bacterial infections with antimicrobials. With respect to the pharmacological properties of the different drugs, the goal of antimicrobial therapy is to either maximize the concentrations of the antimicrobial (e.g., aminoglycosides), to maximize the duration of the exposure to the antimicrobial (e.g., penicillins), or to maximize the amount of antimicrobial (e.g., tetracyclines; 6). Lastly, the antimicrobial concentration at the site of infection must exceed the minimal inhibitory concentration (MIC; 7). The MIC of a particular bacteria-antimicrobial pair represents the minimal concentration of antimicrobial necessary to inhibit that particular bacteria's growth [7]. In clinical settings, the bacteria is considered susceptible when the MIC is less than the breakpoint concentration (i.e., the concentration of antimicrobial possible to accumulate at the site of infection), and resistance occurs when the MIC is greater than the breakpoint concentration [7].

The major classes of antimicrobials can be categorized according to their mechanisms of action (Table 1). Antimicrobials work by employing any of the following actions: inhibition of cell wall synthesis, protein synthesis, or nucleic acid synthesis, and metabolic antagonism [1,4].

The most common class and the least toxic of all antimicrobials act by inhibiting bacterial cell wall synthesis [1,4]. One class of cell wall inhibitors, beta-lactams, have a high degree of selective toxicity because the eukaryotic cell does not contain a cell wall- the target of beta-lactams. Penicillin was the first antibiotic of this class discovered. While the penicillins' defining structural feature is a beta-lactam ring, they differ from one another with respect to the side chains attached to an amino group [1]. The beta-lactam ring is structurally similar to the D-alanyl-D-alanine residue of the peptidoglycan subunit found in the bacterial cell wall. Because of this structural similarity, penicillin works by binding glycopeptide transpeptidase, also called pinicillin-binding protein (PBP), that catalyzes the cross-linking in the peptidoglycan layer [1,4]. The incorporation of penicillin into the PBP active site irreversibly inhibits cell wall synthesis, triggering autolysis and subsequent bacterial cell death [4]. It is important to note that the bactericidal properties of penicillin and its derivates only work on bacteria actively synthesizing new peptidoglycan.

The second largest class of antimicrobials are those that work by inhibiting protein synthesis [4]. Although these drugs discriminate between the prokaryotic 70S ribosome and the eukaryotic 80S ribosome which contributes to a high therapeutic index, the similarity between the eukaryotic mitochondrial chromosomes and prokaryotic chromosomes make these drugs more toxic than the cell wall inhibitors [1]. These drugs can affect initiation of protein synthesis by binding to either the 30S or 50S ribosome, and can also affect elongation by disrupting aminoacyl-tRNA binding, peptide bond formation, mRNA reading, and translocation [1]. Two examples of antimicrobials from this class include aminoglycosides and tetracyclines.

Table 1. Characterization of commonly prescribed antimicrobials

Mechanism of Action	Antimicrobial	Action
Cell Wall Synthesis Inhibition	*β-lactams* (penicillins, cephalosporins, carbapenems, monobactams) *β-lactamase inhibitors* *Glycopeptides* (vancomycin, daptomycin)	Bind transpeptidase→ prevent transpeptidation reaction of peptidoglycan synthesis, Binds β-lactamase Binds D-alanine-D-alanine→ inhibits transglycosylaton and transpeptidation of peptidoglycan
Protein Synthesis Inhibition	*Aminoglycosides* (Streptomycin, kanamycin, gentamicin, neomycin) *Tetracyclines* (Tetracycline, minocycline, doxycycline) *Macrolides* (erythromycin, azithromycin clarithromycin) Clindamycin	Bind 16S in 30S→misread mRNA/blocks 50S from joining 30S→premature protein products Bind 16S in 30S→distorts A site/blocks aminoacyl-tRNA binding to 30S-mRNA complex Bind 23S in 50S→blocks E site/ inhibits polypeptide chain elongation
Nucleic Acid Synthesis inhibition	*Quinolone/Fluoroquinolones* (nalidixic acid, ciprofloxacin, oxolinic acid,levofloxacin, gatifloxican) *Rifampin* Metronidazole	Binds DNA gyrase→inhibits DNA synthesis Binds DNA-dependent RNA Pol→ prevents transcription Nicks bacterial DNA

Adapted from [11].

The defining structural feature of aminoglycosides is a cyclohexane ring linked to amino sugars via glycosidic bonds. The aminoglycosides, such as streptomycin and kanamycin, exhibit their bactericidal properties by irreversibly binding to the 16S ribosomal subunit, inhibiting the completion of translational initiation. These drugs can also cause misreading of mRNA by slowing protein synthesis that has already initiated [1,6]. Also, because these compounds are cationic, they have a high affinity for the lipopolysaccharide (LPS) of the gram-negative bacterial cell wall [6]. Binding of the aminoglycosides to the LPS, or other anionic cellular membrane molecules, contributes to the destabilization of the bacterial cell membrane [8]. These drugs are poorly absorbed from the gut, so are given intramuscularly or intravenously [1, 8]. Furthermore, they are relatively lipid-insoluble resulting in poor penetration of the blood-brain barrier [8].

Tetracyclines, like the aminoglycosides, inhibit protein synthesis by binding to the 30S ribosome [1,4]. Unlike the aminoglycosides, however, tetracyclines reversibly bind to the 30S and are thus bacteriostatic [6]. The drug inhibits aminoacyl-tRNA from entering and binding the acceptor site (A-site) of the 70S ribosome [1,6].

Another class of antimicrobials, the nucleic acid synthesis inhibitors, exert their bactericidal effects by blocking replication or transcription. The selectivity of these drugs result from their ability to differentiate prokaryotic and eukaryotic enzymes involved in nucleic acid synthesis [6]. However, they do have decreased selective toxicity due to some overlap in nucleic acid synthesis machinery between prokaryotes and eukaryotes [6]. Drugs such as rifampin that target DNA gyrase, DNA polymerase, or DNA helicase affect DNA synthesis and function, while those that target RNA polymerase affect RNA synthesis and function [1, 6].

The last class of antimicrobials, that exert bacteriostatic properties by antagonizing metabolic pathways, are often called antimetabolites [1,6]. An example of this class is the sulfonamides. This synthetic antimicrobial is able to exert its bacteriostatic effects because its structural similarity to para-aminobenzoic acid allows it to competitively inhibit the synthesis of folic acid [1, 6]. The selectivity of the sulfa drugs arise from the fact that mammalian cells do not synthesize folic acid; whereas, bacteria must synthesize their own, as they are unable to metabolize supplemented folic acid [1,6].

In the cellular world, any change in genetic information and subsequent cellular functioning will be tolerated only if the costs associated with that change are less than the benefits produced. As mentioned before, plasmids do not confer any genes that are essential for normal functioning. Therefore, plasmids thrive in the bacterial population because the benefits of maintaining them outweigh the costs necessary to express the nonessential genes that they encode. Another way that bacteria can acquire changes to its genetic information, in addition to horizontal gene transfer, is by mutations in the pre-existing DNA.

Antimicrobial resistance genes can be transferred and acquired by a variety of genetic elements such as, chromosomal mutation, resistance transposons, gene cassettes, and resistance integrons [10]. Acquisition of resistance plasmids accounts for the majority of resistance mechanisms employed by bacteria to currently used antibiotics [2, 8]

The antimicrobial resistance mechanism acquired by some bacteria work by targeting the drug in a way to render it ineffective. This could be by directly altering or degrading the antimicrobial, preventing its entry by competitive or noncompetitive inhibition, modification of its target site and extruding it via efflux pumps [1,2]. Table 2 illustrates a list of a few antimicrobials and their corresponding resistance mechanisms.

Resistance to a β-lactam antimicrobial, such as penicillin, works by degrading the drug and was the first antibiotic resistance mechanism to be noticed. Interestingly, right around the same time penicillin was introduced in clinical practice in the 1940s, it was reported that *E. coli* produced a substance that hydrolyzed penicillin [9].

The enzyme, termed penicillinase, belongs to the β-lactamase family and is responsible for hydrolyzing the beta-lactam ring of penicillin. Salmonella resistance to penicillins can be greatly attributed to the production of β-lactamases, one of which is called AmpC enzyme and is encoded by bla_{cmy} to produce resistance to multiple β-lactams [2].

Enzymatic modification by the aminoglycoside phosphotransferases, aminoglycoside acetyltransferases, and aminoglycoside adenyltransferases on the amino and hydroxyl groups of the antimicrobial compromise one of the most important mechanisms of aminoglycoside resistance in bacteria, especially *Salmonella* [1,2,8]. These modifications lessen the affinity for the aminoglycosides to the A-site [2,8]. Kanamycin resistance is due to aminoglycoside phosphotransferase encoded by *aph*A and streptomycin resistance is associated with aminoglycoside adenyltransferase encoded by *aad*A [2].

Table 2. Examples of resistance mechanisms to common antimicrobials

Antibiotic	Resistance Mechanism
β-lactams	Prevent antibiotic-PBP binding Modify antibiotic-PBP binding Hydrolyze antibiotic with beta-lactamase
Aminoglycosides	Mutate ribosomal binding site Decrease uptake of antibiotic (must reach cytoplasm-many points of entry for inhibition) Increase efflux of antibiotic Enzymatic modification of antibiotic
Tetracyclines	Decrease antibiotic penetration into cell wall Efflux antibiotic (most common) Alter ribosomal target site (ribosome protection) Enzymatic modification of antibiotic (oxidation by *tetX* gene product) Mutation of *OmpF* (chromosomal gene that encodes porin protein)
Sulfonamide	Enzymatic modification of enzyme (dihydropteroic acid sythetase) that uses PABA during folic acid synthesis
Quinolones	Mutations in DNA gyrase and topoisomerase type IV structural genes Overexpress efflux pumps Mutations in genes controlling membrane permeability decrease drug uptake

Adapted from [11] and [19].

Tetracycline resistance in *Salmonella* mostly results from efflux pumps encoded by *tet* genes [2]. Resistance to the sulfonamides, is associated with decreased affinity for enzymes to the sulfonamides (e.g. *sul*I or *sul*II); whereas, *dhfr* gene products are altered such that they have a decreased affinity for trimethoprim, resulting in resistance by allowing folic acid biosynthesis in the presence of these drugs [2].

A multidrug-resistant plasmid (MDR)called the IncA/C MDR plasmid, is of particular concern because it is responsible for the dissemination of extended-spectrum beta-lactamase genes among common foodborne pathogens [11]. In *Salmonella enterica*, the AmpC beta-lactamase gene bla_{CMY-2} which hydrolyzes third-generation cephalosporins, is frequently carried on IncA/C or IncI1 plasmids [11,12]. Analysis of a MDR plasmid (pIP1202) isolated from *Yersinia pestis*, the etiological agent of plague, revealed 99-100% nucleotide identity of an IncA/C plasmid backbone with *S.* Newport (pSN254) and *Y. ruckeri* (pYR1; 13). Both the *Y. pestis* and *S.* Newport plasmids contained resistance to eight antibiotics, with five antibiotic resistance phenotypes shared between the two (e.g., ampicillin, chloramphenicol, streptomycin, sulfonamide and tetracycline resistance). MDR plasmid similarity between these two seemingly distant pathogens, one the causative agent of plague that killed millions in 1320 and the other the second most common cause of foodborne illness today, emphasizes the public health concern posed by plasmid-mediated resistance in bacteria [13].

Between 2002 to 2005, 125 MDR *Salmonella* strains were isolated from retail meats in order to determine the occurrence and distribution of the IncA/C plasmid backbone [13]. The backbones were found in 70 of the samples and from all meat types sampled (i.e., chicken, turkey, pork, and ground beef).

Many anthropogenic factors, especially antimicrobial misuse, contribute to antimicrobial resistance [4]. Patients reporting to their doctors of respiratory-associated infections are often given a bacterial diagnosis without culturing, and are prescribed broad-spectrum (i.e., are effective against a broad range of bacteria types) antimicrobials, despite the fact that over 90% of these cases are viral respiratory infections [4]. Other human factors include the self-administration or early termination of treatment [4]. Usually whenever the patient starts feeling better, s/he will discontinue use of the antimicrobial. This causes the drug to have not been in the body for the required amount of time to effectively eliminate all bacteria. Those that were not killed by the antimicrobial due to spontaneous mutation then have the opportunity to reestablish an infection and be resistant to the original antimicrobial used to treat it. Likewise, the self-administration of antimicrobials is very dangerous. Antimicrobials range in their modes of action and pharmacological properties such that expert knowledge of these mechanisms is required to effectively treat a bacterial infection.

A growing body of evidence indicates that selective pressures introduced in medical and animal-production settings greatly contribute to the proliferation of antimicrobial resistance, primarily by plasmid transfer [4]. One study found higher levels of resistant bacteria from patients in intensive care units, which use antibiotics often, than bacteria isolated from patients in other wards and outpatient settings [15]. Animal-production conditions often entail large densities of animals confined to a small area. Cows, who are naturally herbivores and have a neutral rumen (i.e., complex stomach), are often fed corn and corn products instead of grass or hay in livestock warehouses. Because the cow gastrointestinal tract poorly digests starch, undigested grain reaches the colon, where it is then fermented. This increase in fermentation causes acidosis, which can eventually kill the cow, and opens a vulnerability to common feedlot diseases [16]. Antimicrobials such as rumensin and tylosin are given to the animals to acidify the rumen to tolerate the starch diet and to decrease the incidence of liver infection, respectively.

Due to disease-prone constraints and in an effort to promote increased weight gain, sub-therapeutic doses of antimicrobials are regularly given to the animals through the feed or water source prophylactically. In turn, a pressure is placed on those susceptible strains of bacteria to acquire a resistance plasmid and express the resistance gene or otherwise be killed by the antimicrobial. Many studies have shown identical antimicrobial-resistance profiles between animals and infected humans [17]. In order to study how antibiotic use in animal food production could affect human health, the occurrence of *Salmonella* and *Campylocbacter jejuni* in foods of animal origin (i.e., poultry) and the occurrence of human illnesses caused by these two organisms was examined over a twenty month period by the King County Health Department in 1984 [18]. The isolates from infected humans and those from retail poultry had similar antimicrobial susceptibility patterns. This illustrates that the zoonotic transfer of plasmid-encoded resistant bacteria, such as Salmonella, through the food chain can directly affect human health and emphasizes the importance of preserving antimicrobials for human illness.

Even bacteria that are not being directly exposed to an antimicrobial, and thus no selective pressure is placed on them to attain that antimicrobial resistance gene, display resistance genes. However, selective pressures for a particular antimicrobial may confer resistance to other antimicrobials through the acquisition of a gene cassette or MDR plasmid that contains many resistance genes. Interestingly, isolates recovered from the pre-antibiotic era possess resistant genes [19]. These resistance genes serve alternative primary roles in their respective environments, such as metabolic-related advantages and efflux pump mechanisms to extrude toxins [19]. Analysis of some resistance enzymes reveal that they have been plasmid-encoded for millions of years and were largely disseminated by horizontal gene transfer mechanisms [19]. This demonstrates that a direct selective pressure is not always necessary to facilitate the uptake of a resistance plasmid. However, selective pressures for a particular antimicrobial may confer resistance to other antimicrobials through the acquisition of a gene cassette or MDR plasmid that contains many resistance genes. Because of the inherent nature of bacteria to evolve mechanisms to survive and pervade previously uninhabitable niches, antimicrobial resistance poses a serious public health threat. Resistance to all antimicrobials manufactured today and evidence of direct passage of antimicrobial-resistant bacteria through the food chain has been documented. The prudential use of antibiotics should be conserved for human medicine only in order to preserve the effectiveness of these important drugs. Allowing bacteria to be introduced to these antibiotics, through feedlot practices or improper use by humans, only gives them a head-start on evolving molecular strategies to maintain their status as being the oldest form of life on earth [19].

This study aimed to compare the ability of four antibiotics to increase plasmid transfer, as measured by conjugation rates. Thus, a selective pressure (i.e., varying concentrations of four antibiotics) was introduced in order to study the plasmid transfer rates of Salmonella via conjugation in-vitro. The four antimicrobials were selected for their plasmid-encoded resistance genes, activity against gram negative bacteria, and FDA approval for use in animal production. Successful conjugation pairs of *S.* Typhimurium isolates were mated under varying pressure conditions, then cultured on double antibiotic plates to select for transconjugants. Finally, conjugation rates were calculated. Preliminary results indicate a difference in conjugation rates across the four antimicrobials and within antimicrobials of varying concentration. Future work should enlist PCR amplification targeting resistance genes of the transconjugants to ensure that resistance acquisition was plasmid-encoded rather than mutation-acquired. Final results of the study may be useful in identifying antibiotics that may be more or less likely to initiate plasmid transfer between *S.* Typhimurium isolates in-vitro and/or certain concentrations of antibiotics that promote plasmid transfer more or less frequently. By knowing which antibiotics select for plasmid-transfer more frequently, future research can be aimed at the mechanism underlying the increased plasmid-transfer rate.

MATERIALS AND METHODS

Bacterial Strains

Three S. enterica serovar Typhimurium isolates recovered from cattle (n=2) and ground chicken (n=1) between 2001 and 2002 representing multiple states were obtained from diagnostic samples submitted to the USDA National Veterinary Services Laboratory. Isolates were grown on LB agar plates and incubated at 37°C overnight. When not in use, isolates were stored in LB broth and 20% glycerol at -80°C.

Conjugation Experiment

Donors 371/372 and recipients 408/450 were streaked onto an LB plate and incubated overnight at 37. The isolates were then transferred into a 15 mL conical tube containing 5 mL of LB liquid broth and secured in a shaking incubator at 37°C overnight. The donor/recipient pairs (408x371, 408x371, 450x371, and 450x372) were prepared for conjugation the following day by adding 0.2 mL of donor and 1.8 mL of recipient from overnight liquid cultures, as well as 2 mL of LB liquid broth, into a new 15 mL conical tube. The caps were loosely tightened and secured with tape before being incubated in a non-shaking incubator overnight at 37°C.

Transconjugants from each mating pair were plated in triplicates (50μL, 100 μL, and 200 μL) onto dual antibiotic LB plates containing 100 μg/mL of Amp and Rif. Also, both the donors and recipients were plated individually onto dual antibiotic plates. Colonies of the successful transconjugants and their respective donors/recipients were refrozen. Finally, resistance profiles of competent conjugation pairs were determined by Kirby-Bauer disc diffusion assay.

Selective Pressure Plates

The conjugation isolates were mated under varying pressure conditions (Table 3). Each well contained: 100 μL donor cell, 100 μL recipient cell, antibiotic corresponding to the stated concentrations, and LB liquid broth to bring the total well volume to 250 μL. In a 96-well plate, the four antibiotics were serially diluted by ½ for a total of four dilutions for ampicillin (Amp) and tetracycline (Tet), five dilutions for streptomycin (Str), and a six dilutions for kanamycin (Kan).

The first concentration of each antibiotic was one dilution greater than the CLSI resistance breakpoint. Next, 100 μL of donor and recipient were injected into each well. Note, each donor and recipient were grown at 37°C with gentle shaking to an OD_{600} of 0.5 (±0.2) immediately before addition into the well. The total volume of each well was brought to 250 μL by addition of liquid LB broth.

A column containing no antibiotic was implemented to screen for cell viability, while a column containing no bacteria controlled for contamination. The plates were allowed to incubate at 37°C overnight.

After overnight incubation, the presumed transconjugants from the selective pressure plates were spot-inoculated in triplicates onto Amp/Rif LB plates. Three 10 μL drops were inoculated onto the plates for each condition. Note, that the transconjugant samples were serially diluted by 1/10 for a total of four dilutions and that each dilution was spot-inoculated. After overnight incubation at 37°C, the colonies were averaged among the triplicates for each condition.

Table 3. Selective pressure plates

Antibiotic		[Antibiotic] (μg/mL)								
	Row Letter	Column Number								
		1	2	3	4	5	6	7	8	9
Amp	A	64	32	16	8	4	-	-	No abx	No bacteria
Kan	B	128	64	32	16	8	4	2	No abx	No bacteria
Str	C	128	64	32	16	8	4	-	No abx	No bacteria
Tet	D	32	16	8	4	2	-	-	No abx	No bacteria

Amp=ampicillin, Kan=Kanamycin, Str=streptomycin, Tet=Tetracycline.

RESULTS

The successful conjugation pairs were 408x371 and 408x372. The Kirby-Bauer disc diffusion assay resistance profiles are listed in Table 4. 'R' indicate resistant to the specified antibiotic; whereas, 'S' indicates susceptibility and 'I' indicates intermediate resistance.

The averages from the triplicates from all dilutions are reported in Table 5. These data represent conjugation averages of the triplicates per selective pressure condition from the set-up depicted in Figure 2, except that the dilution range for all antibiotics started at 128 μg/mL, regardless of CLSI resistance breakpoint. Under selective pressure of ampicillin, dilutions 2, 4, and 5 produce more transconjugant colonies than the control under no antibiotic pressure.

Table 4. Resistance profiles of donors, recipients, and transconjugants

Iso-late	Antibiotic														
	Amc	AN	AM	CRO	FOX	C	CIP	GM	K	NA	S	G	SXT	Te	XNL
371	R	S	R	S	S	S	S	S	S	S	S	R	S	S	S
372	R	S	R	S	S	R	S	S	S	S	R	R	S	R	S
408	S	S	S	S	S	S	S	S	S	S	S	S	S	S	S
408x 371	R	S	R	S	S	S	S	S	R	S	I	R	R	S	S
408x 372	I	S	R	S	S	S	R	S	R	R	I	R	R	R	S

Amc = Amoxicillin/Clavulonic acid, AN = Amikacin, AM = Ampicillin, CRO = Ceftriaxone, FOX = Cefoxitin,
C = Chloramphenicol, CIP = Ciprofloxacin, GM = Gentamicin, K = Kanamycin, NA = Nalidixic acid,
S = Streptomycin, G = Sulfisoxazole, SXT = Sulfisoxazole/Trimethoprim, Te = Tetricycline, XNL = Ceftiofur.

Table 5. Number of transconjugants produced

Antibiotic	Dilution 1	Dilution 2	Dilution 3	Dilution 4	Dilution 5	Dilution 6	Dilution 7	Control 8	Control 9
Amp	5.0	12.3	6.0	12.0	6.7	1.7	0.0	6.7	0.0
Kan	37.7	25.7	10.0	26.3	25.7	15.3	14.3	17.7	0.0
Str	2.7	15.0	18.7	0.0	18.3	24.3	0.0	0.0	0.0
Tet	1.0	2.0	0.0	0.0	2.0	3.7	4.3	8.3	0.0

Amp = Ampicillin, Kan = Kanamycin, Str = Streptomycin, Tet = Tetracycline.

Table 6. Conjugation Rates*

Antibiotic	Rate With Antibiotic	Rate Without Antibiotic
Amp	$1.23x10^{-4}$	$6.7x10^{-5}$
Kan	$3.77x10^{-4}$	$1.77x10^{-4}$
Str	$1.87x10^{-4}$	N/A
Tet	$4.3x10^{-5}$	$8.3x10^{-5}$

* The highest transconjugant count for a given dilution for each antibiotic was compared to the rate of conjugation of the control (w/o antibiotic). The transconjugant count was multiplied by the dilution factor of 1,000, then divided by the total amount of donor cells at an OD_{600}, which is 10^7.

Under selective pressure of kanamycin, dilutions 1, 2, 4, and 5 produce more transconjugant colonies than the control. The rate of conjugations, reported in units of transconjugants/donor, are reported in Table 6.

CONCLUSION

Results from the conjugation under antibiotic pressure reveal that kanamycin conditions produced the most transconjugants compared to the other antibiotics, while tetracycline conditions produced the least transconjugants.

The highest amount of transconjugants across all conditions was at the CLSI resistance breakpoint of kanamycin (128 µg/mL). Within the ampicillin condition, the highest amount of transconjugants was at ampicillin's CLSI resistance breakpoint of 64 µg/mL.

No dilution of streptomycin or tetracycline tested produced higher transconjugants than the control conditions.

These preliminary results seem to indicate that there are differential rates at which conjugation-mediated plasmid transfers occur in the presence of these four different antibiotics, as well as, at different concentrations of each. After more data collection and subsequent statistical analysis to ensure significant differences among the conjugation rates of the different antibiotics, the next experimental step would be to select for the antibiotic resistance genes by PCR to ensure that plasmid-transfer is responsible for the antibiotic resistance.

Future work could also investigate the molecular mechanism behind these differential rates, perhaps the role and pathway of those particular antimicrobials on the initiation of plasmid transfer in S. Typhimurium.

REFERENCES

[1] Allen, H. K., Donato, J., Wang, H. H., and Cloud-Hansen, K. A. Call of the wild: antibiotic resistance genes in natural environments. *Nature Reviews Microbiology*, doi: 10.1038/nrmicro2312.

[2] Archilbald L, et al.. Antimicrobial resistance in isolates from inpatients and outpatients in the United States: increasing importance of the intensive care unit. *Clinical Infectious Disease*, 1997; (24): 211-215.

[3] Bennett, PM. (2008) Plasmid encoded antibiotic resistance: acquisition and transfer of antibiotic resistance genes in bacteria. *British Journal of Pharmacology*, 153: 5347-5357.

[4] Centers for Disease Control and Prevention 2011. http://www.cdc.gov/salmonella/.

[5] Douard, G; Praud, K; Cloeckaert, A; and Doublet, B. (2010) The Salmonella Genomic Island 1 is specifically mobiolized in trans by the IncA/C multidrug resistance plasmid family. *PLoS ONE,* 5(12): e15302.

[6] Ebert, SC. (2004) Application of pharmacokinetics and pharmacodynamics to antibiotic selection. PandT. 29(4): 244-253.

[7] Foley, SL, and Lynne, A M. (2008) Food animal-associated Salmonella challenges: Pathogenicity and antimicrobial resistance. *Journal of Animal Science*, 86(E. Suppl.): E173-D187.

[8] Freeman, S. Biological Sciences, Volume 1 The Cell, Genetics, and Development. San Francisco: *Pearson Education*; 2008.

[9] Hawkey, PM. (2008) Molecular epidemiology of clinically significant antibiotic resistance genes. *British Journal of Pharmacology*, 153: S406-S413

[10] Mayer, G. Antiobiotics-Protein Synthesis, Nucleic Acid Synthesis and Metabolism. The Board of Trustees of the University of South Carolina 2010. Accessed 2011. http:.//pathmicro.med.sc.edu/mayer/antibiot.htm

[11] Murray P, Rosenthal K, and Pfaller M. Medical Microbiology, 6th edition. Philadelphia: Mosby Elsevier; 2009.

[12] Russell, J. B. (2001) Factors that alter rumen microbial ecology. *Science*, 292(5519): 1119-1122.

[13] Seattle-King County Department of Public Health 1984. Surveillance of the flow of Salmonella and Campylobacter in a community. Food and Drug Administration, Bureau of Veterinary Medicine, Washington, D.C.

[14] Shakil, S, Kahn, R, Zarrilli, R, and Khan, A. (2008). Aminoglycosides versus bacteria-a description of the action, resistance mechanism, and nosocomial battleground. *Journal of Biomedical Sciences*, 15: 5-14.

[15] U.S. Department of Health and Human Services, Food and Drug Administration, and Center for Veterinary medicine. The Judicious use of Medically Important Antimicrobial Drugs in Food-Producing Animals, Draft Guidance. 2010.

[16] United States Government Accountability Office (GAO) Report 2004. Antibiotic Resistance: Federal Agencies Need to Better Focus Efforts to Address risks to Humans from Antibiotic Use in Animals.

[17] Welch, TJ; Fricke, WF; McDermott, PF; White, DG; Rosso, ML; Rasko, DA; Mammel, MK; Eppinger, M; Rosovitz, MJ; Wagner, D; Rahalison, L; LeClerc, JE; Hinshaw, JM; Lindler, LE; Cebula, TA; Carniel, E; and Ravel, J. (2007). Multiple Antimicrobial Resistance in Plague: An Emerging Public Health Risk. *PLoS ONE*, 2(3): e309.

[18] Wiesner, M; Calva, E; Fernandez-Mora, M; Cevallos, M; Campos, F; Zaidi, M; and Silva, C. (2011) Salmonella Typhimurium ST213 is associated with two types of IncA/C plasmids carrying multiple resistance determinants. *BioMed. Central Microbiology*, 11:9.

[19] Willey, JM, Sherwood, LM, and Woolverton, CJ. Prescott's Principles of Microbiology. New York: McGraw-Hill; 2009.

In: Salmonella: Classification, Genetics and Disease Outbreaks ISBN: 978-1-61942-928-4
Editors: Adelaide S. Monte, Paulo Eduardo De Santos © 2012 Nova Science Publishers, Inc.

Chapter 10

MECHANISMS OF COLONIZATION AND SURVIVAL OF *SALMONELLA* WITHIN THE EGG

Avelino Álvarez-Ordóñez[1,2,*], Máire Begley[1], Miguel Prieto[3], Winy Messens[4,†], Mercedes López[3], Ana Bernardo[3] and Colin Hill[1,2]

[1]Department of Microbiology,
University College Cork, Cork, Ireland
[2]Alimentary Pharmabiotic Centre,
University College Cork, Cork, Ireland
[3]Department of Food Hygiene and Technology,
Veterinary Faculty, University of León, León, Spain
[4]Biological Hazards (BIOHAZ) Unit
European Food Safety Authority (EFSA),
Parma, Italy

ABSTRACT

Human salmonellosis infections are usually acquired via the food chain as a result of the ability of *Salmonella* serovars to colonize and persist within the gastrointestinal tract of food-producing animals and the avian reproductive tract, being able to contaminate, survive and grow inside eggs. This review gives an overview of the cellular and molecular processes involved in the colonization of hen's eggs and in *Salmonella* persistence in the harsh conditions of the egg albumen with special focus on serovar Enteritidis, which shows a particular tropism and ability to persist in chicken oviducts and ovaries and to contaminate, survive and grow inside eggs. The trans-ovarian (also referred to as vertical transmission) and the trans-shell (referred to as horizontal transmission) routes of colonization of the egg are briefly described. In addition, several gene candidates involved in bacterial survival in the egg albumen are identified as potential biomarkers, appropriate for the design of ambitious strategies for the prevention of salmonellosis.

---

* E-mail address: a.alvarezordonez@ucc.ie.

† The views and findings in this article are solely those of the author and do not necessarily reflect the views or position of the European Food Safety Authority.

Keywords: *Salmonella*, eggs, colonization, survival strategies, molecular mechanisms

Introduction

Nontyphoidal human salmonellosis is characterised by the acute onset of fever, abdominal pain, nausea, diarrhea, and sometimes vomiting (Hohmann, 2001). The disease is usually self-limiting, lasting a few days. However, in some cases, more serious complications follow, especially in immunocompromised people, pregnant women, elderly and children. Dehydration due to vomiting and diarrhea can lead to electrolyte imbalance and hypovolemic shock. In addition, approximately 5% of the individuals having gastrointestinal illness will develop bacteremia which is often accompanied by focal infections such as meningitis, septic arthritis, osteomyelitis, pneumonia and arteritis, and about 2% of *Salmonella* infections are followed by reactive arthritis (Mead *et al.*, 1999). In 2009, salmonellosis was the second only to campylobacteriosis in terms of reported zoonotic disease in the European Union. A total of 108,614 confirmed cases (23.7 per 100,000 population) were reported from 27 Member States. A 17.4% decrease in the notification rate was observed since 2008 and a decreasing trend was noted for the fifth consecutive year (EFSA, 2011); however, due to significant underreporting this number represents only a portion of the actual number of illnesses (EFSA, 2008). The two most commonly reported *Salmonella* serovars were *S. enterica* serovar Enteritidis and *S. enterica* serovar Typhimurium, representing 52.3% (11.8 per 100,000 population) and 23.3% (5.3 per 100,000 population), respectively, of all reported serovars in salmonellosis confirmed cases. Human *S.* Enteritidis cases were most commonly associated with the consumption of contaminated eggs and poultry meat, while *S.* Typhimurium cases were mostly associated with the consumption of contaminated pig, poultry and bovine meat (EFSA, 2011).

In order to cause the foodborne disease in humans, *Salmonella* spp. must colonize the gastrointestinal or reproductive tract of their reservoir host, survive in the food chain and cross the species gap to colonize the human. In contrast to mammals, the avian embryo does not develop in the safe environment of the womb, and, for this reason, the egg has an impressive arsenal of antimicrobial protective mechanisms, including non-specific physical barriers and bactericidal compounds such as lysozyme and ovotransferrin. Consequently, *Salmonella* has evolved adaptive networks to cope with the challenges of a changing environment. A better understanding of the mechanisms involved in *Salmonella* spp. colonization and survival in the egg may help to optimize salmonellosis control programs. This review provides an overview of host–pathogen interactions in the hen reproductive tract and eggs at the cellular and molecular level. Hence, the main routes of colonization of the egg by *Salmonella* spp. are described, and the most relevant research studies carried out in the last few years in order to elucidate the primary cellular systems of defense employed by *Salmonella* spp. to protect them against stress conditions prevailing within the egg are compiled.

S. Enteritidis shows a particular tropism and ability to persist in hen oviducts and ovaries and to contaminate, survive and grow inside eggs. The silent infection and colonization of different parts of the reproductive organs can lead to eggs contaminated with *S.* Enteritidis cells in either yolk or albumen (De Buck *et al.*, 2004). The natural capacity to infect and colonize the reproductive tract is seemingly shared by other serovars, such as *S.* Typhimurium, and *S.* Gallinarum (Keller *et al.*, 1997; De Buck *et al.*, 2004), and additionally, many *Salmonella* serovars can be isolated from the on-farm environment or the egg shell. But *S.* Enteritidis is the only serovar routinely isolated from egg contents. Therefore, if not specifically stated, the information given in this review refers to experiments performed with the most frequent serovar responsible for egg-linked foodborne infection, *S.* Enteritidis.

STRATEGIES FOR PENETRATION/COLONIZATION OF THE EGG (VERTICAL *VS* HORIZONTAL TRANSMISSION)

Contamination of intact eggs by *Salmonella* can occur by two routes. In the transovarian route (also referred to as vertical transmission), yolk, albumen, eggshell membranes or eggshells are directly contaminated as a result of *Salmonella* infection of the reproductive organs. In the trans-shell route (referred to as horizontal transmission), egg interiors are contaminated by *Salmonella* penetration through the eggshell from the colonized gut or from contaminated faeces during or after oviposition. Both transmission routes have been extensively reviewed by Gantois *et al.* (2009a) and Messens *et al.* (2005a), respectively. There is no agreement as to the most important route for *Salmonella* contamination of eggs. While some (Gast & Beard, 1990; Guard-Petter, 2001) believe vertical transmission to be the most important route, others (Barrow & Lovell, 1991; Bichler *et al.*, 1996) suggest horizontal transmission to be of primary importance. According to Cogan & Humphrey (2003) vertical transmission of *S.* Enteritidis is more common. With salmonellae other than *S.* Enteritidis, horizontal transmission is probably the most important route (Humphrey, 1994).

Vertical Transmission

The deposition of *Salmonella* inside eggs is thus most likely a consequence of reproductive tissue colonization in infected laying hens. The oviduct can be subdivided into five functional regions (Figure 1). Starting from the ovary, there are the infundibulum, magnum, isthmus, uterus and vagina. The infundibulum captures the ovulatory follicles, the magnum produces the albumen, the isthmus deposits the eggshell membranes, the uterus forms the eggshell and the vagina is involved in oviposition. *Salmonella* colonizing the oviduct could be incorporated into the albumen, the eggshell membranes or the eggshell itself, depending on the site of colonization (magnum, isthmus and uterus, respectively) (Gantois *et al.*, 2009a). Given that *S.* Enteritidis can be isolated from all sites in the hen reproductive tract contamination of any part of the egg is possible.

Colonization of the reproductive organs is a consequence of systemic spread of *Salmonella* from the intestine (Vázquez-Torres *et al.*, 1999). Upon colonization of the intestinal lumen, bacteria invade the intestinal epithelial cells. Macrophages are attracted to the site of invasion and enclose the *Salmonella* bacteria, enabling their survival and multiplication in the intracellular environment of the macrophage. These macrophages then migrate to the internal organs such as the reproductive organs (systemic spread). *Salmonella* pathogenicity island-2 (SPI-2) is essential in this process (Gantois *et al.*, 2009a). A thorough overview of host–pathogen interactions in the hen reproductive tract at the cellular and molecular level is given in a recent review article by Gantois *et al.* (2009a).

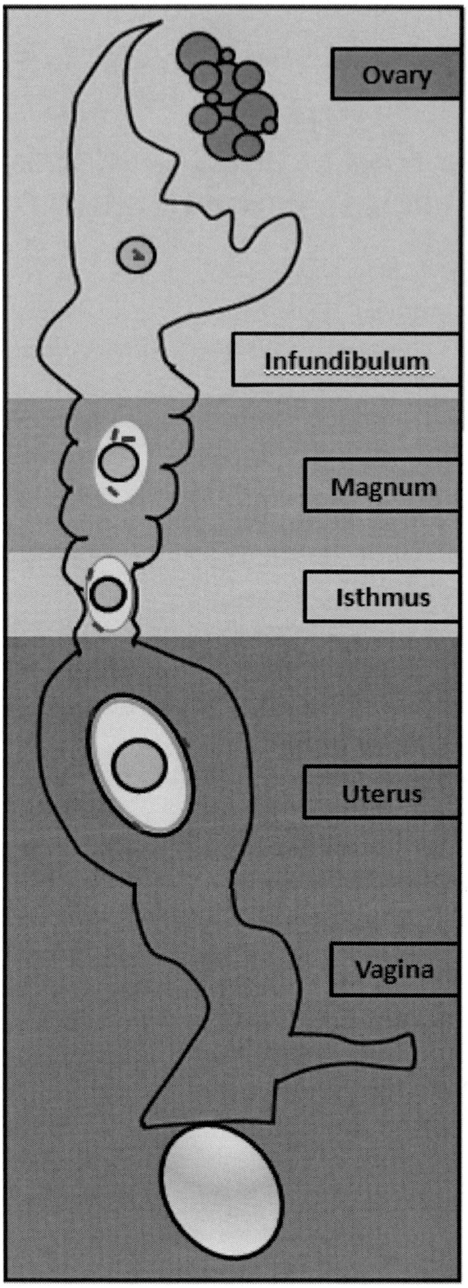

Figure 1. Pathogenesis of egg contamination by *Salmonella* through the transovarian route (vertical transmission). Direct contamination of the yolk, albumen, shell membranes and egg shell is originated from infection of the infundibulum, magnum, isthmus and uterus, respectively.

Horizontal Transmission

The egg possesses three physical barriers to bacterial penetration: the cuticle, the eggshell and the membranes.

The Cuticle

The cuticle is the hydrophobic proteinaceous layer covering the eggshell, and is considered the egg's first defence against bacterial infection. Shortly after oviposition, the eggshell is more susceptible to bacterial penetration as the cuticle is immature and usually moist (Miyamoto *et al.*, 1998) and a positive temperature differential is present at that moment as the egg is warmer (42°C) than the environment (Bruce & Drysdale, 1994).

When mature the cuticle functions as an effective barrier to bacterial invasion as it closes the eggshell pores and impedes the movement of bacteria (Berrang *et al.*, 1999a). This has been shown in an early study (Board *et al.*, 1979) in which the cuticle was intentionally removed by abrasion or by EDTA treatment of the shell. However cuticle effectivity may be affected by at least two phenomena. First, aging of the egg leads to drying of the cuticle and results in shrinkage, leaving the pores more exposed (Mayes & Takeballi, 1983). Second, the cuticle is not considered to be an intrinsic component of the true shell. One study (Board & Halls, 1973) showed that 3.5% of eggs lacked a demonstrable cuticle, while 8.0% had no cuticle on the egg poles. Later on, Nascimento (1992) demonstrated by scanning electron microscopy (SEM), that the cuticle of most eggs (> 98%) was absent or patchy. In the study by Messens *et al.* (2005b) the cuticle deposition of eggs was not correlated with trans-shell penetration by *Salmonella*. Other studies (Messens *et al.*, 2005b; De Reu *et al.*, 2006) reported a lower mean cuticle deposition of penetrated eggs compared to unpenetrated eggs. Eggs from various sources were included in the latter study. This was later confirmed by Messens *et al.* (2007) and it was concluded that trans-shell penetration by *S.* Enteritidis was enhanced to a great extent in the absence of cuticle, yet, when cuticle was present, its degree of deposition apparently did not significantly affect trans-shell penetration.

The Eggshell

The effect of the shell thickness on the ability of *Salmonella* to penetrate is not yet established. One study indicated that thinner eggshells were more likely to be penetrated by *Salmonella* (Sauter & Petersen, 1974), but other studies could not confirm this (Smeltzer *et al.*, 1979; Messens *et al.*, 2005b; De Reu *et al.*, 2006). The construction of the eggshell is more crucial according to Nascimento *et al.* (1992): eggs with a visually judged poorer eggshell ultrastructure were more sensitive to trans-shell penetration by *S.* Enteritidis.

The numerous pores in the hen's eggshell, ranging from 7,000-17,000 per egg, enable the ingress of bacteria through the eggshell to the shell membranes (Mayes & Takeballi, 1983). Most of these pores are blocked in the presence of an undamaged cuticle, but at least 10 to 20 pores lack an adequate cover or plug of cuticle (Board & Tranter, 1995). Current evidence

(Nascimento *et al.*, 1992; Messens *et al.*, 2005b; De Reu *et al.*, 2006) suggests that the number of pores does not influence trans-shell penetration by *S.* Enteritidis.

Eggs with hairline cracks were subjected to extensive trans-shell penetration by *S.* Enteritidis: 93% of the eggshells with cracks were penetrated (Messens *et al.*, 2005b). Microcracks are much smaller (less than 5 μm in length) than hairline cracks and can be generated by routine egg handling since eggs collide with each other or with a part of the collecting machinery (Macleod *et al.*, 2006). The influence of the presence or absence of microcracks on trans-shell penetration by *S.* Enteritidis seemed to depend on strain, age and management system in the study by Leleu *et al.* (submitted). Thermal microcracks can be formed when eggs are rapidly cooled. Fajardo *et al.* (1995) reported that thermally induced microcracks influenced the ability of *S.* Enteritidis to penetrate into the egg contents. However this was subsequently refuted by Thompson *et al.* (2000) and by Chen *et al.* (2002).

The Shell Membranes

The shell membranes, separating the eggshell and the albumen, are built up of three distinct layers: the inner and outer membranes which consist of a network of randomly oriented fibres and a homogeneous third layer of electron-dense material called the limiting membrane (Bruce & Drysdale, 1994). These membranes act like filters and pose a temporary barrier to the inward movement of bacteria (Berrang *et al.*, 1999a). Of the two membranes, the inner membrane offers the greatest resistance to bacterial penetration, possibly because its inner surface is clothed with a limiting membrane (Board & Tranter, 1995).

Penetration of the shell membranes by *S.* Enteritidis is an infrequent process according to Chen *et al.* (1996) and cells remain trapped in the shell pores and/or shell membranes. Berrang *et al.* (1999b) suggested that the meshwork of the inner membrane might relate more with bacterial penetration than its density. Alternatively, the likelihood of bacterial penetration of these membranes might be more affected by other factors, such as the charge of the chemical structure of the membrane. It is worth mentioning that proteins with antibacterial properties have been associated with eggshell and shell membranes: lysozyme (Hincke *et al.*, 2000), ovotransferrin (Gautron *et al.*, 2001), and ovocalyxin-36 (Gautron *et al.*, 2006).

SURVIVAL WITHIN THE EGG

The albumen has many antimicrobial substances such as enzyme inhibitors (ovoinhibitor, ovostatin), vitamin sequesters (avidin), antibacterial proteins (lysozyme), and iron-limiting compounds (ovo-transferrin), and therefore is considered a stressful environment for *Salmonella* bacteria. When the egg is laid, the pH of the albumen ranges between 7.6-7.8, but it increases to 9.1-9.6 after three days of storage at ambient temperature due to loss of carbon dioxide. During storage, progressive changes occur also in albumen viscosity and vitelline membrane integrity. The survival and persistence of *S.* Enteritidis in egg albumen is not completely understood. Some studies have probed the ability of different *Salmonella* serovars to survive in albumen at chicken body temperature. Serovars Enteritidis, Typhimurium and Heidelberg were able to survive in the albumen for 24 h, while serovars Virchow and Hadar were much more susceptible to the albumen, and almost all bacteria were killed after 24 h (Gantois *et al.*, 2008a). Most studies have shown an improved survival of serovar Enteritidis in the albumen at 37ºC (Lu *et al.*, 2003; Clavijo *et al.*, 2006), while no remarkable differences in albumen survival were found between several Enteritidis phagotypes (Gast & Holt, 2001).

Clavijo *et al.* (2006) used transposon-mediated mutagenesis to identify genes important for association of *S.* Enteritidis with chicken eggs. A transposon mutant library was screened for mutants impaired in their ability to survive in egg albumen after 24h of incubation at 37°C. Thirty-six of the 2,850 mutants screened were consistently more susceptible to egg albumen than the wild-type strain. Their results suggest that genes involved in cell wall integrity and nucleic acid and amino acid metabolism are important for persistence in egg albumen (Table 1). Two regions unique to *S.* Enteriditis were identified, SEN4287 and Prot6E gene, which may encode a restriction endonuclease and a fimbrial biosynthesis protein respectively. Cloning SEN4287 into *S.* Typhimurium enhanced its survival in egg albumen compared to the parent (Clavijo *et al.* 2006).

Gantois and co-workers (2008b) employed an *in-vivo* expression technology (IVET) promoter trap strategy to identify genes expressed during oviduct colonization and egg contamination with *S.* Enteritidis. Twenty-five clones with *in-vivo* induced promoters were isolated from the oviduct tissue and from laid eggs, seven of which were isolated from both oviducts and eggs. Sequence analysis revealed that promoters included those of genes involved in cell membrane and cell wall integrity (*murA*, *peg-yohN*, *hflK*, *tatA*), stress responses (*uspBA*, *yrfI*), motility (*flgG*) and amino acid and nucleic acid metabolism (*lysC*, *glyA*, *gmpA* etc).

The lipopolysaccharide (LPS) structure seems to be a major factor determining *S.* Enteritidis survival because of its protective function against the bactericidal components present in albumen. The Enteritidis serovar is phenotypically pleomorphic with regard to LPS structure with variable ability to contaminate eggs (Guard-Petter *et al.*, 1999). The LPS has different degrees of glucosylation in the O-chain region displaying an unusual degree of intra-serovar diversity (Guard-Petter, 2001). The LPS O-chain glucosylation in *S.* Enteritidis is quickly lost in response to environmental conditions (Parker *et al.*, 2001). The glucosylated LPS O-chain appears to contribute to an extracellular matrix or biofilm rich in flagella and fimbriae. *S.* Enteritidis strains seem more prone to produce a glucosylated high-molecular-mass variant of LPS (HMM LPS), and this is apparently correlated with high cell-density growth, swarm cell differentiation and a high incidence of egg contamination (Guard-Petter, 2001). In contrast the LPS O-chain from *S.* Typhimurium is more homogeneous with a low degree of diversity, and has usually low molecular mass (LMM) LPS (Parker *et al.*, 2001; Guard-Bouldin *et al.*, 2004). Another fact that demonstrates the importance of the LPS in survival in the albumen is the participation of the *rfbH* gene, involved in lipopolysaccharide O-antigen synthesis. The *rfbH* gene was found to be transcriptionally induced during growth in whole eggs at room temperature (Gantois *et al.*, 2009a,b), and *Salmonella* cells deficient in *rfbH* were immediately killed after inoculation in albumen at 42ºC, while the wild-type strain was able to survive in albumen for 24h.

Table 1. Main *S.* Enteritidis genes implicated in survival in the egg and oviduct colonization

Link to survival in the EGG	Functional category	Genes	Reference
Mutants affected in growth in egg albumen	Cell wall structure or function	SEN3892, *prgH*, *glnH*, *prgJ*, *proY*, *modF*, *bcfC*, *spaP*, *waaJ*, *yijC*	Clavijo *et al.* 2006
	Putative cell wall proteins	SEN1188, *yigQ*, SEN1861, STM3980, SEN0784, SEN1204	Clavijo *et al.* 2006
	Metabolism	*ordL*, *tdk*, *yejD*, *ydiB*, *ybdL*, *tyrR*, *cadA*, *lysC*	Clavijo *et al.* 2006
	Unknown function	SEN2128, SEN2997, *ygdI*, SEN2263, *ybbN*, *rssC*	Clavijo *et al.* 2006
	S. Enteritidis specific genes	SEN4287, Prot6E	Clavijo *et al.* 2006
	Nucleases involved in DNA repair	*yafD*, *xthA*	Lu *et al.*, 2003
	Motility proteins	*fliC*, *motAB*	Baron *et al.* 1997; Cogan *et al.*, 2004
	Fimbria protein	*agfA*	Cogan *et al.*, 2004;
	Iron acquisition proteins	*entF*, *feoAB*	Kang *et al.* 2006
	LPS synthesis	*rfbH*	Gantois *et al.* 2009b
Promoters induced in oviduct tissue and laid eggs	Metabolic	*folC*, *lysC*, *asnS*, *glyA*, *leuS*, *valS*, *serS*, *aceA*, *purA*, *tmk*, *ndkD*, *dnaX*, *rpoZ*, *gpmA*	Gantois *et al.* 2008b
	Motility	*flgG*	Gantois *et al.* 2008b
	Cell membrane and cell wall integrity	*tatA*, *hflK*, *peg-yohN*, *murA*	Gantois *et al.* 2008b
	Regulator	*lrp*	Gantois *et al.* 2008b
	Stress	*uspBA*, *yrfI*	Gantois *et al.* 2008b
	Virulence plasmid	*repB*, *tap*, *repA*	Gantois *et al.* 2008b
	Unknown function	STY3802, *ygfA*	Gantois *et al.* 2008b

The role of the *yafD* and *xthA* genes in conferring protection against the bactericidal activity of egg albumen has also been demonstrated (Lu *et al.*, 2003). Both YafD and XthA are nucleases involved in repairing DNA lesions generated by egg albumen. *S.* Enteritidis mutants lacking either gene were more susceptible to egg albumen. Another *S.* Enteritidis-specific endonuclease supposedly conferring improved survival in comparison to *S.*

Typhimurium is SEN4287 (Clavijo *et al.* 2006). Flagella are also important determinants and contribute to survival in albumen and growth in yolk as they can facilitate *Salmonella* migration towards the vitelline membrane (Cogan *et al.*, 2004). Non-motile mutants, such as Δ*fliC* and Δ*motAB* mutants, were not able to move through the albumen and growth did not occur (Cogan *et al.*, 2004). This inability to grow is also observed in non-motile serovars such as *S.* Gallinarum and *S.* Pullorum. Curli fimbriae are adhesive cellular appendages expressed by *Salmonella* which bind a variety of components, such as the glycoproteins (fibronectin) present in the vitelline membrane. Curli fimbriae-deficient strains (Δ*agfA* mutants) were less efficient in yolk invasion and displayed high-level growth in significantly fewer eggs than those able to express curli (Cogan *et al.*, 2004).

Salmonella has iron-acquisition systems for both ferric and ferrous iron to overcome iron chelation by ovotransferrin. The *ent* operon is responsible for the synthesis of enterobactin, the main siderophore of *Salmonella* (*ent*F encodes a subunit of enterobactin synthase; *ton*B encodes part of the TonB–ExbB–ExbD complex, required for the transport of ferric siderophores; *feo*A and *feo*B genes encode the ferrous uptake system). Iron-acquisition mutants of *S.* Enteritidis (Δ*ent*F and Δ*feo*AB) also showed decreased survival in egg albumen (Kang *et al.*, 2006).

The exact basis of the increased resistance of *S.* Enteriditis to egg albumen is unknown. It is possible that *S.* Enteriditis may have unique "egg-resistant genes" that are absent in *S.* Typhimurium. Comparison of the entire genome sequences of *S.* Typhimurium LT2 and *S.* Enteritidis PT4 revealed that while they share 3,991 "core genes", there are 399 LT2-specific genes and 266 PT4-specific genes (Wang et al 2010). It is also possible that genes may be differentially regulated between the serovars. Wang *et al.* (2010) recently examined the transcriptomic responses of *S.* Enteriditis and *S.* Typhimurium to chlorine treatments and found that while the majority of the genes whose expression changed are "core genes" the serovars differed in the responses of 33 stress-related genes and 19 virulence associated genes. Similar microarray analyses with egg albumen would reveal whether genes necessary for survival in eggs are differentially regulated in serovars Enteriditis and Typhimurium.

CONCLUSIONS

The natural defences of the egg are not entirely sufficient to prevent penetration and survival of *Salmonella enterica* serovars. *S.* Enteritidis is the most relevant serovar linked to human salmonellosis cases caused by consumption of eggs and egg products. This serovar is unique in the way that it can pass into the egg and multiply inside it without inducing noticeable changes. This review compiles the main research articles published in the last decades to understand the mechanisms by which *S.* Enteritidis contaminates chicken eggs much more successfully than any other *Salmonella* serovar.

Salmonella serovars must be able to cope with stresses encountered in their various ecological niches as well as in their hosts in order to persist and cause disease. In the case of avian salmonellosis, following the systemic dispersion and the colonization of the reproductive tract, *S.* Enteritidis cells are faced to the complex antimicrobial machinery of the egg. Therefore, in addition to the "true" virulence factors (e.g. invasins and toxins), other factors involved in environmental stress management are essential and may also be considered as directly influencing the outcome of the infection. However, these are not strictly 'virulence factors' and may be more correctly regarded as 'niche factors'. The recent availability of numerous genome sequences and the development of novel molecular methodologies have lead to an increasing number of genomics-driven transcriptomics and proteomics studies, from which the functions of different genes and macromolecules have been predicted. As a result, several response and regulatory systems have been identified as part of the defensive strategies used by pathogenic bacteria to cope with the harsh conditions of the host. During the last few years the search for biomarkers for bacterial resistance and virulence has emerged as an indispensable tool for the design of rational therapeutic and diagnostic strategies, as they can be used to predict the state of biological systems or processes. This review article identifies those genes essential for *S.* Enteritidis colonization of hen's eggs and persistence in the harsh conditions of the egg albumen, which could be considered as biomarkers appropriate for the design of ambitious strategies for the prevention of salmonellosis.

Acknowledgements

Álvarez-Ordóñez A. gratefully acknowledges the financial support from the "Alfonso Martín Escudero" Foundation.

References

Baron F, Gautier M & Brule G (1997) Factors involved in the inhibition of growth of *Salmonella enteritidis* in liquid egg white. *J Food Prot* 60: 1318-1323.

Barrow PA & Lovell MA (1991) Experimental infection of egg-laying hens with *Salmonella enteritidis* phage type 4. *Avian Pathol* 20: 335-348.

Berrang ME, Cox NA, Frank JF & Buhr RJ (1999a) Bacterial penetration of the eggshell and shell membranes of the chicken hatching egg: A review. *J Appl Poultry Res* 8: 499-504.

Berrang ME, Frank JF, Buhr RJ, Bailey JS & Cox NA (1999b) Eggshell membrane structure and penetration by *Salmonella* Typhimurium. *J Food Prot* 62: 73-76.

Bichler LA, Nagaraja KV & Halvorson DA (1996) *Salmonella enteritidis* in eggs, cloacal swab specimens, and internal organs of experimentally infected White Leghorn chickens. *Am J Vet Res* 57: 489-495.

Board RG & Halls NA (1973) The cuticle: a barrier to liquid and particle penetration of the shell of hen's eggs. *Brit Poultry Sci* 14: 69-97.

Board RG & Tranter HS (1995) The microbiology of eggs. *Egg Science and Technology* (Stadelman WJ & Cotterrill OJ, eds), pp. 81-104. The Haworth Press, London, UK.

Board RG, Loseby S & Miles VR (1979) A note on microbial growth on hen egg-shells. *Brit Poultry Sci* 20: 413-420.

Bruce J & Drysdale EM (1994) Trans-shell transmission. *Microbiology of the Avian Egg* (Board RG & Fuller R, eds), pp. 63-91. Chapman & Hall, London, UK.

Chen J, Clarke RC & Griffiths MW (1996) Use of luminescent strains of *Salmonella enteritidis* to monitor contamination and survival in eggs. *J Food Prot* 59: 915-921.

Chen HQ, Anantheswaran RC & Knabel SJ (2002) Effect of rapid cooling of shell eggs on microcrack development, penetration of *Salmonella enteritidis*, and eggshell strength. *J Food Process Pres* 26: 57-73.

Clavijo RI, Loui C, Andersen GL, Riley LW & Lu S (2006) Identification of genes associated with survival of *Salmonella enterica* serovar Enteritidis in chicken egg albumen. *Appl Environ Microbiol* 72: 1055–1064.

Cogan TA & Humphrey TJ (2003) The rise and fall of *Salmonella* Enteritidis in the UK. *J Appl Microbiol* 94: 114S-119S.

Cogan TA, Jørgensen FH, Lappin-Scott M, Benson CE, Woodward MJ & Humphrey TJ (2004) Flagella and curli fimbriae are important for the growth of *Salmonella enterica* serovars in hen eggs. *Microbiol* 150: 1063-1071.

De Buck J, Van Immerseel F, Haesebrouck F & Ducatelle R (2004) Colonization of the chicken reproductive tract and egg contamination by *Salmonella*. *J Appl Microbiol* 97: 233-245.

De Reu K, Grijspeerdt K, Messens W, Heyndrickx A, Uyttendaele M, Debevere J & Herman L (2006) Eggshell factors influencing eggshell penetration and whole egg contamination by different bacteria, including *Salmonella enteritidis*. *Int J Food Microbiol* 112: 253-260.

EFSA (2008) A quantitative microbiological risk assessment on *Salmonella* in meat: Source attribution for human salmonellosis from meat. *EFSA J* 625: 1–32.

EFSA (2011) The European Union Summary Report on Trends and Sources of Zoonoses, Zoonotic agents and food-borne outbreaks in 2009. *EFSA J* 9: 2090.

Fajardo TA, Anantheswaran RC, Puri VM & Knabel SJ (1995) Penetration of *Salmonella enteritidis* into eggs subjected to rapid cooling. *J Food Prot* 58: 473-477.

Gantois I, Eeckhaut V, Pasmans F, Haesebrouck F, Ducatelle R & Van Immerseel F (2008a). A comparative study on the pathogenesis of egg contamination by different serotypes of *Salmonella*. *Avian Pathol* 37: 399–406.

Gantois I, Ducatelle R, Pasmans F, Haesebrouck F & Van Immerseel F (2008b). *Salmonella enterica* Serovar Enteritidis Genes Induced during Oviduct Colonization and Egg Contamination in Laying Hens. *Appl Environ Microbiol* 74: 6616-6622.

Gantois I, Ducatelle R, Pasmans F, Haesebrouck F, Gast R, Humphrey TJ & Van Immerseel F (2009a) Mechanisms of egg contamination by *Salmonella* Enteritidis. *FEMS Microbiol Rev* 33: 718-738.

Gantois I, Ducatelle R, Pasmans F, Haesebrouck F & Van Immerseel F (2009b). The *Salmonella* Enteritidis lipopolysaccharide biosynthesis gene *rfbH* is required for survival in egg albumen. *Zoonoses Public Hlth* 56: 145–149.

Gast RK & Beard CW (1990) Production of *Salmonella* Enteritidis contaminated eggs by experimentally infected hens. *Avian Dis* 34: 438-446.

Gast RK & Holt PS (2001) Multiplication in egg yolk and survival in egg albumen of *Salmonella enterica* serotype Enteritidis strains of phage types 4, 8, 13a, and 14b. *J Food Prot* 64: 865-8.

Gautron J, Hincke MT, Panheleux M, Garcia-Ruiz JM, Boldicke T & Nys Y (2001) Ovotransferrin is a matrix protein of the hen eggshell membranes and basal calcified layer. *Connect Tissue Res* 42: 255-267.

Gautron J, Nys Y, McKee MD & Hincke M (2006) Ovocalyxin-36 is a novel chicken eggshell protein related to lipopolyssaccharide-binding proteins (LBP) bactericidal permeability-increasing proteins (BPI), and Plunc family proteins. *Poultry Sci* 85: 21-21.

Guard-Bouldin J, Gast RK, Humphrey TJ, Henzler DJ, Morales C & Coles K (2004) Subpopulation characteristics of egg-contaminating *Salmonella enterica* serovar Enteritidis as defined by the lipopolysaccharide O chain. *Appl Environ Microbiol* 70: 2756-63.

Guard-Petter J (2001) The chicken, the egg and *Salmonella enteritidis*. *Environ Microbiol* 3: 421-430.

Guard-Petter J, Parker CT, Asokan K & Carlson RW (1999) Clinical and veterinary isolates of *Salmonella enterica* serovar Enteritidis defective in lipopolysaccharide o-chain polymerization. *Appl Environ Microbiol* 65: 2195–2201.

Hincke MT, Gautron J, Panheleux M, Garcia-Ruiz J, McKee MD & Nys Y (2000) Identification and localization of lysozyme as a component of eggshell membranes and eggshell matrix. *Matrix Biol* 19: 443-453.

Hohmann EL (2001) Nontyphoidal salmonellosis. *Clin Infect Dis* 32: 263-269.

Humphrey TJ (1994) Contamination of egg-shell and contents with *Salmonella* Enteritidis - a review. *Int J Food Microbiol* 21: 31-40.

Kang H, Loui C, Clavijo RI, Riley LW & Lu S (2006) Survival characteristics of *Salmonella enterica* serovar Enteritidis in chicken egg albumen. *Epidemiol Infect* 134: 967-976.

Keller LH, Schifferli DM, Benson CE, Aslam S & Eckroade RJ (1997) Invasion of chicken reproductive tissues and forming eggs is not unique to *Salmonella enteritidis*. *Avian Dis* 41: 535-539.

Leleu S, Bain M, Herman L, *et al.* (submitted) The effect of microcracks and cuticle deposition on the trans-shell penetration of *Salmonella enterica* serovar Enteritidis through hen's eggs.

Lu S, Killoran PB & Riley LW (2003) Association of *Salmonella enterica* serovar Enteritidis yafD with resistance to chicken egg albumen. *Infect Immun* 71: 6734-6741.

Macleod N, Bain MM & Hancock JW (2006) The mechanics and mechanisms of failure of hens' eggs. *Int J Fracture* 142: 29-41.

Mayes FJ & Takeballi MA (1983) Microbial contamination of the hens egg - a review. *J Food Prot* 46: 1092-1098.

Mead P, Slutsker L, Dietz V, McCaig LF, Bresee JS, Shapiro C,Griffin PM & Tauxe RV (1999) Foodrelated illness and death in the United States. *Emerg Infect Dis* 5: 607-625.

Messens W, Grijspeerdt K & Herman L (2005a) Eggshell penetration by *Salmonella*: a review. *World Poultry Sci J* 61: 71-85.

Messens W, Grijspeerdt K & Herman L (2005b) Eggshell characteristics and penetration by *Salmonella enterica* serovar Enteritidis through the production period of a layer flock. *Brit Poultry Sci* 46: 694-700.

Messens W, Grijspeerdt K, De Reu K, De Ketelaere B, Mertens K, Bamelis F, Kemps B, De Baerdemaeker J, Decuypere E & Herman L (2007) Eggshell penetration of various types of hens' eggs by *Salmonella enterica* serovar Enteritidis. *J Food Prot* 70: 623-628.

Miyamoto T, Horie T, Baba E, Sasai K, Fukata T & Arakawa A (1998) *Salmonella* penetration through eggshell associated with freshness of laid eggs and refrigeration. *J Food Prot* 61: 350-353.

Nascimento VP (1992) The ease of translocation of *Salmonella enteritidis* through the eggshell wall: an immunocytochemical/ultrastructural study. Thesis, University of Glasgow, Glasgow.

Nascimento VP, Cranstoun S & Solomon SE (1992) Relationship between shell structure and movement of *Salmonella enteritidis* across the eggshell wall. *Brit Poultry Sci* 33: 37-48.

Parker CT, Liebana E, Henzler DJ & Guard-Petter J (2001). Lipopolysaccharide O-antigen microheterogeneity of *Salmonella* serotypes Enteritidis and Typhimurium. *Environ Microbiol* 3: 332-342.

Sauter EA & Petersen CF (1974) Effect of egg-shell quality on penetration by various salmonellae. *Poultry Sci* 53: 2159-2162.

Smeltzer TI, Orange K, Peel B & Runge G (1979) Bacterial penetration in floor and nest box eggs from meat and layer birds. *Aust Vet J* 55: 592-593.

Thompson JF, Knutson J, Ernst RA, Kuney D, Riemann H, Himathongkham S & Zeidler G (2000) Rapid cooling of shell eggs. *J Appl Poultry Res* 9: 258-268.

Vázquez-Torres A, Jones-Carson J, Baumler AJ, Falkow S, Valdivia R, Brown W, Le M, Berggren R, Parks WT & Fang FC (1999) Extraintestinal dissemination of *Salmonella* by CD18-expressing phagocytes. *Nature* 401: 804-808.

Wang S, Phillippy AM, Deng K, Rui X, Li Z, Tortorello ML & Zhang W (2010) Transcriptomic responses of *Salmonella enterica* serovars Enteritidis and Typhimurium to chlorine-based oxidative stress. *Appl Environ Microbiol* 76: 5013-5024.

In: Salmonella: Classification, Genetics and Disease Outbreaks ISBN: 978-1-61942-928-4
Editors: Adelaide S. Monte, Paulo Eduardo De Santos

Chapter 11

GENOME COMPARISONS OF SALMONELLA: FUNCTIONAL CONSERVATION OF GENES WITHIN PATHOGENICITY ISLANDS

Alison Garner, Anish Bavishi, Cole Anderson, Madhusudan Choudhary and Aaron M. Lynne*

Department of Biological Sciences, Sam Houston State University, Huntsville, TX, US

ABSTRACT

Members of *Salmonella* are able to infect a wide range of hosts with some subspecies and serovars being host-specific while others are wide host range organisms. Salmonella is most commonly associated with humans, food animals (bovine, swine and poultry) and reptiles such as turtles, lizards, and iguanas. The exact nature of this diversity towards host susceptibility is still unclear. In the present study, whole genomes and subsequent protein homologues from Salmonella Pathogenicity Islands 1 and 2 of several *Salmonella* serovars were analyzed for their structure-function constraints to identify evolutionary pressures. Whole genome alignment showed no explicit pattern of rearrangement, phylogenetic trees of pathogenicity islands genes revealed that the branch lengths were very small, and functional constraint analysis revealed that most of these genes were operating under negative selection. The results indicate that genes of Salmonella Pathogenicity Island 1 and 2 are functionally conserved across serovars, regardless of host range. Thus, the present result suggests that genes located in the pathogenic islands may not be sufficient solely for host specificity and pathogenesis, and other accessory proteins from different strains as well as host factors may play an important role in influencing the severity of the outcome of the diseases.

Keywords: *Salmonella enterica,* Salmonella Pathogenicity Islands, Genome, Functional Constraints

---

* Correspondence Address: Department of Biological Sciences, Sam Houston State University, Huntsville, TX 77341. Email: aaronlynne@shsu.edu.

1. INTRODUCTION

It is accepted that, following divergence from a common ancestor with *E. coli* 120-160 million years ago, the ancestors of current S*almonellae* remained associated with reptiles until acquisition of the *inv/spa* genes allowed them to become intracellular pathogens (Li et al., 1995). Most studies suggest that, after divergence into species and subspecies adapted to either warm-blooded or cold-blooded animals, additional virulence genes were then acquired by horizontal transfer from other microorganisms, resulting in the plethora of subspecies and serovars extant today. Previous studies have demonstrated that approximately half of the putative horizontally acquired genes in Salmonella were acquired prior to the divergence of *Salmonella enterica* and *Salmonella bongori* from a common ancestral species; three-fourths of these genes are thought to be unique to serovars of *Salmonella enterica* subspecies. In addition, relatively recent transfer events are thought to consist predominantly of acquisition of prophage elements demonstrating comparable base composition due to host adaptation rather than amelioration (Vernikos et al., 2007).

It has been shown that typical *Salmonella* serovars have between 80 and 100% genetic relatedness, despite a high degree of variability in both host adaptability and pathogenesis (Bakowski et al., 2008). Additionally, Salmonella shares many genes with *E. coli*, having 80% to 85% identity between homologous genes (Edwards et al., 2002). Analysis of orthologous genes, similar genetic sequences occurring in different species as a result of common ancestry, has shown divergence in *Salmonella* serovar nucleotide sequences of only 3.8% to 4.6 % (Baumler et al. 1998). Such overall similarity implies that small genomic differences must initiate the significant variability observed in host adaptation and virulence.

Much of the virulence capability of S*almonella* is attributed to large chromosomal genetic elements called Salmonella Pathogenicity Islands (SPI's), which harbor numerous virulence factor genes (Amavisit et al., 2003). The genes on these islands are involved in adherence, invasion, intracellular survival, and toxicity (Eswarappa et al., 2008). Of the five definitively identified islands, SPI-1 and SPI-2 are most highly characterized. The genes of SPI-1 function in initial invasion into host intestinal epithelial cells; genes of SPI-2 are implicated in intracellular survival, replication and systemic spread (Foley et al, 2008).*Salmonella* Pathogenicity Island 1 is a well-characterized 40-kb island located at centisome 63 on the bacterial chromosome. Research suggests that SPI-1 functions are crucial in the initial intestinal phase of all *Salmonella* infections, whether they remain gastrointestinal in nature or progress to systemic disease (Lostroh and Lee, 2001). Principal functions of SPI-1 include encoding of regulatory genes, production of components required for formation of a Type Three Secretion System (T3SS) and numerous effector proteins subsequently secreted by the Type One Secretion System (T1SS). These effector proteins function as virulence factors that facilitate uptake of the bacteria into intestinal epithelial cells (Hansen-Wester and Hensel, 2001). *Salmonella* Pathogenicity Island 2 is another large genomic region located at centisome 30 of the chromosome. Like, SPI-1, *Salmonella* Pathogenicity Island 2 genes encode a Type Three Secretion System; however, the SPI-2 system functions primarily in the systemic spread of the disease through facilitation of survival in host cells and intramacrophage growth and lymphatic spread. Most importantly, SPI-2 proteins aid in formation of Salmonella Containing Vacuoles (SCV's), membranous compartments inside the host cell epithelial intestinal cells that harbor *Salmonella* after it has entered the cell, thus allowing it to replicate (Bakowski et al., 2008).

The exact physiological mechanisms by which such genetically similar organisms as the *Salmonella enterica* serovars develop host-specificity or promiscuity, as well as create such a wide variety of disease symptoms in respective hosts, remains a perplexing puzzle in *Salmonella* research (Kingsley and Baumler, 2000). *S.* Typhimurium, *S.* Enteritidis and *S.* Heidleberg are typically wide-host range organisms, whereas *S.* Cholearaesuis is primarily a disease of swine, *S.* Gallinarum prefers poultry, *S.* Dublin has adapted to cattle and *S.* Typhi affects only humans (Eswarapp et al, 2008). Observed symptoms in hosts may range from self-limiting gastroenterititis to focal infections, flu-like typhoid and bacterimia (Foley et al., 2008). Host-specific serovars may occasionally infect novel hosts, causing a wide array of symptoms. As an example, *S.* Choleraesuis causes a range of diseases in swine, such as cholera-like enterocolitis, respiratory illness, septicemia and reproductive disorders; however, infection in humans commonly results in endovascular infection, leading to an infective aneurysm (Chiu et al., 2005).

Since several subspecies and serovars of *Salmonella* have recently been completely sequenced and fully annotated, a comprehensive DNA sequence analysis has become possible.

The goal of the present study is analyze whole genomes of *Salmonella enteric* representing serotypes that either have a wide or narrow host range for insights into the evolution host adaptation and virulence. Genomes were analyzed for gross levels of DNA sequence alterations and sequence identity using Mauve 2.20. Several protein homologues from corresponding pathogenic islands (SPIs) were examined for their evolutionary relationships using phylogenetic analysis. Also, the whole genome sequences were analyzed in order to identify the regions that have possibly been acquired by horizontal gene transfers (HGTs). In addition, gene homologues were further analyzed for their structure-function constraints in order to identify the evolutionary pressures experienced by these gene homologues. Results were discussed for the origin and evolution of these strains as well as the evolution of genes located in pathogenic island that would help identify genes for further molecular characterization.

2. Materials and Methods

2.1. Global Genome Alignments

Global genome comparisons can provide insight in to the differences and variability among *Salmonella enterica* serovars. Several pairwise comparisons of the complete genome sequences of five *Salmonella enterica* serovars (S. Cholerasuis str. SC-B67, S. Dublin str. CT_ 02021853, S. Enteritidis str. P125109, S. Typhi str. CT18, S. Typhimurium str. LT2) were conducted using Mauve 2.2.0 (Darling et al., 2004). Whole genome sequence data was obtained from the National Center for Biological Information (NCBI) Database. A summary of characteristics including Accession number, host range, chromosome size and G+C content for the *Salmonella* strains used in this study can be found in Table 1.

Table 1. Salmonella enterica serovar characteristics

Salmonella enterica subsp. enterica serovar	Accession #	Host	Chromosome Size (bp)	Chromosome G+C Content (%)
S. Choleraesuis str. SC-B67	NC_006905.1	Swine	4,755,700	52.1
S. Dublin str. CT_02021853	NC_011205.1	Cattle	4,842,908	52.2
S. Enteritidis str. P125109	NC_011294.1	Wide	4,685,848	52.0
S. Gallinarum str. 287/91	NC_011274.1	Poultry	4,740,000	52.2
S. Heidelberg str. SL476	NC_011083.1	Wide	4,888,768	53.0
S. Typhi str. CT18	NC_003198.1	Human	4,809,037	51.9
S. Typhimurium str. LT2	NC_003197.1	Wide	4,857,432	53.0

Mauve is a global alignment software that can be used to identify regions of similarity throughout entire genome sequences (Darling et al., 2004). As it detects features such as inversions and translocations, it is able to align genomes that have significantly diverged from one another.Its algorithm determines regions of similarity known as Multiple Maximal Unique Matches (multi-MUMs) and then classifies these areas into Local Collinear Blocks (LCBs). These LCBs possesses homologous nucleotide sequences shared by the genomes under comparison and therefore serve as anchors for an alignment. An initial seed size of 15 was utilized. Seed size essentially represents the minimum number of matching nucleotides that Mauve will recognize. Since an LCB weight that is at least 3 times the initial seed length guards against false collections and matches (Darling et al., 2004), a minimum LCB weight of 45 was used. The minimum LCB weight is an important factor because higher minimum LCB weights facilitate the identification of rearrangements that have a higher likelihood of existence while lower minimum weights are more sensitive to smaller genome rearrangements. Since Mauve aligns sequences only once from one genome to each of the others, the algorithm deals only with orthologous regions. Orthologous regions are those that have descended from a common ancestor and are in contrast to paralogous regions, which are related across duplication events. The number of common LCBs (CLCBs), the number of deletions within the CLCBs, the total length of the CLCBs, and the identity retained within the CLCBs were extracted for each Mauve alignment. The total length of the CLCBs was obtained by summing the length of all of the nucleotide strands contained within each CLCB while the identity retained within the CLCBs was computed by dividing the common nucleotide strands by the total length of the CLCBs.

2.2. Phylogenetic Analysis

Analysis of individual virulence genes in *Salmonella* serovars can provide insight into the roles of certain genes and can reveal differences between gene rates of evolution..

As such, key genes in SPI-1 and SPI-2 were phylogenetically analyzed to determine their rates of evolution in different serovars. Gene sequences were obtained for seven serovars: S. Choleraesuis str. SC-B67, S. Dublin str. CT_02021853, S. Enteritidis str. P125109, S. Gallinarum str. 287/91, S. Heidelberg str. SL476, S. Typhi str. CT18, and S. Typhimurium str. LT2. Only genes that had been annotated in the serovars or for which a reliable homolog match was available were used for reliability and to avoid inconsistent alignments. In particular, if a gene was not found to be annotated or outlined in the NCBI Database for a particular serovar, genes in other serovars coding for the desired functions were used to search these genomes by BLASTN (Altschul et al., 1990) and the necessary gene homologs were derived accordingly.

For SPI-1, trees for *hilA, invA, invC, invE, invH, orgA, prgH, prgJ, sipA, sipB, spaN, spaO, spaP, spaR,* and *spaS* were constructed. For SPI-2, trees for *sifA, ssaC, ssaH, ssaL, ssaM, ssaO, ssaP, ssaS, ssaV, sseA, sseB, sseC, ssrA, ttrA,* and *ttrB* were constructed.

Geneious 4.8, a multipurpose bioinformatics suite, was used to obtain and align the sequences (Drummond et al., 2010). The nucleotide sequences of the genes were aligned using MUSCLE (Edgar, 2004), a robust algorithm that is both quick and particular. PhyML (Guindon et al., 2009; Guindon et al., 2010; Guindon and Gascuel, 2003) was used to construct maximum likelihood (ML) trees for the gene alignments.

The Tamura-Nei substitution model was utilized as it incorporates features such as excess transitions, substitution rate variance, and dissimilar nucleotide frequencies (Tamura and Nei, 1993). Trees were optimized for length, rate, and topology.

2.3. Functional Constraints Analysis

In the evolution of organisms, point mutations of nucleotide bases in the genome may be more or less significant based on whether or not they result in insertions of a different amino acid into the translated protein, leading to subsequent changes in function. A synonymous substitution involves a change in a nucleotide within a codon that does not result in translation to a different amino acid. Nucleotide substitutions that resulting in replacement of the original amino acid with a different one are known as nonsynonymous substitutions. K_aK_s_Calculator is a software package that calculates nonsynonymous (K_a) and synonymous (K_s) rates and the nonsynonymous-synonymous ($\omega = K_a/K_s$) ratio (Zhang et al., 2006b). This program was used to explore the nature of functional constraints operating on several key virulence genes in SPI-1 (*hilA, invA, invC, invE, invH, orgA, prgH, prgJ, sipA, sipB, spaN, spaO, spaP, spaR, spaS*) and SPI-2 (*sifA, ssaC, ssaH, ssaL, ssaM, ssaO, ssaP, ssaS, ssaV, sseA, sseB, sseC, ssrA, ttrA, ttrB*). Nucleotide sequences for each gene were downloaded from the NCBI Database and were pairwise aligned against orthologous genes in other serovars using MUSCLE (Edgar, 2004). The alignments were transformed into the original DNA sequences and then each pair of DNA sequences was subjected to the K_aK_s_ Calculator (Zhang et al., 2006b). The rate ratio, ω, was calculated using the Modified Yang-Nielsen (MYN) method and under this method values of ω = 0.3, 1.0, and 3.0 were used as delineations for negative, neutral, and positive selection, respectively (Yang and Nielsen, 2000; Zhang et al., 2006a).

2.4. Horizontal Gene Transfer Analysis

Horizontal gene transfer estimates for the seven *Salmonella* serovars in this study were determined using three methods: Alien_hunter (Vernikos and Parkhill, 2006), Island-DIMOB

(Hsiao et al., 2003; Hsiao et al., 2005), and SIGI-HMM (Waack et al., 2006). Alien_hunter uses an interpolated variable order motif (IVOM) method to discover areas of compositional bias and probable HGT origin within genomes. Putative HGT regions are those that possess enough compositional bias to cross threshold level determined by the Alien_hunter algorithm. The original algorithm and software was developed for and used in several *Salmonella* serovars including comparisons with three serovars examined in this study: S.gallinarum 287/91, S.typhi CT18, and S.typhimurium LT2 (Vernikos and Parkhill, 2006). The Island-DIMOB method takes into account compositional features to determine regions of putative HGT origin (Hsiao et al., 2003; Hsiao et al., 2005) while the SIGI-HMM method employs hidden Markov models to expose potential HGT areas (Waack et al., 2006). Although Alien_hunter possesses high recall, it is imprecise as it presents many false positives whereas Island-DIMOB and SIGI-HMM are comparatively more accurate and precise but posses lower recall (Azad and Lawrence, 2007; Langille et al., 2008; Langille et al., 2010). The Island-DIMOB and SIGI-HMM estimates were provided through IslandViewer, a public web-based resource that provides HGT island information on a range of completed genomes in NCBI (Langille and Brinkman, 2009).

3. Result and Conclusion

3.1. Global Genome Analysis Reflects High Level of Genetic Identity

Figure 1 contains four example Mauve alignments for four different comparisons. Each alignment image depicts different genome patterns, as Figure 1A possesses no inversion while the other alignments possess one (Figure 1B), two (Figure 1C), or three (Figure 1D) inversions. There does not appear to be an explicit pattern, such as increased rearrangements, in the comparisons between wide-host range and narrow host-range serovars. However, genomic rearrangements do occur in SPI regions as evidenced in a comparison between host-adapted serovar, *S.* Typhi str. CT18, and host-promiscuous serovar, *S.* Typhimurium str. LT2. More specifically, as seen in Figure 1C, there are notable inversions in *S.* Typhi in relation to the homologous regions on *S.* Typhimurium that encompass Salmonella Pathogenicity Islands (SPIs) 2 and 5.

A summary of the Mauve data comparisons is located in Table 2. These Mauve pairwise comparisons revealed fairly high identity retention among the serovars with an average identity retention of 90.22%. Once again, no explicit pattern of divergence was found between host-adapted and host-promiscuous strains comparisons. However, the comparisons with *S.* Typhi str. CT18 seem to possess the lowest levels of identity retention – less than 87% - and a fairly high number of deletions among the organisms. It may be that *S.* Typhi is comparatively faster evolving than the other strains as an adaptation to its host (human) or by acquisition of prophage elements demonstrating comparable base composition due to host adaptation rather than amelioration (Vernikos et al., 2007).

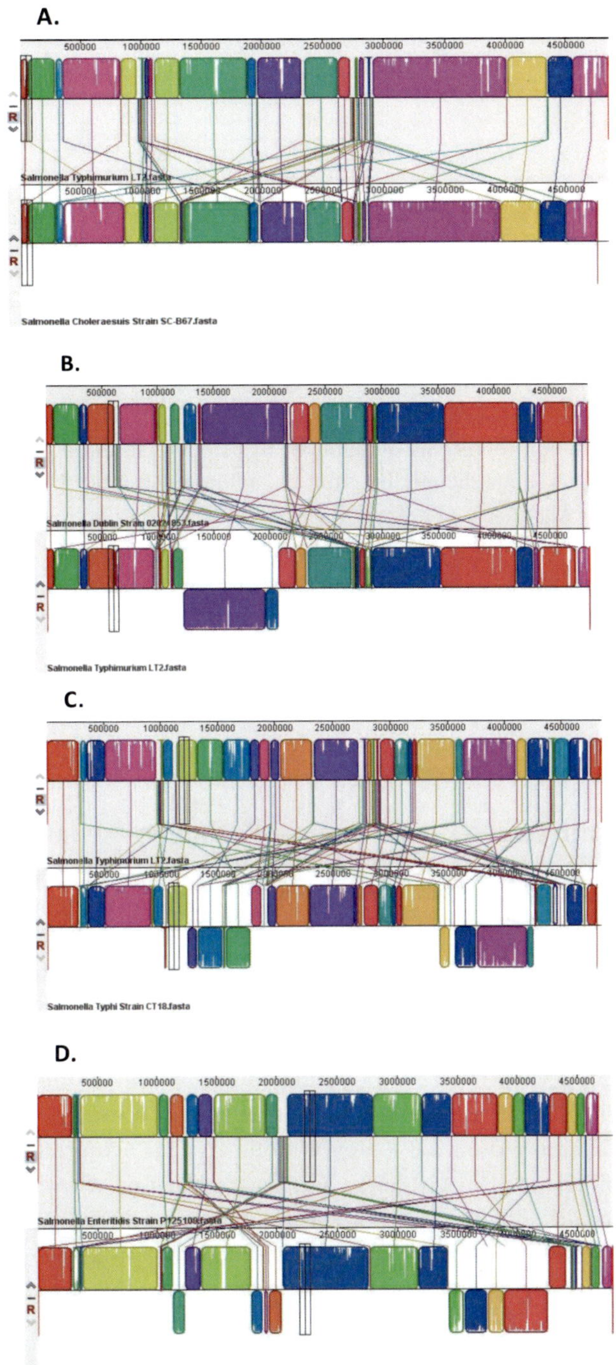

Figure 1. Four visual depictions of Mauve global genome alignments. The linked colored blocks represents local collinear blocks (LCBs) that are used to anchor the alignment. Inside the LCBs are similarity plots between the homologous regions. These provide a visual measure of the identity between the linked regions. Figure 1B, 1C, and 1D depict one, two, and three inversions, respectively. These inversions are readily identifiable as they are present on the opposite side of the line running horizontally for the second genome in each of the comparisons. The organism names for the compared genomes are visible beneath the horizontal line upon which the whole genome sequences rest.

Talbe 2. Summary of Mauve Data Comparisons

Serovar Comparison	# of CLCBs[1]	Deletions in CLCBs[2]	Length of CLCBs	% Identity Retained in CLCBs
S. Dublin str. CT_ 02021853 / S. Enteritidis str. P125109	26	32696:134046	4,805,234	96.01
S. Dublin str. CT_ 02021853 / S. Choleraesuis str. SC-B67	76	143869:206949	4,855,172	91.42
S. Enteritidis str. P125109 / S. Choleraesuis str. SC-B67	61	187419:185115	4,808,481	91.01
S. Typhi str. CT18 / S. Dublin str. CT_ 02021853	72	326913:235041	4,916,509	86.90
S. Typhi str. CT18 / S. Enteritidis str. P125109	57	266071:329715	4,890,669	86.24
S. Typhimurium str. LT2 / S. Choleraesuis str. SC-B67	65	190877:264318	4,955,990	89.61
S. Typhimurium str. LT2 / S. Dublin str. CT_ 02021853	72	155636:181232	4,887,128	91.98
S. Typhimurium str. LT2 / S. Enteritidis str. P125109	75	132636:211170	4,824,855	91.81
S. Typhimurium str. LT2 / S. Typhi str. CT18	80	224552:334353	4,912,439	86.98

[1] CLCBs = Common Local Collinear Blocks.

[2] The number before the colon represents the number of deletions in the organism before the forward slash in the first column while the number after the colon represents the number of deletions in the organism after the forward slash.

Also given that the lengths of the common LCBs (CLCBs) are larger than the genome lengths of the serovars in many cases, there is a sizeable level of horizontal gene transfer or gene duplication occurring in these organisms. This is especially noteworthy given the fairly highly level of deletions within these organisms that offsets the insertion or acquisition of new genetic material.

3.2. Horizontal Transferred Genes within Pathogenic Island Are Highly Conserved

Table 3 details the HGT estimates for the *Salmonella* serovars by three different methods. Results revealed that approximately 5% of genomic regions representing pathogentic islands resulted from horizontal gene transfer from other species. This level of horizontal gene transfer is not unusual in many bacterial species, however this low level of gene transfer resulted pathogenic properties. This result validated the earlier finding that less than 10% of core genes show evidence of homologous recombination; however, positive selection and homologous recombination may drive the evolution of genes acquired by horizontal transfer, leading to the variability noted in virulence and host restriction (Soyer et al., 2009). Finally, relatively recent transfer events are thought to consist predominantly of acquisition of prophage elements demonstrating comparable base composition due to host adaptation rather than amelioration (Vernikos et al., 2007). These islands are assumed to been acquired by horizontal transfer since their average G+C content of 42% is generally lower than that of the typical *Salmonella* genome of approximately 52-53%. Although G+C content is not the definitive characteristic for the HGTs, functional conservation of these regions may be an important factor for keeping these genes integrity.

Phylogenetic trees illustrate the topographical relationships and evolutionary distances between selected virulence genes. Figure 2 depicts an example phylogenetic tree for a gene (*invH*) in an SPI. Analysis of phylogenetic trees revealed that the branch lengths were very small (almost 0 in some cases), thus they do not demonstrate significant evolutionary relationships among these subspecies. The small branch lengths reflected the low level of amino acid changes between protein sequences that may have resulted by different mechanisms. These genes were originated relatively recent, and gene sequences have not yet diverged enough to show high level of genetic divergence. Alternatively, these gene homologues have been functionally constrained, and are possibly under purifying selection.

The functional constraints analysis for genes in SPI-1 (Figure 3) and genes in SPI-2 (Figure 4) revealed that most genes in these islands are operating under negative or purifying selection.

Many alignments did not give an ω value either because they were unalignable for some reason or no divergence between the gene sequences had occurred to provide usable substitution rate information.

Table 3. Horizontal GeneTransfer Estimates Among Serovars.

Salmonella enterica subsp. enterica serovar	Alien_hunter Estimates		Island-DIMOB Estimates		SIGI-HMM Estimates	
	Total Length of HGT Regions	% of Total Genome	Total Length of HGT Regions	% of Total Genome	Total Length of HGT Regions	% of Total Genome
S. Choleraesuis str. SC-B67	687,571	14.46	248,902	5.23	281,621	5.92
S. Dublin str. CT_02021853	827,986	17.10	226,574	4.68	230,918	4.77
S. Enteritidis str. P125109	818,421	17.47	158,844	3.39	249,350	5.32
S. Gallinarum str. 287/91	666,261	14.06	172,762	3.64	238,446	5.03
S. Heidelberg str. SL476	991,356	20.28	237,363	4.86	322,684	6.60
S. Typhi str. CT18	980,086	20.38	291,251	6.06	239,428	4.98
S. Typhimurium str. LT2	827,585	17.04	195,023	4.01	245,983	5.06

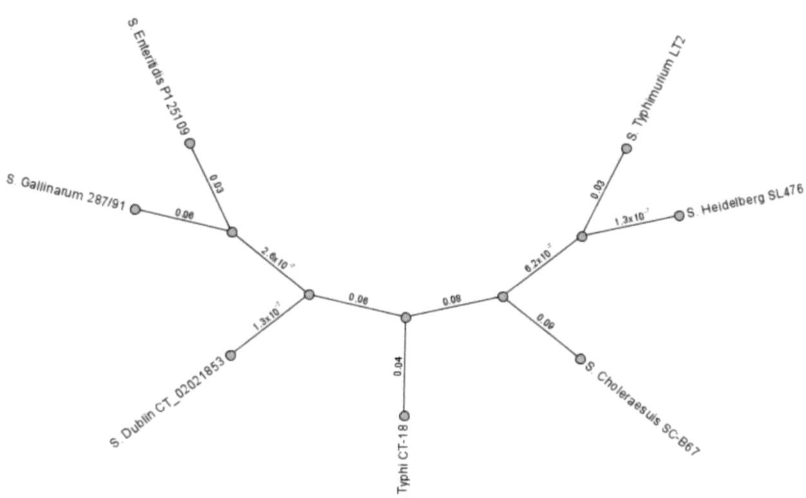

Figure 2. An example maximum likelihood phylogenetic tree for the gene *invH* located in SPI-1. The numbers on the branches represent substitutions per site. This gene is fairly conserved among serovars as evidenced by the low substitution rates.

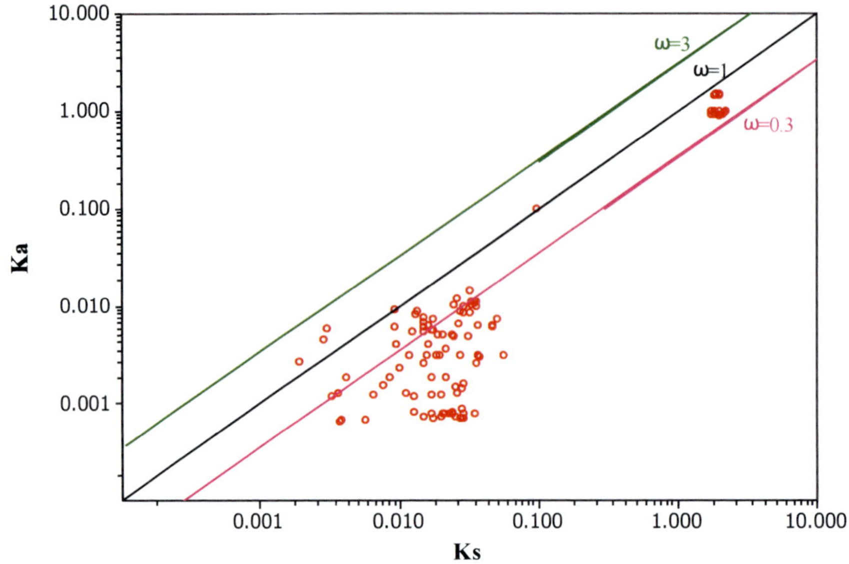

Figure 3. K_a-K_s correlation of genes in Pathogenicity Island 1 (SP-1) among different *Salmonella* serovars. K_a and K_s values were estimated using the MYN (Modified Yang-Nielsen) algorithm. ω = 0.3, 1, and 3 were used for negative, neutral, and positive selection, respectively.

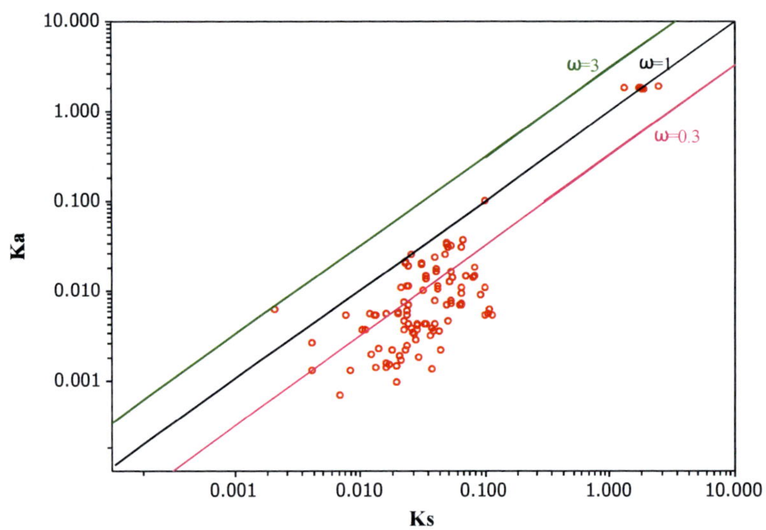

Figure 4. K_a-K_s correlation of genes in Pathogenicity Island 2 (SP-2) among different *Salmonella* serovars. K_a and K_s values were estimated using the MYN (Modified Yang-Nielsen) algorithm. ω = 0.3, 1, and 3 were used for negative, neutral, and positive selection, respectively.

Those were removed from the dataset and only those with ω values were analyzed. SPI-1 genes had an average ω = 0.2 while SPI-2 genes had an average ω = 0.4. Given the high similarity among the serovars and the genes themselves, such constraints should be expected. This would indicate that the majority of genes in SPI-1 and SPI-2 are functionally constrained regardless of host range. However, some comparisons revealed that a few genes in both islands did not follow this paradigm and may be operating under neutral or positive selection in certain serovars. More specifically, in SPI-1, comparisons revealed two genes possibly operating under neutral selection: *sipA* and *spaN*. In SPI-2, *sseA* possessed ω values greater than one in two comparisons, but more notably, a comparison with *sseC* almost neared a ω = 3, indicating near positive selection. As such, these genes may operate under these relaxed selection mechanisms because they play roles in adaption or niche specialization. Further experiment will be required to test whether these genes play important roles in host adaptation.

ACKNOWLEDGEMENTS

We thank Lin Lin for her help on the construction of phylogenetic and functional constraint analyses.

REFERENCES

Altschul, SF; Gish, W; Miller, W; Myers, EW; Lipman, DJ; (1990). Basic local alignment search tool. *J. Mol. Biol.*, 215, 403-410.

Amavisit, P., Lightfoot, D; Browning, GF; and Markham, PF. (2003). Variation between Pathogenic Serovars within Salmonella Pathogenicity Islands. *J. Bacteriol.*, 185:3624-3635.

Azad, RK and Lawrence, J.G. (2007). Detecting laterally transferred genes: use of entropic clustering methods and genome position. *Nucleic Acids Res.*, 35, 4629-4639.

Bakowski, M; Braun V; and Brumell, J. (2008). *Salmonella*-Containing Vacuoles: Directing Traffic and Nesting to Grow. *Traffic*, 9:2022-2031.

Beltran, P; Musser, JM; Helmuth, R; Farmer, JJ; Frerichs, WM; Wachsmuth, IK; Ferris, K; McWhorter, AC; Wells, JG and Cravioto, A. (1988). Toward a population genetic analysis of Salmonella: genetic diversity and relationships among strains of serotypes S. choleraesuis, S. derby, S. dublin, S. enteritidis, S. heidelberg, S. infantis, S. newport, and S. typhimurium. *Proc. Natl. Acad. Sci. USA*, 85:7753-7757.

Chiu, CH; Tang, P; Chu, C; Hu, S; Bao, Q; Yu, J; Chou, YY; Wang, HS; and Lee, YS. (2005). The genome sequence of Salmonella enterica serovar Choleraesuis, a highly invasive and resistant zoonotic pathogen. *Nucl. Acids Res.*, 33:1690-1698.

Darling, AC; Mau, B; Blattner, FR; and Perna, NT. (2004). Mauve: multiple alignment of conserved genomic sequence with rearrangements. *Genome Res.*, 14, 1394-1403.

Drummond, A; Ashton, B; Buxton, S; Cheung, M; Heled, J; Kearse, M; Moir, R; Stones-Havas, S; Thierer, T; and Wilson, A. (2010). *Geneious*, v4.8, 4.8 ed.

Edgar, RC. (2004). MUSCLE: multiple sequence alignment with high accuracy and high throughput. *Nucleic Acids Res.*, 32, 1792-1797.

Eswarappa, SM; Janice, J; Nagarajan, AG; Balasundaram, SV; Karnam, G, Dixit, NM; and Chakravortty, D. (2008). Differentially Evolved Genes of Salmonella Pathogenicity Islands: Insights into the Mechanism of Host Specificity in Salmonella. *PLoS ONE* 3:e3829.

Foley, SL; Nayak, R; and Lynne, AM. (2008). Food animal-associated Salmonella challenges: Pathogenicity and antimicrobial resistance. *J. Anim. Sci.*, 86:E173-187.

Guindon, S; Delsuc, F; Dufayard, JF; and Gascuel, O. (2009). Estimating maximum likelihood phylogenies with PhyML. *Methods Mol. Biol.*, 537, 113-137.

Guindon, S; Dufayard, JF; Lefort, V; Anisimova, M; Hordijk, W; and Gascuel, O. (2010). New algorithms and methods to estimate maximum-likelihood phylogenies: assessing the performance of PhyML 3.0. *Syst. Biol.*, 59, 307-321.

Guindon, S. and Gascuel, O. (2003). A simple, fast, and accurate algorithm to estimate large phylogenies by maximum likelihood. *Syst. Biol.*, 52, 696-704.

Hansen-Wester, I. and Hensel, M. (2001). Salmonella pathogenicity islands encoding type III secretion systems. *Microbes and Infection*, 3:549-559.

Hsiao, WW; Wan, I; Jones, SJ; and Brinkman, FS. (2003). IslandPath: aiding detection of genomic islands in prokaryotes. *Bioinformatics*, 19, 418-420.

Hsiao, WW; Ung, K; Aeschliman, D; Bryan, J; Finlay, BB; and Brinkman, FS. (2005). Evidence of a large novel gene pool associated with prokaryotic genomic islands. *PLoS Genet*, 1, e62.

Kingsley, RA; and Bäumler AJ. (2000). Host adaptation and the emergence of infectious disease: the Salmonella paradigm. *Mol. Microbiol.*, 36:1006-1014.

Langille, MG; and Brinkman, FS. (2009). IslandViewer: an integrated interface for computational identification and visualization of genomic islands. *Bioinformatics*, 25, 664-665.

Langille, MG; Hsiao, WW; and Brinkman, FS. (2008). Evaluation of genomic island predictors using a comparative genomics approach. *BMC Bioinformatics*, 9, 329.

Langille, MGI; Hsiao, WW; and Brinkman, FSL. (2010). Detecting genomic islands using bioinformatics approaches. *Nat. Rev. Micro.*, 8, 373-382.

Li, J; Ochman, H; Groisman, EA; Boyd, EF; Solomon, F; Nelson, K; and Selander, RK. (1995). Relationship between evolutionary rate and cellular location among the Inv/Spa invasion proteins of Salmonella enterica. *Proc. Natl. Acad. Sci. USA*, 92:7252-7256.

Lostroh, CP and Lee, CA. (2001). The Salmonella pathogenicity island-1 type III secretion system. *Microbes and Infection*, 3:1281-1291.

Soyer, Y; Orsi, R; Rodriguez-Rivera, L; Sun, Q; and Wiedmann, M. (2009). Genome wide evolutionary analyses reveal serotype specific patterns of positive selection in selected Salmonella serotypes. *BMC Evolutionary Microbiology*, 9:264.

Tamura, K and Nei, M. (1993). Estimation of the number of nucleotide substitutions in the control region of mitochondrial DNA in humans and chimpanzees. *Mol. Biol. Evol.*, 10, 512-526.

Vernikos, G; Thomson, N; and Parkhill, J. (2007). Genetic flux over time in the Salmonella lineage. *Genome. Biol.*, 8:R100.

Vernikos, GS and Parkhill, J. (2006). Interpolated variable order motifs for identification of horizontally acquired DNA: revisiting the *Salmonella* pathogenicity islands. *Bioinformatics*, 22, 2196-2203.

Waack, S; Keller, O; Asper, R; Brodag, T; Damm, C; Fricke, WF; Surovcik, K; Meinicke, P; and Merkl, R. (2006). Score-based prediction of genomic islands in prokaryotic genomes using hidden Markov models. *BMC Bioinformatics*, 7, 142.

Yang, Z and Nielsen, R. (2000). Estimating synonymous and nonsynonymous substitution rates under realistic evolutionary models. *Mol. Biol. Evol.*, 17, 32-43.

Zhang, Z; Li, J; and Yu, J. (2006a). Computing Ka and Ks with a consideration of unequal transitional substitutions. *BMC Evol. Biol.*, 6, 44.

Zhang, Z; Li, J; Zhao, X.-Q; Wang, J; Wong, GKS; and Yu, J. (2006b). KaKs_Calculator: Calculating Ka and Ks Through Model Selection and Model Averaging. Genomics, *Proteomics and Bioinformatics*, 4, 259-263.

In: Salmonella: Classification, Genetics and Disease Outbreaks ISBN: 978-1-61942-928-4
Editors: Adelaide S. Monte, Paulo Eduardo De Santos

Chapter 12

HAPPY BIRTHDAY: FORTY YEARS OF *SALMONELLA*/MICROSOME ASSAY

***Flavio Manoel Rodrigues da Silva Júnior*[1] *and Vera Maria Ferrão Vargas*[2]**

[1]Laboratório de Ensaios Farmacológicos e Toxicológicos, Instituto de Ciências Biológicas, Universidade Federal do Rio Grande - FURG, Rio Grande, RS, Brazil

[2]Programa de Pesquisas Ambientais, Divisão de Biologia, Fundação Estadual de Proteção Ambiental – FEPAM, Porto Alegre, RS, Brazil

ABSTRACT

The *Salmonella*/microsome assay is a technique for detection of mutagens based on the principle that mutagens can cause the the reversion of genetic engineered mutations that suppress biosynthesis of histidine in strains of *Salmonella typhimurium*. It started and has been employed since the beggining of the 70's to investigate chemical and biological samples (urine, feces and plasma) and is currently the most used to evaluate the presence of mutagenic compounds in environmental samples (soil, water, atmospheric material and sediment). Due to its importance, it is nowadays included in environmental legislation in several countries. Several improvements were introduced to enhance the sensibility of the test and broaden its applicability and reliability. Even about to complete its forty-year birthday, the assay keeps receiving improvements, including the development of new sensitive strains for detection of groups of compounds and new ways of evaluation and interpretation of the results. This chapter brings a brief review covering the forty years of the *Salmonella*/microsome assay studies and future perspectives and trends of this important mutagenicity assay.

Keywords: Mutagenicity, Ames test, prokaryotic system, short-term bioassay

1. Historical Elements

The development of the *Salmonella*/microssoma assay or "Ames test" by Dr. Bruce Ames and co-workers (Ames, 1971; Ames, 1972; Ames et al., 1973) is the milestone of the studies in the field of mutagenesis. The evaluation of mutagenicity of chemicals, pharmaceutical products ans environmental samples begins with this invaluable bioassay in procaryotic system of the bacteria *Salmonella typhimurium,* which completes forty years of existence this decade.

The ability of this test in identifying the presence of mutagenic compounds in a sample is related to their capacity to promote reverse mutagenesis in mutant strains of *S. typhimurium* that had been genetically engineered to be defective in the biosynthetic pathway of the amino acid histidine. Bacteria from these strains do not grow in the absence of this amino acid in culture media (auxotrophy), but in the presence of a mutagen this condition can be reverted (wild type like - prototrophic). These revertents are then able to synthesize histidine and grow in minimum culture media (without this amino acid). The principle of this test is schematized in figure 1.

The studies that preceded the construction of the mutant strains of *S. typhimurium* are related to the elucidation of the biosynthetic pathway of histidine, among them the Ph.D. thesis of Dr. Bruce N. Ames (Ames, 1953), which investigated the biosynthesis of histidine in the fungus *Neurospora crassa*. Deeper studies considering genes organization and their regulation in the operon of histidine in *S. typhimurium* are more recent (Schmid & Roth, 1983; Alifano et al., 1996). The histidine operon is composed of 8 genes (*hisG*, *hisD*, *hisC*, *hisB*, *hisH*, *hisA*, *hisF* e *hisI*). Three of these genes (*hisD*, *hisB* e *hisI*) codify bifunctional enzymes and two (*hisH* e *hisF*) codify polypeptidic chains that compose a molecule of the enzyme that catalyzes the only step of the pathway (Alifano et al., 1996). The biosynthetic pathway of histidine is schematized in figure 2.

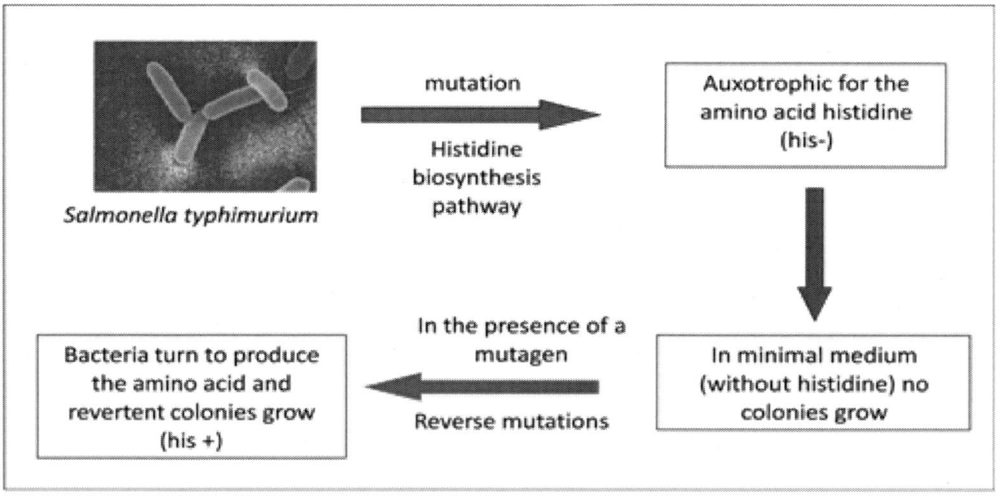

Figure 1. The principle of the *Salmonella*/microsome test.

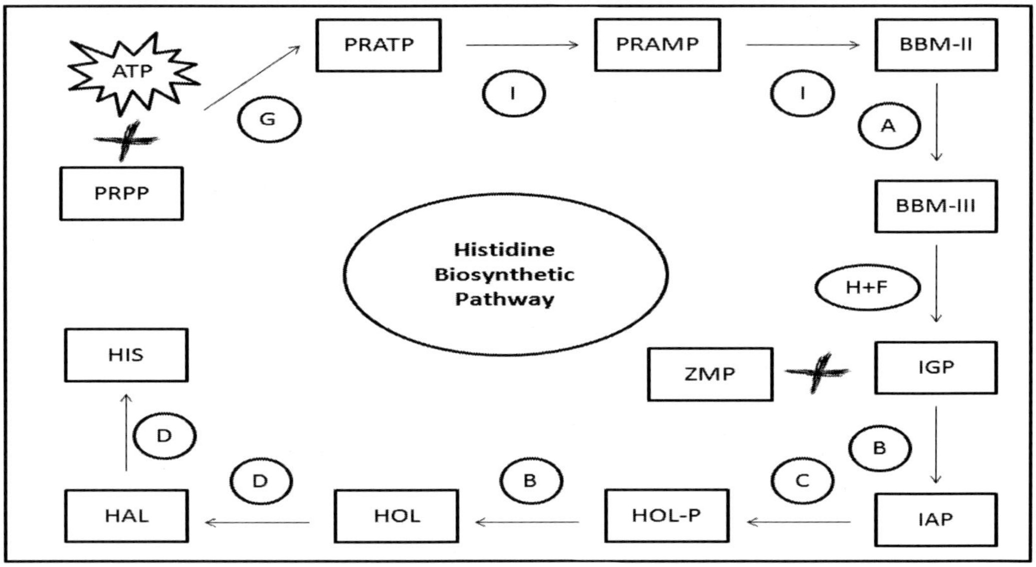

Figure 2. The histidine biosynthetic pathway. PRPP- 5-phosphoribosyla-1-pyrophosphate; PRATP - N9-59-phosphoribosyl-ATP; PRAMP - N9-59-phosphoribosyl-AMP; BBM-II - (59-ProFAR), N9-[(59-phosphoribosyl)-formimino]-5 aminoimidazole-4 carboxamide ribonucleotide; BBM-III - (59-PRFAR), N9-[(59-phosphoribulosyl)-formimino]-5-aminoimidazole-4-carboxamide-ribonucleotide; IGP - imidazole glycerol-phosphate; ZMP (AICAR) - 59-phosphoribosyl-4-carboxamide-5-aminoimidazole; IAP - imidazole acetol-phosphate; HOL-P - L-histidinol-phosphate; HOL - L-histidinol; HAL - L-histidinal (not found as a free intermediate); HIS - L-histidine. Enzymes: N9-59-phosphoribosyl-ATP transferase (G); Cyclohydrolase - carboxyl-terminal domain – (I); Cyclohydrolase - amino-terminal domain (I); *hisA* gene product (A); IGP synthase holoenzyme (H+F); *hisB* gene product – carboxyl-terminal domain (B); pyridoxal-P-dependent aminotransferase (C); IGP synthase - amino-terminal domain (B); L-histidinol dehydrogenase (D).

The several strains that are available for the Ames test were created from mutation points in different genes of the histidine operon, with emphasis on studies at the end of the 60's and beginning of the 70's (see Martin, 1967; Pierre, 1968 and Yourno et al., 1971). The main strains employed and their genotypes are listed in tables 1 and 2.

Besides the histidine mutation, the standardized strains have other alterations that augment the sensibility of the assay for the detection of mutagenic agents. One of them (*rfa* mutation) causes loss of the lipopolysaccharide membrane that covers the bacterial surface. This allows large molecules to pass through the bacterial cell membrane. Another mutation was the deletion of the gene (*uvr*b), which causes loss of the excision repair by impeding the enzymes of this type of repair to act. For technical reasons, the deletion of this gene also caused the disruption of the biotin gene (Maron & Ames, 1983). Later on, it was also pointed that other genes, besides these two mentioned, were also affected by this excision. The number varies according to the strain, but this deletion affected, for example, 119 genes in the TA98 strain (Porwollik et al., 2001). Another alteration was the introduction of the plasmid pKM101, known as R-factor, which endows the cell with increased error-prone repair system and resistence to ampicilin marker. The strain TA102 also possesses the multicopy plasmid pAQ1 that carries the mutation *his*G428 which in turn increases the mutation targets. This plasmid has also the marker for tetracycline resistence (Maron & Ames, 1983).

Table 1. Genotypes of the strains used for mutagenesis testing

Strain	LPS	Repair	R-factor	*oat* and *nfs* gene overexpression
TA1538	*rfa*	Δ*uvr*B	- R	-
TA98	*rfa*	Δ*uvr*B	+ R	-
YG1021	*rfa*	Δ*uvr*B	+ R	*nfs*
YG1024	*rfa*	Δ*uvr*B	+ R	*oat*
YG1041	*rfa*	Δ*uvr*B	+ R	both
TA98NR	*rfa*	Δ*uvr*B	+ R	*Nfs* deficient
TA98 1,8DNP$_6$	*rfa*	Δ*uvr*B	+ R	Transacetylase deficient
TA1535	*rfa*	Δ*uvr*B	- R	-
TA100	*rfa*	Δ*uvr*B	+ R	-
YG1026	*rfa*	Δ*uvr*B	+ R	*nfs*
YG1029	*rfa*	Δ*uvr*B	+ R	*oat*
YG1042	*rfa*	Δ*uvr*B	+ R	both
TA100NR	*rfa*	Δ*uvr*B	+ R	*Nfs* deficient
TA100 1,8DNP$_6$	*rfa*	Δ*uvr*B	+ R	Transacetylase deficient
TA97	*rfa*	Δ*uvr*B	+ R	-
TA1537	*rfa*	Δ*uvr*B	- R	-
TA102	*rfa*	Δ*uvr*B	+ R	-

According to Maron & Ames (1983), the confirmation of the maintenance of the genotype must be done (1) right after the acquisition of the culture of *S. typhimurium*, (2) when creating a new set of permanent lyophilized or frozen cultures, (3) when the number of spontaneous revertent colonies is out of the normal interval, or (4) when there is loss of sensibility to the standard mutagens.

In order to investigate the mutagenicity of compounds that are biologically active after metabolization (for example, polycyclic aromatic hydrocarbons), the assay uses a microsomal fraction (S9 fraction). This system, also called Metabolic Oxidation System based on cytochrome P450, is present mainly in the liver, but also in lungs and kidneys, and is capable of metabolizing a great number of chemicals to electrophilic forms that react with DNA. This system works in the presence of NADP and co-factors for the oxidation supported by NADPH (Mortelmans & Zeiger, 2000). This S9 fraction is obtained normally through the induction by PCBs (polychlorinated biphenyls) Aroclor 1254 in mice or rats. All these elements served as foundation for the insertion of the *Salmonella*/microsome at the baseline of fundamental bioassay for the mutagenic agents evaluation.

2. Application

The applicability of this bioassay is directly related to its versatility and to the diversity and specificity of bacterial strains existent. The *Salmonella*/microsome assay can be used for the investigation of mutagenicity of biological samples, chemical substances and environmental samples with slight modifications in the original protocol.

Table 2. DNA sequence specificity on the Salmonella tester strains

Strain	Mutation point	Mutation	Reversion event
TA1538	*his*D3052	-1pb –C-G-C-G-C-G-C-G-	Frameshift mutation
TA98	*his*D3052	-1pb –C-G-C-G-C-G-C-G-	Frameshift mutation
YG1021	*his*D3052	-1pb –C-G-C-G-C-G-C-G-	Frameshift mutation
YG1024	*his*D3052	-1pb –C-G-C-G-C-G-C-G-	Frameshift mutation
YG1041	*his*D3052	-1pb –C-G-C-G-C-G-C-G-	Frameshift mutation
TA98NR	*his*D3052	-1pb –C-G-C-G-C-G-C-G-	Frameshift mutation
TA98 1,8DNP$_6$	*his*D3052	-1pb –C-G-C-G-C-G-C-G-	Frameshift mutation
TA1535	*his*G46	-GGG- (pro) > -GAG- (leu)	Base pair substitution
TA100	*his*G46	-GGG- (pro) > -GAG- (leu)	Base pair substitution
YG1026	*his*G46	-GGG- (pro) > -GAG- (leu)	Base pair substitution
YG1029	*his*G46	-GGG- (pro) > -GAG- (leu)	Base pair substitution
YG1042	*his*G46	-GGG- (pro) > -GAG- (leu)	Base pair substitution
TA100NR	*his*G46	-GGG- (pro) > -GAG- (leu)	Base pair substitution
TA1001,8DNP$_6$	*his*G46	-GGG- (pro) > -GAG- (leu)	Base pair substitution
TA97	*his*D6610	+1pb –C-C-C-C-C-C-	Frameshift mutation
TA1537	*his*C3076	+1pb –C-C-C-C-C-C-	Frameshift mutation
TA102	*his*G428	-TAA- > –ATT- (stop codon)	Transition/transversion

Spot test – this test is based on the application of the sample on a paper filter disc of approximately 6 mm that is placed inside a plate inoculated with the bacteria in top agar minimum medium. It is fast and is indicated for an initial screening of a large number of compounds. It can be employed with unsterile samples and with solid cristals of mutagens. However, it is a basically qualitative assay and useful for water soluble samples. A negative result does not necessarily indicate the absence of mutagenicity in *Salmonella* and a positive result must be confirmed with another protocol that employs a dose-response curve (Maron & Ames, 1983; Mortelmans & Zeiger, 2000).

Standard plate incorporation assay – in this procedure, it is added a mixture of buffer or S9 mix, bacteria (approximately 10^8 mL^{-1}) and the sample to be tested in top agar containing traces of histidine and biotine to the plate. After solidification, the plates must be incubated at 37 °C for 48 h and then it is counted the number of revertant colonies. This trace of histidine and biotine is important to promote a few initial cell divisions, necessary for the action of the mutagenic compounds, since most of them act on replicating DNA. Additionally, it is possible to inoculate the same mixture (buffer or S9 mix + bacterial suspension + sample) in a nutritive culture medium and investigate the toxicity of the samples from the decreasing of the growth of colonies in relation to the negative control (Vargas et al., 1993; Mortelmans & Zeiger, 2000).

Pre-incubation assay or liquid incubation assay - incorporates another step prior to the inoculation in minimum agar medium: the incubation of the mixture (buffer or S9 mix + bacterial suspension + sample) in water bath for 37 °C for 20-30 minutes. Commonly, this procedure is more sensible than the plate incorporation assay, because the time of reaction between the mutagens and the bacteria is increased (Maron & Ames, 1983; Mortelmans & Zeiger, 2000).

Microsuspension assay - this procedure was proposed in order to increase the sensibility of the *Salmonella*/microsome assay to detect low levels of mutagens in urine. The strategy of increasing the concentration of urine per plate is not efficient because of the presence of histidine in urine that can lead to false positive results_(Maron & Ames, 1983). Kado and co-workers (1983) introduced slight modifications to the liquid incubation assay: they increased the concentration of bacterial cells (from 10^8 para 10^9 por mL^{-1}) and reduced the volume of the sample and the buffer (or S9) mix (from 5- to 10-fold less). Their results showed that this procedure were 13 times more sensible than the liquid incubation assay protocol.

Desiccator assay – recommended to test volatile chemicals and gases (Maron & Ames, 1983; Mortelmans & Zeiger, 2000).

Mutagenic glycosides assay – plants may contain mutagens in inactive, conjugated forms, like glycosides. The mutagenic portion (aglycone) may act through the presence of bacterial glycosidases in the intestine. Assays have demonstrated the absence of mutagenic induction because these substances are not hydrolyzable by the microsomal enzymes of the liver. The protocol to investigate the mutagenicity of glycosides must incorporate enzimes able to hydrolyze these compounds (e.g. fecalase) or fecal extracts from rats (Maron & Ames, 1983).

Ames fluctuation test – this is a modification of the protocol and is carried in microtiter plates (e.g. 384 wells). The volume of the sample used is substantially smaller and the possibility of automation offers advantages over the microsuspension protocol (Green et al., 1976).

Spiral Salmonella assay – this protocol also brings some advantages in relation to the microsuspension protocol because it can also be automatized and uses a small number of plates (Claxton et al., 2001).

Besides the choice of the experimental protocol, the treatment of the samples is of paramount importance to the trustability of the results. Samples can be used in *Salmonella*/microsome without any special treatment (like isolated chemical substances); with just filter sterilization (0.22 μm), as in the case of groundwater; or another more ellaborated treatment like the use of resins, or aqueous/acid/organic extraction (biological samples, superficial water, sediment or soil) (Stierum et al., 1993; Tagliari et al., 2004; Da Silva-Júnior et al., 2009).

The great number of options for this assay makes the *Salmonella*/microsome assay the most commonly used biosassay for the investigation of the presence of mutagens in samples from different origins.

The early works evaluated the mutagenic potential of chemicals (McCann & Ames, 1976; De Flora et al., 1984, among others) and the concern was the relationship with the carcinogenicity of the same elements. The first data demonstrated a high (85%) proportion of carcinogens that responded positively to the *Salmonella*/microsome assay (Ames et al., 1975). Another line of investigation employed the Ames test to evaluate the exposition of humans (smokers and occupationally exposed) to mutagenic agents using urine (Kado et al., 1983; Stierum et al., 1993; Smith, 1996).

At the same time emerged the first works that used the *Salmonella*/microsome assay in the investigation of complex environmental matrices (surface water, air, sediment and soil), preoccupied in detecting the presence of mutagens in the environment, becoming the most employed for this purpose (see reviews in Chen & White, 2004; White & Claxton, 2004, Ohe et al.,2004; Claxton et al.,2004).

3. Recent Advances

The dinamism of the *Salmonella*/microsome assay has followed the main scientific developments in the areas of molecular biology, statistics and environmental chemistry. These correlated sciences have been acting as useful tools for the comprehension of some mechanisms or increasing the specificity of the assay. The amplification of genes of enzymes involved in bioactivation or the disruption of these genes are some of the most common processes for the elaboration of new specific strains for the detection of some compounds (see Espinosa-Aguirre et al., 1999; Kokubo et al., 2005; Matsui et al., 2006).

Efforts have been made in several parts of the world for the incorporation of the *Salmonella*/microsome assay as a parameter in environmental monitoring by environmental protection agencies. In countries like Brazil, the bioassay is present in the legislation of some states (São Paulo e Rio Grande do Sul) (Rio Grande do Sul, 2007) and some works have been made aiming at incorporating the test in legal devices for the monitoring of surface water and groundwater (Vargas et al., 1993, 1995, 2008; Umbuzeiro et al., 2001; Valente-Campos et al., 2009). More recently, compartments like soil (Da Silva Júnior & Vargas, 2009; Da Silva Júnior et al., 2009; Costa et al., 2012), sediment (Horn et al., 2004; Tagliari et al., 2004) and atmosphere (Vargas et al., 1998; Vargas, 2003; Coronas et al., 2008; Pereira et al., 2010) have also been target of the same efforts.

The utilization of this assay when related to chemical analyses has promoted the investigation of the dispersion of contaminants among different environmental compartments (FEPAM, 2008; Da Silva Júnior, 2009; Cappi et al., 2012), and when related to other tests of ecotoxicological evaluation has allowed to define acute, chronic and genotoxic effects of complex mixtures (Cardozo et al., 2006; Vargas et al., 2008). It has still allowed measuring human exposure to genotoxic agents associated with biomarkers like the comet assay in periferic lymphocytes and micronucleus in oral exfoliation cells (Coronas et al., 2009). These more recent strategies, like studies *in silico* comprise useful tools in environmental monitoring programs and in the environmental risk evaluation of new chemical substances (Hayashi et al., 2005; McCarren et al., 2011).

4. Perspectives

Even after 40 years of existence, the *Salmonella*/microsome assay has not fallen into disuse as a bioassay for the detection of agents with mutagenic potential. On the other side, it has undergone improvements and adequacies to expand the types of fractions/samples and increase the specificity of the response. Although the number of chemical substances already tested through the *Salmonella*/microsome assay is high, new substances have been synthetized every day and there is the need to evaluate their mutagenic potential, including emergent polutants like pharmaceutical products, endocrine disuptors and nanocompounds. Beyond that, the consequences generated by the interaction of these compounds should still be the target of intensive studies in the area of mutagenesis.

The strategy of fractioning of complex environmental samples and the utilization of specific strains for the detection of the mutagenicity of groups of compounds and specific types of DNA mutations can highlight important details concerning the mutagenic potential of this type of material, contributing with information in environmental monitoring programs.

Hence, the utilization of the *Salmonella*/microsome assay is a good choice for the investigation of mutagenic agents and even after 40 years still remains as an importante short-term bioassay.

REFERENCES

Alifano, P.; Fani, R.; Lio, P.; Lazcano, A.; Bazzicalupo, M.; Carlomagno, M.S.; Bruni C.B. Histidine Biosynthetic Pathway and Genes: Structure, Regulation, and Evolution. *Microbiological reviews,* 1996, 60, 44-69.

Ames, B. N. *Chemical Mutagens: Principles and Methods for their Detection,* ed. Hollaender, A. (Plenum Press, New York), 1971, 1, 267-282.

Ames, B.N. The biosynthesis of histidine in *Neurospora crassa. Doctoral thesis,* 1953. 42p.

Ames, B.N. The detection of chemical mutagens with enteric bacteria In: Hollaender, A. *Chemical Mutagens: Principles and Methods for their detection,* vol. I. New York: Plenum, 1972.

Ames, B.N; Durston, WE; Yamasaki, E.; Lee, FD. Carcinogens are mutagens: a simple test system combining liver homogenates for activation and bacteria for detection. *Procediment Natural Academic Science,* 1973, 70, 2281-2285.

Ames, B.N; Mccann, J; Yamasaki, E. Methods for detecting carcinogens and mutagens with the *Salmonella*/mammalian-microsome mutagenicity test. *Mutation Research,* 1975, 31, 347-364.

Cardozo, T.R.; Rosa, D. P.; Feiden, I. R.; Rocha, J.A.V.; Pereira, T.S.; Pastoriza, T.F.; Lemos, C.T.; Terra, N.R.; Vargas, V.M.F.; Marques, D.M. Genotoxicity and toxicity assessment in urban hydrographic basins. *Mutation Research,* 2006, 603, 83-96.

Chen, G; White, PA. The mutagenic hazards of aquatic sediments: a review. *Mutation Research,* 2004, 567, 151-225.

Claxton, L.D.; Houk,V.S.; Warren, S. Methods for the spiral *Salmonella* mutagenicity assay including specialized applications. *Mutation Research,* 2001, 488, 241–257.

Claxton, LD; Matthews, PP.; Warren, SH. The genotoxicity of ambient outdoor air, a review: *Salmonella* mutagenicity. *Mutation Research,* 2004, 567, 347-399.

Coronas, M.V.; Horn, R.C.; Ducatti, A.; Rocha, J.A.V.; Vargas, V.M.F. Mutagenic activity of airborne particulate matter in a petrochemical industrial area, *Mutation Research,* 2008, 650, 196-201.

Coronas, M.V; Pereira, T.S. Rocha, J.A. Lemos, A.T. Fachel, J.M.G.; Salvadori, D.M.F.; Vargas, V.M.F. Genetic biomonitoring of an urban population exposed to mutagenic airborne pollutants. *Environment International*, 2009, 35, 1023–1029.

Costa,T.C.; Tagliari de Brito, K.C.; Rocha, J.A.V.; Leal, K.A.; Kolowski Rodrigues, M.L.; Minella, J.P.G.; Matsumoto, S.T.; Vargas, V.M.F. Runoff of genotoxic compounds. *Ecotoxicology and Environmental Safety*, 2012, 75 63-72.

Da Silva Júnior, FMR; Vargas, VMF. Using the *Salmonella* assay to delineate the dispersion routes of mutagenic compounds from coal wastes in contaminated soil. Mutation Research, 2009, 673, 116-123.

Da Silva Júnior, FMR; Rocha, JAV; Vargas, VMF. Extraction parameters in the mutagenicity assay of soil samples. *Science of the Total Environment,* 2009, 407, 6017-23.

De Flora, S.; Zanacchi, P.; Camoirano, A.; Bennicelli, C. Badolat, G.S. Genotoxic activity and potency of 135 compounds in the Ames reversion test and in a bacterial DNA-repair test. *Mutation Research,* 1984, 133, 161-198.

Espinosa-Aguirre, J.J.; Yamada, M. Matsui, K.; Watanabe, M; Sofuni, T; Nohmi, T. New O-acetyltransferase-deficient Ames *Salmonella* strains generated by specific gene disruption. *Mutation Research,* 1999, 439, 159–169.

FEPAM Fundação Estadual de Proteção Ambiental Henrique Luís Roessler. Atlas Ambiental: Estratégias ecotoxicológicas para avaliaçaão de risco aplicado à Bacia Hidrográfica do Rio Caí. [The Henrique Luis Roessler State Environmental Protection Foundation: Ecotoxicological strategies for risk evaluation applied to a Cai River hydrographic basin]. In: V.M.F. Vargas, N.R. Terra, E.C. Sarmento, (Org.), FEPAM, Porto Alegre, 164 pp., 2008.

Green, M.H.L; Muriel, W.J; Bridges, B.A. Use of a simplified fluctuation test to detect low levels of mutagens, *Mutation Research,* 1976, 38, 33-42.

Hayashi, M.; Kamata, E.; Hirose, A.; Takahashi, M.; Morita, T.; Ema, M. *In silico* assessment of chemical mutagenesis in comparison with results of *Salmonella* microsome assay on 909 chemicals. *Mutation Research,* 2005, 588, 129–135.

Horn, R. C.; Rocha, J.A.; Vargas, V.M.F. Determination of sediment mutagenicity and cytotoxicity in an area subject to petrochemical contamination, *Mutagenesis,* 2004, 19, 445-451.

Kado, N.Y., Langley, D., Eisentadt, E. A simple modification of the Salmonella liquid incubation assay: increased sensitivity for detecting mutagens in human urine. *Mutation Research,* 1983, 121, 25-32.

Kokubo, K. Yamada, M.; Kanke, Y.; Nohmi, T. Roles of replicative and specialized DNA polymerases in frameshift mutagenesis: Mutability of *Salmonella typhimurium* strains lacking one or all of SOS-inducible DNA polymerases to 26 chemicals. *DNA Repair,* 2005, 4, 1160–1171.

Maron, DM; Ames, BN. Revised methods for the *Salmonella* mutagenicity test. *Mutation Research,* 1982, 11, 173-215.

Martin, R.G. Frameshift Mutants in the Histidine Operon of *Salmonella typhimurium*. *Journal of Molecular Biology,* 1967, 26,311-328.

Matsui, K; Yamada, M.; Imai, M.; Yamamoto, K. Nohmi, T. Specificity of replicative and SOS-inducible DNA polymerases in frameshift mutagenesis: Mutability of *Salmonella typhimurium* strains overexpressing SOS-inducible DNA polymerases to 30 chemical mutagens. *DNA Repair,* 2006, 5, 465–478.

McCann, J.; Ames, B. N. Detection of Carcinogens as Mutagens in the *Salmonella*/Microsome Test: Assay of 300 Chemicals: Discussion. *PNAS* 1976, 73, 950-954.

McCarren, P.; Bebernitz, G.R; Gedeck, p.; Glowienke, S.; Grondine, M.S.; Kirman, L.C.; Klickstein, J.; Schuster, H.F.; Whitehead. L. Avoidance of the Ames test liability for aryl–amines via computation. *Bioorganic & Medicinal Chemistry,* 2011, 19, 3173–3182.

Mortelmans, K. Zeiger, E. The Ames *Salmonella*/microsome mutagenicity assay. *Mutation Research,* 2000, 455, 29-60.

Ohe, T; Watanabe, T; Wakabayashi, K. Mutagens in surface waters: a review. *Mutation Research,* 2004, 567, 109-149.

Pereira, T.S.; Rocha, J.A.V.; Duccatti, A.; Silveira, G.A.; Pastoriza, T.F.; Bringuenti, L. Vargas, V.M.F. Evaluation of mutagenic activity in supply water at three sites in the state of Rio Grande do Sul, Brazil. *Mutation Research.* 2007, 629, 71–80.

Pierre St, M.L. Mutations Creating a New Initiation Point for Expression of the Histidine Operon in *Salmonella typhimurium. Journal of Molecular Biology,* 1968, 35, 71-82.

Porwollik, S.; Wong, R.M. S. H. Sims, S.; Schaaper, R.M.; DeMarini, D.M.; McClelland, M. The ΔuvrB mutations in the Ames strains of *Salmonella* span 15 to 119 genes. *Mutation Research,* 2001, 483, 1–11.

RIO GRANDE DO SUL, CONSELHO ESTADUAL DO MEIO AMBIENTE. Resolução CONSEMA N ° 129/2006. Dispõe sobre a definição de critérios e padrões de emissão para toxicidade de efluentes líquidos lançados em águas superficiais do Estado do Rio Grande do Sul. Porto Alegre, 2006. Disponível em: <http: www.sema.rs.gov.br>. Acesso em: 6 de Fevereiro de 2007.

Schmidt, M.B.; Roth, J.R. Internal Promoters of the his Operon in *Salmonella typhimurium. Journal of bacteriology,* 1983, 153, 1114-1119.

Smith, D.W.E. Mutagenicity of cycasin aglycone (methylazoxymethanol) a naturally occurring carcinogen, *Science,* 1966, 192, 1273–1274.

Stierum, R.H.; Hageman, G.J.; Welle, I.J.; Albering, H.J.; Schreus, J.G.M.; Kleinjans, J.C.S. Evaluation of exposure reducing measures on parameters of genetic risk in a population occupationally exposed to coal fly ash. *Mutation Research,* 1993, 319, 245-255.

Tagliari, K.C.; Cecchini, R.; Rocha, J.A.V.; Vargas, V.M.F. Mutagenicity of sediment and biomarkers of oxidative stress in fish from aquatic environments under the influence of tanneries. *Mutation Research,* 2004, 561, 101-117.

Umbuzeiro, G.A.; Roubicek, D.A.; Sanchez, P.S.; Sato,M.I.Z. The *Salmonella* mutagenicity assay in a surfacewater quality monitoring programbased on a 20-year survey, *Mutation Research,* 2001, 491, 119–126.

Valente-Campos, S.; Diasb, C.L.; Barbourb, E.D.A.; Nascimento, E.S.; Umbuzeiro, G. The introduction of the Salmonella/microsome mutagenicity assay in a groundwater monitoring program. *Mutation Research,* 2009, 675, 17–22.

Vargas, V.M.F.; Motta, V.E.P.; Henriques, J.A.P. Mutagenic activity detected by the Ames test in river water under the influence of petrochemical industries. *Mutation Research,* 1993, 319, 31-45.

Vargas, V.M.F.; Guidobono, R.R;, Henriques, J.A.P. Use of two short term test to evaluate genotoxicity of river water treated with different concentration extraction procedure. *Mutation Research,* 1995, 343, 31-52.

Vargas, V.M.F. Mutagenic activity as a parameter to assess ambient air quality for protection of the environment and human health, *Mutation Research*, 2003, 544, 313–319.

Vargas, V.M.F.; Migliavacca, S.B.; Horn, R.C.; Terra, N.R. Comparative temporal ecotoxicological . *Science of the Total Environment,* 2008, 392, 79-92.

White, PA; Claxton, L.D. Mutagens in contaminated soil: a review. Mutation Research, 2004, 567, 227–345.

Yotjrno, J.; Ino, I.; Kohno, T. A Hotspot for Spontaneous Frameshift Mutations in the Histidinol Dehydrogenase Gene of *Salmonella typhimurium. Journal of Molecular Biology,* 1971, 62, 233-240.

In: Salmonella: Classification, Genetics and Disease Outbreaks ISBN: 978-1-61942-928-4
Editors: Adelaide S. Monte, Paulo Eduardo De Santos

Chapter 13

SALMONELLA IN SUB-ANTARCTICA AND ANTARCTICA

Vigo Germán
Cátedra de Microbiología, Facultad de Ciencias Veterinarias, Universidad Nacional de La Plata, Buenos Aires, Argentina

ABSTRACT

Salmonella enterica subspecies *enterica* has been isolated from every region around the world and is considered as a potential pathogen for many animal species. The epidemiology, reservoirs and transmission of *Salmonella* is very complex owing to humans, animals and environment are involved. The purpose of this work was to review the current knowledge of *Salmonella* in the wildlife of sub-Antarctic and Antarctic region. For a long time Antarctic was a region that remained isolated from human contact, but in recent years the human presence has notably increased and as consequence, the danger of introduction of microorganisms to the Antarctic fauna. One of the most extensively studied bacterial species in the region is *Salmonella*, because of its characteristics mentioned above. *Salmonella* infections in Antarctic wildlife were first reported in 1970. Since then, several studies have been conducted, which showed that *Salmonella enterica* subspecies *enterica* isolated from sub-Antarctic and Antarctic fauna belonged to the most prevalent serovars in humans and domesticated animals, with the exception of few rare or exotic serovars. Some of *Salmonella* serovars found in Antarctic wildlife were: Enteritidis, Typhimurium, Newport, Infantis which are among the main serovars isolated from salmonellosis cases in humans and animals in the world. *Salmonella* infections in sub-Antarctic and Antarctic wildlife were reported in the following animals: *Adelie* penguins (*Pygoscelis adelie*), south polar skuas (*Catharacta maccormicki*), gentoo penguins (*Pygoscelis papua*), fur seal (*Arctocephalus gazelle*), black-browed albatross (*Diomedea melanophrys*), sea lions (*Phocarctos hookeri*), southern petrels (*Macronectes giganteus*), kelp gulls (*Larus dominicanus*), Weddell seals (*Leptonychotes weddelli*), emperor penguin (*Aptenodytes forsteri*). All of these animal species were *Salmonella* carriers and none of them had clinical signs of salmonellosis. Different routes of introduction of *Salmonella* to Antarctic region have been proposed: by human carriers, by contaminated foods, by infected birds, sewage from some land-based operations or from discharge of this material from ships sailing in waters of the region. One of the most possible routes of introduction is by birds, because many Antarctic birds have long routes of migration. Studies on *Salmonella* carried out in Antarctic region allow the scientific community to know the sanitary status of Antarctic fauna and also, they can be used as an indicator to know the local ecosystem status. Up to now, in spite of the different studies that have been performed in sub-Antarctic and Antarctic, it was impossible to determine if *Salmonella* was introduced or was and indigenous bacterium in the Antarctic ecosystem.

ISOLATION OF ANTARCTIC WILDLIFE

It is likely that many of the diseases found even on the southern continents will not be found in Antarctic species because of the geographical isolation of Antarctica. The nearest continent, South America, is 1500 km to the north, South Africa is 4100 km and Australia 3600 km. This isolation which has existed for long periods of geological time coupled with epochs of glacial advance and retreat has limited the colonization to those vertebrate species (seals and birds) which are able to cross the southern ocean by swimming or flying. The southern ocean forms a barrier across which very few avian species cross, a consequence of this separation is that seals and birds in the Antarctic and on sub-Antarctic Islands have evolved in relative isolation. Distance limits contact with disease and inhibits the introduction of vectors or intermediate hosts, this factor may well have protected these species from the major diseases found in birds and other species to the north. However, the speed of modern transport to Antarctica and sub-Antarctic and the numbers of people visiting the south polar regions as scientists or tourist have increased enormously and these changes may increase the possibility of unwitting introduction of diseases. Transport around the Antarctic continent has increased, particularly from tourist ventures, and this increases the risk of disease spread regardless of whether the disease is endemic or introduced. The sub-Antarctic Islands are similarly isolated. They form a ring approximately half way between the Antarctic Continent and the other southern continents and straddle the south polar front. Some Islands are heavily glaciated, for example, South Georgia and Heard Island but all share a maritime climate and are to some degree vegetated with flowering plants which on the northernmost Islands are woody. All support large colonies of sea birds and seals which range widely to forage particularly during the non-breeding season. Several species of birds, for example the wandering albatross and the giant petrel, feed in the coastal waters of the continents to the north. The milder climate means that arthropod vectors of infectious disease such as ticks and fleas are likely to be present and are able to complete their life-cycle. It is possible therefore that disease may be introduced into the wildlife of these Islands more readily than the Antarctic and that they in turn may also play a role in the transmission of disease into Antarctic wildlife. (Kerry, 1999).

Enzootic diseases are those that are widespread, although they may be of low incidence, in a population. Exotic diseases are those that are not present in the population or are sufficiently localized to be eradicable. The terms enzootic and exotic do not convey any information on whether humans were involved in their introduction or spread of disease. Those diseases which may be present in a population, but those introduction or spread were not mediated by humans, are referred to as native or indigenous diseases. Virtually nothing is known of endemic diseases in Antarctic populations of seals and birds and or whether any non-indigenous diseases are present. A few cases of bacterial infections leading to death have also been reported. This low incidence of reported disease does not mean that Antarctic wildlife is disease free. It is likely that agents capable of causing disease are present among the population but their expression in terms of diseased individuals has not been observed because of the small human presence in Antarctica (Kerry, 1999)

FACTORS THAT COULD INTRODUCE AND SPREAD *SALMONELLA* SPP

The avifauna of sub-Antarctica and Antarctica consists (among others) of the following species: Adelie penguin (*Pygoscelis adeliae*), chinstrap penguin (*Pygoscelis Antarctica*), gentoo penguin (*Pygoscelis papua*), emperor penguin (*Aptenodytes forsteri*), king penguin (*Aptenodytes patagonicus*), rockhooper penguin (*Eudyptes crestatus*), macaroni penguin (*Eudyptes chrysolophus*), southern fulmar (*Fulmaras glacialoides*), southern giant fulmar (*Macronectes giganteus*), cape pigeon (*Daption capense*), snow petrel (*Pagodroma nivea*), Wilson´s storm petrel (*Oceanites oceanicus*), blue-eyed shag (*Phalacrocorax atriceps*), American sheathbill (*Chionis alba*), South polar skua (*Catharacta maccormicki*), brown polar skua (*Catharacta lonnbergi*), southern black-backed gull (*Larus dominicanus*), Antarctic tern (*Sterna vittata*), wandering albatross (*Diomedea exulans*), black-browed albatross (*Diomedea melanophrys*), Antarctic petrel (*Thalassoica Antarctica*). The marine mammals present in sub-Antarctic and Antarctic zone are the following: Antarctic fur seal (*Arctocephalus gazella*), leopard seal (*Hydrurga leptonyx*), Weddell seal (*Leptonichotes weddelli*), crabeater seal (*Lobodon carcinophagus*), Ross seal (*Ommatophoca rossii*), southern elephant seal (*Mirounga leonina*). Many of these animals have long routes of migration, where they could acquire *Salmonella* and introduce the microorganism into the Antarctic ecosystem.

Antarctic krill has the capacity to act as an intermediate host for pathogenic organisms and krill swarms exposed to factory ships and convergent wildlife provide a marine staging post and vehicle for the spread of *Salmonella* infections to penguin chicks and seal pups during the breeding season (Iveson, 2009).

HUMAN ACTIVITY

Human activity in Antarctica could be the cause of disease outbreaks by a number of direct and indirect mechanisms. People could be act as vectors for infectious agents, either by bringing non-indigenous pathogens into the region or by translocating indigenous pathogens. In addition stress caused by human activity could reduce immunity, increase pathogenicity and could cause the expression of a disease that might otherwise not have revealed itself. Stress may be the result of direct human disturbance, food shortage, exposure to pollutants and possible, in the long term, as a result of climate change. Travel between countries is recognized as one of the major factors causing the rapid spread of disease around the globe, visits to different countries and different environments increase the chance of coming into contact with a variety of diseases.

Sewage is often discharged into the ocean from Antarctic stations and sometimes illegally by ships. Untreated sewage is likely to contain some organisms pathogenic to humans and may also pose threat to susceptible indigenous wildlife (Kerry, 1999).

Environment

Stress is a major contributing factor to the outbreak of disease and may have many causes. It may be induced by climatic conditions beyond the normal range, food shortage, catastrophic natural events, habitat destruction and fragmentation, environmental contaminants, direct human disturbance and other more subtle forms of human interference. Antarctic species are well adapted to survive under conditions that would be extreme to species that have evolved elsewhere and they exhibit many remarkable features that enable them occupy their particular niches.

However, their success is at least in part attributable to the absence of land based mammalian predators or niche competition from more competitive species. Although tolerant of the natural environment they are not necessarily immune to environmental stress by particularly sever conditions, particularly those that limit access to food such as unusually extensive, or limited, sea ice and unusual snow cover on nest sites. Species breeding at the northern edge of their range at the Antarctic Peninsula region may at times also suffer from thermal stress. This stress will increase in the advent of further global warming when temperatures on land are higher and less sea ice is present. The absence of predators makes species less prepared for humans, when they are disturbed by people the response is a rise in heart rate indicative of mild to severe stress and behavioral changes (Kerry, 1999). Polar regions also represents the low-temperature extremes for coastal marine environments, with seawater frequently poised at, or near, its freezing point. Survival of enteric bacteria in these environments is generally enhanced by reduced grazing rates of heterotrophic nanoflagellates and larvae, in addition to the effects of lower seawater temperatures (Patt, 1990; Rivkin, 1991). Several studies describing the persistence of human enteric bacteria in aquatic environments have demonstrated that many of these microorganisms enter an altered physiological state termed viable but nonculturable (VBNC) (Kaprelyants, 1993; Roszak, 1987). This is commonly defined as the inability to form colonies on a given solid medium while remaining active by direct-viable-count methods (Smith, 1994).

Animal Behavior

Animal behavior will influence the potential for introduction and spread infectious disease-causing agents in several ways. The tendency to form aggregations will increase the opportunities for infectious agents to be spread within a population. The mode of feeding will influence the probability of coming into contact with the body fluids of other species. Of all feeding types, scavengers and carrion feeders are probably the ones most likely to be in contact with tissues of infected animals or human food. Migration patterns will affect the chance that a species may translocate a disease-causing agent. Many species travel between Antarctica and other regions and may be exposed to diseases by contact with wildlife or as a consequence of human activity, such as waste disposal, in these regions. The animals most likely to come into contact with pathogens as a result of human activity are those that will feed on waste generated by people given the opportunity. Species that also scavenge at aggregations, such as breeding colonies, are most likely to be agents of disease transfer to other Antarctic species. (Kerry, 1999)

ROUTES OF INFECTION

Different routes of introduction of *Salmonella* to Antarctic region have been proposed: by human carriers, by contaminated foods, by infected birds, sewage from some land-based operations or from discharge of this material from ships sailing in waters of the region. One of the most possible routes of introduction is by birds, because many Antarctic birds have long routes of migration.

Isolation of *Salmonella* in sub-Antarctica and Antarctica

Campaigns with negative results: Sieburth collected samples from skua, gull, sheathbill, giant fulmar, Adelie, emperor, gentoo penguin from sub-Antarctica and Antarctica during 1957-1958 (Sieburth, 1959). Soucek and Mushin analysed Adelie, emperor, chinstrap, king, royal rockhopper and gentoo penguin, leopard, crabeater, Weddell, Ross and elephant seal and skua in sub-Antarctica and Antarctica during 1962-1965 (Soucek and Mushin, 1970). Bonnedal collected samples from eight bird species on the Antarctic Peninsula during the Antarctic Summer 2001-2002 (Bonnedal, 2005). This author explained the negative result owing to a failure to detect the microorganism could be due to the prolonged time or a too low prevalence in the population. Furthermore, accounting for the sample size of this study, the true population prevalence must have been less than 1,6% to not have been detected.

Table 1. shows the isolation of Salmonella in sub-Antarctic and Antarctic region

Host animals and location	*Salmonella* serovar	Year	Reference
Adelie penguin and south polar skua, Ross Island, sub-Antarctica	Blockey, Johannesburg, Panama, Typhimurium, Infantis	1970-1971	Oelke and Steineger, 1973
Adelie penguin, Cape Denison, Antarctica	Enteritidis	1985	Iveson et al., 2009
King penguin	Oranienburg	1986	Iveson et al., 2009
Gentoo penguin, Bird Island, sub-Antarctica	Enteritidis	1995-1996	Olsen et al., 1996
Antarctic fur seal, gentoo penguin, black-browed albatross, Bird Island, sub-Antarctica	Havana, Typhimurium, Enteritidis, Newport	1996, 1998	Palmgren et al., 2000
Sea lion, Dundas Island, Enderly Island, sub-Antarctica	Cerro, Derby, Enteritidis, Newport	1998	Fenwick et al., 2004
Southern giant petrel, Adelie penguin, skua, kelp gull, Weddell seal, Potter Peninsula and Hope Bay, Antarctica	Newport, Enteritidis	2000, 2003	Vigo et al., 2011
Emperor penguin	Antarctica	2009	Iveson et al., 2009

CONCLUSIONS

Up to now, any study carried out on sub-Antarctica and Antarctica in the wildlife population has isolated *Salmonella* spp. from an animal with clinical signs of salmonellosis.

All *Salmonella* isolates from Antarctica analysed in different studies were susceptible to all the antimicrobial agents tested. This would indicate that Antarctic isolates were not exposed to antimicrobial selection pressure and neither acquired resistance from other microorganisms circulating in the Antarctic ecosystem.

Salmonella enterica subspecies *enterica* isolated from sub-Antarctic and Antarctic fauna belonged to the most prevalent serovars in humans and domesticated animals, with the exception of few rare or exotic serovars. Some of the *Salmonella* serovars found in Antarctic wildlife were: Enteritidis, Typhimurium, Newport, Infantis which are among the main serovars isolated from salmonellosis cases in humans and animals in the world.

There are few reports of molecular epidemiology carried out with *Salmonella* isolates from sub-Antarctica and Antarctica. Palmgren, in 1996, in Bird Island, sub-Antarctica, reported the isolation of *S.* Havana, *S.* Typhimurium and *S.* Enteritidis from gentoo penguins and fur seals. In 1998, fur seals were infected with *S.* Havana, *S.* Enteritidis and *S.* Newport. All isolates, except one, showed identical pulsed-field gel electrophoresis-patterns within each serotype, irrespective of sampling year and animal reservoir (Palmgren, 2000). Vigo, in summer 2000 in Potter Peninsula, Antarctica, reported the isolation of *S.* Newport and *S.* Enteritidis from southern giant petrels. In summer 2003, *S.* Enteritidis was isolated from Adelie penguins, skuas, kelp gulls and Weddell seals. All the isolates belonging to the same serovar showed indistinguishable genomic profiles by pulsed-field gel electrophoresis and by random amplified polymorphic DNA (RAPD-PCR) (Vigo, 2011). These two studies had very similar results and the same conclusion: the very low heterogeneity in the *Salmonella* isolates found could be either indicate a high genetic adaptation of the bacteria to the environment or a recent introduction of *Salmonella* into the area (Palmgren, 2000).

Studies on *Salmonella* carried out in Antarctic region allow the scientific community to know the sanitary status of Antarctic fauna and also, they can be used as an indicator to know the local ecosystem status.

Nowadays, in spite of some studies performed in sub-Antarctica and Antarctica, it was impossible to know if *Salmonella* was introduced or was an indigenous bacterium in the Antarctic ecosystem. The epidemiology of *Salmonella* in the Antarctic fauna needs to be further investigated.

REFERENCES

Kerry K, Riddle M, Clarke J. Diseases of Antarctic wildlife. *A report for The Scientific Committee on Antarctic Research* (SCAR) and The Council of Managers of National Antarctic programs (COMNAP), September 1999.

Patt M, Borsheim K, Miceli G, Stoecker D. 1990. Seasonal changes in cell size and abundance of bacterioplankton during the *Phaeocystis* sp. bloom in McMurdo Sound. *Antarct. J. U.S.* 25:199-201.

Kaprelyants A, Gottschal J, Kell D. 1993. Dormancy in non-sporulating bacteria. *FEMS Microbiol. Rev*. 104:271-286.

Roszak D, Colwell R. 1987. Survival strategies of bacteria in the natural environment. *Microbiol. Rev*. 51:356-379.

Rivkin R, Anderson M, Gustafson D. 1991. Ingestion of phytoplankton and bacterioplankton by polar and temperate echinoderm larvae. *Antarct. J. U. S*. 26:156-158.

Smith J, Howington J, McFeters G. 1994. Survival, physiological response, and recovery of enteric bacteria exposed to a polar marine environment. *Appl. Environm. Microbiol.* 60:2977-2984.

Oelke H and Steiniger F. 1973. *Salmonella* in Adélie penguins (*Pygoscelis adeliae*) and south polar skuas (*Catharacta maccormicki*) on Ross Island, Antarctica. *Avian Dis*. 17: 568-573.

Iveson J, Shellam G, Bradshaw S, Smith D, Mackenzie J, Mofflin R. 2009. *Salmonella* infections in Antarctic fauna and island populations of wildlife exposed to human activities in coastal areas of Australia. *Epidemiol. Infect*. 137:858-870.

Olsen B, Bergstrom S, McCafferty D, Sellin M, Wistrom J. 1996. *Salmone*lla Enteritidis in Antarctica: zoonosis in man or humanosis in penguins? *Lancet*, 348:1319-1320.

Palmgren H, McCafferty, Aspán A, Broman T, Sellin M, Wollin, Bergstrom S, Olsen B. 2000. *Salmonella* in sub-Antarctica: low heterogeneity in *Salmo*n*ella* serotypes in South Georgian seals and birds. *Epidemiol. Infect*. 125:257-262.

Fenwick S, Duignan P, Nicol C, Leyland M, Hunter J. 2004. A comparison of *Salmonella* serotypes isolated from New Zealand Sea Lions and Feral Pigs on the Auckland Islands by pulsed-field gel electrophoresis. *J. Wild. Dis*. 40:566-570.

Vigo G, Leotta G, Caffer M, Salve A, Binsztein N, Pichel M. 2011. Isolation and characterization of *Salmonella enterica* from Antarctic wildlife. *Polar Biol.* 34:675-681.

Sieburth J. Gastrointestinal microflora of Antarctic birds. *J. Bacteriol*. 1959, 77:521-531.

Soucek Z and Mushin R. 1970. Gastrointestinal bacteria of certain Antarctic birds and mammals. *Appl. Microbiol.* 20:561-566.

Bonnedal J, Broman T, Waldenstrom J, Palmgren H, Niskanen T, Olsen B. 2005. In search of human-associated bacterial pathogens in Antarctic wildlife: report from six penguin colonies regularly visited by tourists. *Ambio*. 24:430-432.

INDEX

B

C

D

E

I

N

O

P

Q

R

S